Clinical Manual of Addiction Psychopharmacology

Second Edition

Edited by

Henry R. Kranzler, M.D.

Domenic A. Ciraulo, M.D.

Leah R. Zindel, R.Ph., M.A.L.S.

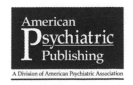

American Psychiatric Publishing
A Division of American Psychiatric Association

Washington, DC
London, England

Copyright © 2014 American Psychiatric Association
ALL RIGHTS RESERVED

Manufactured in the United States of America on acid-free paper
17   16   15   14   13   5   4   3   2   1
Second Edition

Typeset in Adobe Garamond and Helvetica.

American Psychiatric Publishing

A Division of American Psychiatric Association
1000 Wilson Boulevard
Arlington, VA 22209-3901
www.appi.org

Library of Congress Cataloging-in-Publication Data
Clinical manual of addiction psychopharmacology / edited by Henry R. Kranzler, Domenic A. Ciraulo, Leah R. Zindel.—2nd edition.
    p. ; cm.
Includes bibliographical references and index.
ISBN 978-1-58562-440-9 (pbk. : alk. paper)
I. Kranzler, Henry R., 1950– editor of compilation. II. Ciraulo, Domenic A., editor of compilation. III. Zindel, Leah R., 1959– editor of compilation. IV. American Psychiatric Association, issuing body.
[DNLM: 1. Substance-Related Disorders—drug therapy. 2. Psychopharmacology—methods. 3. Psychotropic Drugs—therapeutic use. WM 270]
RC564.15
616.89'18—dc23

2013036961

British Library Cataloguing in Publication Data
A CIP record is available from the British Library.

Contents

Contributors

Domenic A. Ciraulo, M.D.
Professor and Chair of Psychiatry, Boston University School of Medicine; Psychiatrist-in-Chief, Boston Medical Center, Boston, Massachusetts

Steven Epstein, M.D.
Professor and Chairman, Department of Psychiatry, Georgetown University, Washington, D.C.

Tony P. George, M.D., F.R.C.P.C.
Professor of Psychiatry and Co-Director, Division of Brain and Therapeutics, Department of Psychiatry, University of Toronto; Medical Director, Complex Mental Illness Program, and Chief, Schizophrenia Division, Centre for Addiction and Mental Health, Toronto, Ontario, Canada

John H. Halpern, M.D.
Assistant Professor of Psychiatry, Harvard Medical School; Director of the Laboratory for Integrative Psychiatry, Psychiatrist-in-Charge of Division Coverage, and Medical Director of the McLean Residence at the Brook Division of Alcohol and Drug Abuse, McLean Hospital, Belmont, Massachusetts

Carlos Hernandez-Avila, M.D., Ph.D.
Assistant Professor, Department of Psychiatry, University of Connecticut School of Medicine, Farmington, Connecticut

Kyle M. Kampman, M.D.
Professor, Department of Psychiatry, Perelman School of Medicine, University of Pennsylvania, Treatment Research Center, Philadelphia, Pennsylvania

Clifford M. Knapp, Ph.D.
Associate Professor of Psychiatry, Boston University School of Medicine, Boston, Massachusetts

Henry R. Kranzler, M.D.
Professor of Psychiatry, Perelman School of Medicine of the University of
Pennsylvania and VISN4 MIRECC, Philadelphia Veterans Affairs Medical
Center, Philadelphia, Pennsylvania

David M. Ledgerwood, Ph.D.
Associate Professor, Department of Psychiatry and Behavioral Neurosciences,
Wayne State University School of Medicine, Detroit, Michigan

Frances R. Levin, M.D.
Kennedy-Leavy Professor of Clinical Psychiatry, Columbia University, New
York, New York

John J. Mariani, M.D.
Assistant Professor of Clinical Psychiatry, Columbia University, New York,
New York

James R. McKay, Ph.D.
Professor of Psychology in Psychiatry, Perelman School of Medicine, University of Pennsylvania, and Philadelphia Veterans Affairs Medical Center, Philadelphia, Pennsylvania

Cheryl A. Oncken, M.D., M.P.H.
Professor of Medicine and Obstetrics and Gynecology, and Program Director,
Clinical Research Center, University of Connecticut Health Center, Farmington, Connecticut

Torsten Passie, M.D., M.A.
Visiting Professor, Department of Psychiatry, Harvard Medical School, Boston, Massachusetts; Professor of Psychiatry and Psychotherapy, Hannover
Medical School, Hannover, Germany

Nancy M. Petry, Ph.D.
Professor of Medicine, University of Connecticut School of Medicine, Farmington, Connecticut

John A. Renner Jr., M.D.
Professor of Psychiatry, Boston University School of Medicine; Associate Chief of Psychiatry, Boston VA Healthcare System, Boston, Massachusetts

Richard N. Rosenthal, M.D.
Arthur J. Antenucci Professor of Psychiatry, Columbia University College of Physicians & Surgeons; Chairman, Department of Psychiatry, St. Luke's Roosevelt Hospital Center, New York, New York

Ramon Solhkhah, M.D.
Chairman, Department of Psychiatry, Jersey Shore University Medical Center; Corporate Medical Director, Meridian Behavioral Health Services; Associate Clinical Professor and Vice Chairman, Department of Psychiatry, Rutgers—Robert Wood Johnson Medical School, New Jersey

Leah R. Zindel, R.Ph., M.A.L.S.
Freelance medical writer and editor, Philadelphia, Pennsylvania

Disclosure of Interests

The following contributors to this book have indicated a financial interest in or other affiliation with a commercial supporter, a manufacturer of a commercial product, a provider of a commercial service, a nongovernmental organization, and /or a government agency, as listed below:

Domenic A. Ciraulo, M.D.   *Research grant/contract:* Catalyst Pharmaceuticals

Tony P. George, M.D., F.R.C.P.C.   *Data monitoring committee:* Novartis; *Contract and grant support:* Pfizer; *Speaking fees:* Pfizer; *Grant support:* National Institutes of Health, Canadian Institutes of Health Research

Henry R. Kranzler, M.D.   Dr. Kranzler is a consultant or member of an advisory board for the following companies: Alkermes, Lilly, Lundbeck, Pfizer, Roche. Dr. Kranzler is also a member of the American Society of Clinical Psychopharmacology's Alcohol Clinical Trials Initiatives, which is supported by Lilly, Lundbeck, Abbott, and Pfizer.

David M. Ledgerwood, Ph.D.   *Research funding sources:* National Institutes of Health, State of Michigan, Ontario Problem Gambling Research Centre. Dr. Ledgerwood has no corporate funding sources to disclose.

Cheryl A. Oncken, M.D., M.P.H.   Dr. Oncken has received free medication supplies of nicotine inhaler and placebo to conduct a trial of nicotine replacement therapy for smoking cessation during pregnancy.

John A. Renner Jr., M.D.   Dr. Renner is Professor of Psychiatry at Boston University School of Medicine (nonsalaried) and full-time staff psychiatrist at the Department of Veterans Affairs. *Minority stockholder:* Johnson & Johnson, General Electric

Ramon Solhkhah, M.D.   *Speaker's bureau:* Bristol-Myers Squibb, Janssen Pharmaceuticals, Merck

The following contributors to this book have indicated no competing interests to disclose during the year preceding manuscript submission:

Steven Epstein, M.D.; John H. Halpern, M.D.; Carlos Hernandez-Avila, M.D., Ph.D.; Kyle M. Kampman, M.D.; Clifford M. Knapp, Ph.D.; Frances R. Levin, M.D.; John J. Mariani, M.D.; James R. McKay, Ph.D.; Torsten Passie, M.D., M.A.; Nancy M. Petry, Ph.D.; Richard N. Rosenthal, M.D.

Preface

Dramatic advances in neuroscience since the 1990s have substantially improved our understanding of the biology of addictive disorders and their pharmacological treatment. For example, knowledge obtained from neurogenetics and neuroimaging has provided new insights into the etiology and pathophysiology of addiction, prompting a renewed interest in the pharmacological treatment of substance use disorders. Through efforts initially driven by the National Institutes of Health in the United States, pharmaceutical companies have shown greater interest in developing new medications to treat addictive disorders, particularly dependence on alcohol, tobacco, and opioids. Nonetheless, the high prevalence of these and other addictive disorders contrasts sharply with the limited pharmacological options that exist to treat them. There are also many more medications to treat other psychiatric conditions than there are for addictive disorders, and neither prevalence rates nor personal or economic costs explains this discrepancy.

Given these circumstances, the market potential for efficacious medications to treat addictions is enormous. Interest on the part of the pharmaceutical industry could be a harbinger of continued progress in the identification of candidate compounds and their evaluation for the treatment of addictions. Medications development for addictive disorders is important to the care of patients with addictive disorders and thus of public health significance.

If past experience in the treatment of major depression is an indicator, one important effect of the greater availability of efficacious treatments for addictive disorders will be decreased stigma associated with addiction. This, along with provisions of the Affordable Care Act and the Mental Health and Substance Abuse Parity Act of 2010, will increase the number of addicted individuals seeking treatment and the number of practitioners willing to provide such treatment. The identification and treatment of tobacco dependence, which occurs commonly in primary care settings, was driven by the availability of efficacious medications for smoking cessation and a greater awareness of the serious health consequences of smoking. As treatment options grow and societal views change, the care of patients with other addictive disorders may also become the province of primary care practitioners.

The chapters in this volume are ordered according to a combination of prevalence of use and availability of pharmacotherapy options. Recently, the American Psychiatric Association published the Diagnostic and Statistical Manual of Mental Disorders, 5th Edition (DSM-5), which combines the DSM-IV categories of substance abuse and substance dependence into a single substance use disorder measured on a continuum from mild to severe. The chapters in this manual focus largely on DSM-IV dependence, as the extant literature is based heavily on that diagnosis. Despite coverage of the different DSM-5 classes of addictive drugs, developments in the pharmacotherapy of the addictive disorders have not occurred uniformly across substances. As mentioned above, multiple medications are approved by the U.S. Food and Drug Administration (FDA) to treat tobacco dependence, including some that are now available over the counter. A growing number of FDA-approved treatments for opioid and alcohol dependence are also available. However, despite promising developments, there are no FDA-approved treatments for dependence on other substances discussed in this volume, notably cocaine and other stimulants and cannabis. There clearly remains a great deal to do to identify and test new agents for these indications. The substantial insights into the pharmacology of the various addictive substances, which are discussed in detail in this volume, provide a solid basis for medications development across the spectrum of addictive disorders.

Converging with these trends are developments in human genetics and genomics, which have accelerated the pace of discovery of variants that affect the risk of addiction. This has provided new targets for medications development and identified novel genetic variants that moderate medication response. The application of pharmacogenetics to the treatment of addictive disorders is, however, still in its early stages, with most studies based on small samples using secondary analysis. Prospective studies of large samples are essential to the advancement of this field. Ultimately, pharmacogenetics can be expected to provide a basis for the personalized treatment of addiction by matching specific medications to patients based on their genetic and epigenetic characteristics, enhancing treatment efficacy and reducing the risk of adverse effects. We look forward to the new age of addiction psychopharmacology.

Henry R. Kranzler, M.D.
Domenic A. Ciraulo, M.D.
Leah R. Zindel, R.Ph., M.A.L.S.

Alcohol

Henry R. Kranzler, M.D.

Clifford M. Knapp, Ph.D.

Domenic A. Ciraulo, M.D.

Alcohol affects a wide variety of neurotransmitter systems, including virtually all of the major systems associated with psychiatric symptoms (Lovinger and Roberto 2013). This diversity of effects explains, at least in part, why chronic heavy drinking is commonly associated with many different psychiatric symptoms (Kranzler and Tinsley 2004). Alcohol alters the absorption and metabolism of nutrients, and chronic heavy drinking can disturb intermediary metabolism and produce a variety of deficiency states. Alcohol abuse also results in both psychological and physiological dependence, with abrupt cessation causing withdrawal states. Although the most common effect of abrupt cessation of drinking is an uncomplicated alcohol withdrawal syndrome, severe effects also may result. In a medically compromised patient, severe withdrawal—which can include tonic-clonic seizures, hallucinations, and delirium tremens—can be lethal.

Epidemiology of Drinking, Heavy Drinking, and Alcohol Use Disorders

Alcohol consumption occurs along a continuum, and drinking patterns vary considerably among individuals, with no clear demarcation between "social" or "moderate" drinking and "problem" or "harmful" drinking (Babor et al. 1987). However, as the average amount of drinking and the frequency of intoxication increase, associated medical and psychosocial problems also increase (Kranzler et al. 1990). In DSM-IV (American Psychiatric Association 1994), the most commonly identified group of people affected by alcohol problems are those with alcohol abuse or dependence. A less prominent, but more numerous, group consists of individuals referred to as problem drinkers or harmful drinkers who do not meet criteria for alcohol dependence. In DSM-5, alcohol dependence and abuse have been replaced with a single category of alcohol use disorder (American Psychiatric Association 2013). This is likely to result in "diagnostic orphans" (e.g., individuals with alcohol-related problems but no DSM-IV diagnosis) receiving an alcohol use disorder diagnosis in DSM-5 (Peer et al. 2012).

In the 2009 National Survey on Drug Use and Health (NSDUH; Substance Abuse and Mental Health Services Administration 2010), a majority of the U.S. population age 12 years and older (51.9%, or 130.6 million people) reported consuming alcohol during the month before the interview. Nearly a quarter of such individuals (23.7%, or 59.6 million people) engaged in binge drinking (five or more drinks on the same occasion) at least once during this time. Heavy drinking (five or more drinks on five separate occasions during the month) was reported by 6.8% of the population, or 17.1 million people. The prevalence of current alcohol use increased with age up to the age group of 21–25 years, where it reached a peak of 70.2%. This is also the age group for which the rates of both binge drinking (46.5%) and heavy drinking (16%) peaked.

The 2009 NSDUH (Substance Abuse and Mental Health Services Administration 2010) also showed that men were more likely than women to drink (57.6% vs. 46.5%). Drinking behavior also differed by race/ethnicity. Fifty-six percent of white persons reported drinking during the past month, followed by individuals reporting two or more races (47.6%), African American persons (42.8%), Hispanic persons (41.7%), Asian persons (37.6%), and American Indian/Alaska Native persons (37.1%). Binge drinking was most common among Hispanic individuals (25.0%), followed by white (24.8%), American Indian/Alaska Native (22.2%), African American (19.8%), and Asian (11.1%) individuals.

Several large-scale community studies conducted since 1980 have provided estimates of the lifetime and past-year prevalence of alcohol use disorders in the general population. For example, the National Comorbidity Survey (NCS), a representative household survey of more than 8,000 individuals ages 15–54 years, was conducted to assess lifetime and past-year alcohol use disorders using DSM-III-R criteria (American Psychiatric Association 1987). The NCS estimated the lifetime prevalence of alcohol abuse and alcohol dependence for adults ages 18–54 years to be 9.4% and 14.1%, respectively. Together, these data indicate that more than one in five young to middle-aged adults in the United States met the criteria for a lifetime alcohol use disorder (Kessler et al. 1997). The 12-month prevalence rates for alcohol abuse and dependence were 2.5% and 4.4%, respectively (Kessler et al. 1997).

The 1992 National Longitudinal Alcohol Epidemiologic Survey (NLAES), based on interviews with a national probability household sample of more than 43,000 adults age 18 and older, showed the 1-year prevalence of a DSM-IV alcohol use disorder to be 7.4% (i.e., 3.0% with alcohol abuse and 4.4% with alcohol dependence) (Grant 1994, 2000). The National Epidemiologic Survey on Alcohol and Related Conditions (NESARC), also a community-based survey of more than 43,000 individuals (Grant et al. 2004a), permitted an evaluation of trends in alcohol use disorder prevalence and characteristics, because it used a methodology very similar to that of the 1992 NLAES. The NESARC showed a 12-month prevalence of alcohol abuse and dependence of 4.7% and 3.8%, respectively, so that an estimated total of 17.6 million adult Americans had an alcohol use disorder during 2001–2002. The prevalence of alcohol abuse in the NESARC was significantly increased over that seen in the NLAES, whereas the prevalence of alcohol dependence decreased significantly over the 10-year period between the two surveys.

Consistent with drinking behavior, national prevalence data also show that rates of alcohol use disorders vary by age, gender, race/ethnicity, socioeconomic status, and geographic location. The prevalence of alcohol use disorders has consistently been higher among men than among women, by at least twofold (Grant 1994; Grant et al. 2004a; Kessler et al. 1997; Substance Abuse and Mental Health Services Administration 2010). The highest prevalence rates of alcohol abuse and dependence occur among young adults, with rates declining gradually with increasing age.

Pharmacology of Ethanol and Its Relation to Medication Development

Pharmacokinetics of Ethanol

Absorption and Distribution

Alcohol, or more specifically ethanol, is absorbed from both the stomach and the duodenum. When an alcoholic beverage is consumed with food, it dilutes the ethanol concentration in the stomach and delays passage into the duodenum, slowing absorption and decreasing the subjective effects of alcohol. Food delays and lowers peak blood ethanol concentrations and lowers the total amount of ethanol reaching the systemic circulation. Ethanol absorption is fastest when the stomach empties quickly, as in the fasting state, but high-concentration alcoholic beverages, such as distilled spirits, may cause pylorospasm and delay emptying.

Ethanol distributes rapidly, with concentrations in body water 10 times higher than in body fat. Tissues with the greatest blood supply equilibrate most rapidly with arterial blood circulation. Shortly after alcohol ingestion, the ethanol concentration in the brain is higher than the venous concentration.

Approximately 5%–10% of ethanol is excreted unchanged in the breath and urine. The blood-to-breath ratio of ethanol is 2,000:1, an important relation that permits blood alcohol determination from expired air, providing the basis for the use of breath alcohol measurement for clinical, research, and forensic applications.

Metabolism

The primary route of hepatic ethanol metabolism is oxidation to acetaldehyde and then acetic acid (Figure 1–1). Acetic acid enters the Krebs citric acid cycle as acetyl coenzyme A to supply the cell with a source of energy. Three different enzyme systems are capable of oxidizing ethanol: alcohol dehydrogenase (ADH), catalase, and the microsomal ethanol oxidizing system (particularly cytochrome P450 enzyme 2E1 [CYP2E1] in heavy drinkers). Aldehyde dehydrogenase (ALDH) is the enzyme responsible for metabolizing acetaldehyde,

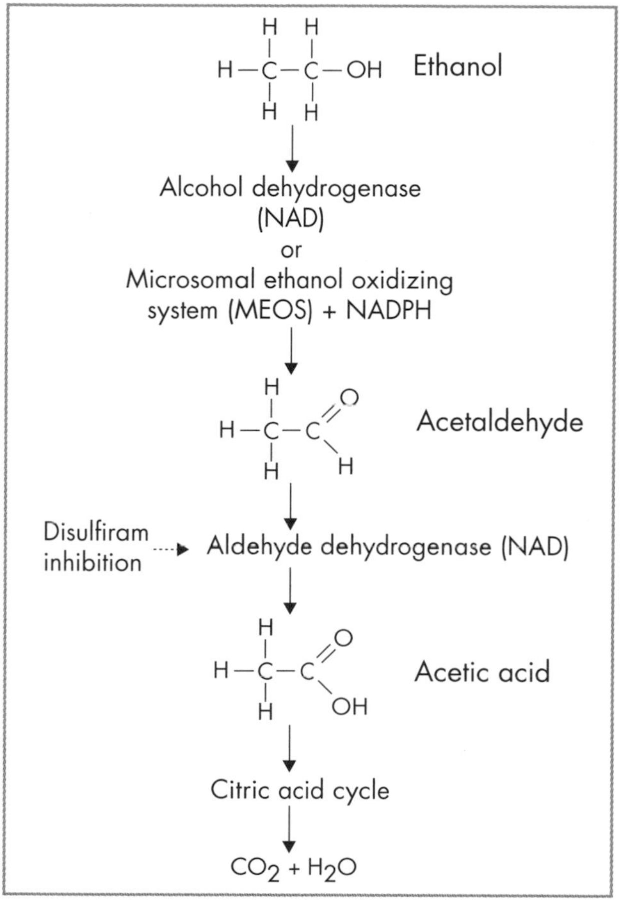

Figure 1–1. Primary route of ethanol metabolism.

Ethanol is oxidized by alcohol dehydrogenase (in the presence of nicotinamide adenine dinucleotide [NAD]) or the microsomal ethanol oxidizing system (MEOS) (in the presence of reduced nicotinamide adenine dinucleotide phosphate [NADPH]). Acetaldehyde, the first product in ethanol oxidation, is metabolized to acetic acid by aldehyde dehydrogenase in the presence of NAD. Acetic acid is broken down through the citric acid cycle to carbon dioxide (CO_2) and water (H_2O). Impairment of the metabolism of acetaldehyde to acetic acid is the major mechanism of action of disulfiram for the treatment of alcoholism.

the first product in ethanol oxidation. Functional polymorphisms of the genes encoding ADH, ALDH, and CYP2E1 are important in altering the risk for the development of alcohol dependence and ethanol-associated illnesses.

Gastric ADH also metabolizes ethanol, and lower levels of this enzyme in women may account for higher blood ethanol concentrations in women than in men given equivalent amounts of alcohol (Frezza et al. 1990), although a study by Lai et al. (2000) did not replicate the finding. In addition, men may have higher hepatic ADH activity than do women (Chrostek et al. 2003). In one study, the absolute elimination rate of alcohol (grams per hour) was higher in men than in women, but the rates were similar for men and women when adjusted for liver weight (Dettling et al. 2007).

ADH classes I–III are present in the liver, and class IV is in the stomach; subtypes of each class exist. Different molecular forms of ADH vary considerably in their kinetic properties and, along with ALDH subtypes, have been among the first genetic risk factors associated with alcohol dependence. The kinetic properties of the enzymes influence the rate of metabolism. Rapid metabolism of ethanol to acetaldehyde and impaired metabolism of acetaldehyde to acetic acid result in accumulation of that metabolite, leading to unpleasant physiological effects ("the flushing reaction").

The prevalence of enzymes with different kinetic properties varies among individuals and racial groups, serving as genetically determined protective factors. The variant allele of the ADH enzyme, *ADH1B*2,* protects against the development of alcohol dependence (Chen et al. 2009). This variant is common among East Asian individuals, including Han Chinese, Japanese, and Korean individuals. In contrast, the *ADH1B*1* allele is prevalent in white and Native American individuals. The *ALDH2*2* allele occurs in between 16% and 24% of East Asian populations but is rare in white, African American, and Native American individuals (Chen et al. 2009). Individuals who have this allele cannot oxidize acetaldehyde rapidly, so that levels of acetaldehyde accumulate in the blood, leading to aversive effects after ethanol consumption, including general discomfort and intense heart palpitations. These aversive effects of alcohol may act as protective factors in preventing alcohol dependence.

One fascinating aspect of the effect of genetic polymorphisms described earlier is that acculturation can partially overcome the protective factor, and Asian groups born in North America may have only partial protection (Goldman 1993; Tu and Israel 1995). In individuals who consume small amounts of alcohol over time, the aversive effects diminish—an effect similar to that described in clinical reports of patients who developed "a resistance" to the effects of disulfiram.

ADH also has clinical significance in the metabolism of methanol and ethylene glycol, two substances with toxic metabolites. Methanol is oxidized by ADH to formaldehyde, which damages the retina and can cause blindness. Ethylene glycol is metabolized by ADH to oxalic acid, which has renal toxicity. The toxic effects of both methanol and ethylene glycol can be reduced by ethanol administration, which inhibits their metabolism by competing for the oxidizing enzymes and allows elimination of the intact parent compounds. The treatment for intoxication with these agents, which occurs with some regularity in emergency departments, is intravenous ethanol.

Catalase is a liver enzyme that uses hydrogen peroxide to oxidize other substances. The catalase system does not play a significant role in ethanol metabolism in the body overall, probably because the quantities of hydrogen peroxide available are insufficient for ethanol metabolism. However, in animal studies, catalase in the brain contributes to the metabolism of ethanol to acetaldehyde (Zimatkin and Buben 2007).

The microsomal ethanol oxidizing system is another mechanism of ethanol metabolism. CYP2E1 may be an important enzyme in the metabolism of ethanol in heavy drinkers, who may have a 10-fold increase in activity. Two allelic variants in the gene (i.e., c1 and c2) have different enzymatic activity. Approximately 40% of Japanese people have the more active c2 allele, which is rare in individuals of European heritage (Sun et al. 2002). Although the c2 allele is not believed to affect risk for the development of alcoholism, current studies are examining its relation to the severity of a variety of ethanol-related diseases.

Acetaldehyde

Acetaldehyde is the first metabolic product of ethanol. The most important hepatic enzymes involved in its metabolism are mitochondrial ALDH2 and cytosolic ALDH1 (Chen et al. 1999), although only variation in the gene encoding ALDH2 appears to be a genetic risk factor for alcoholism. The *ALDH2*2* allele is a null mutant that encodes a protein with little capacity to metabolize acetaldehyde. The inactive allele (Lys487) may be dominant, because even individuals heterozygous for this allele experience the flushing reaction to ethanol, and the risk of alcoholism is reduced 4- to 10-fold in this group (Radel and Goldman 2001; Thomasson et al. 1994).

Acetaldehyde in the brain is synthesized from alcohol partly through reactions that are mediated by brain catalase enzymes (Zimatkin and Buben 2007). The role of acetaldehyde in the production of the reinforcing effects of ethanol is controversial (Quertemont et al. 2005). Animal studies indicate that acetaldehyde may increase the activity of dopaminergic neurons within the ventral tegmental area (VTA) of the brain and may enhance dopamine release in the nucleus accumbens, consistent with the activation of the brain's mesolimbic reward system (Diana et al. 2008). Voluntary consumption of ethanol is decreased by selective inhibition of the expression of catalase in the VTA (Karahanian et al. 2011). These more recent findings tend to support the contention that the generation of acetaldehyde from alcohol may be important in the production of ethanol's reinforcing effects, but a definitive role for this substance in mediating the reinforcing effects of ethanol in humans has not been clearly established.

Pharmacodynamics of Ethanol

Ethanol may act directly to augment the inhibitory effects of γ-aminobutyric acid type A (GABA$_A$) receptors while inhibiting the excitatory effects of activation of N-methyl-D-aspartate (NMDA) and other glutamate receptors. Many of the behavioral effects of ethanol, including its antianxiety, anticonvulsant, locomotor stimulant, motor-coordination-impairing, and sedative-hypnotic effects, may be mediated by interactions with GABA$_A$ receptors (Grobin et al. 1998; Kumar et al. 2009). Ethanol-induced inhibition of NMDA receptor activity may be involved in both the cognitive and the motor impairments produced by alcohol administration. Adaptations of both the GABA$_A$ and the NMDA receptors have been implicated in the development of alcohol dependence and tolerance. A variety of neurotransmitters, endogenous neuropeptides, neurosteroids, and intracellular second-messenger systems also appear to modulate the effects of ethanol.

GABA and Glycine

GABA is the most abundant inhibitory neurotransmitter in the central nervous system (CNS). The development of medications targeting the GABA system is based on the known effects of ethanol on GABA, the effectiveness of GABA agonists (e.g., benzodiazepines) in the treatment of alcohol withdrawal, and the observed actions of GABA agonists and antagonists in animal models of alcoholism. Acute doses of ethanol increase GABA activity, whereas chronic dosing decreases GABA receptor activity.

The acute administration of ethanol enhances the effects of GABA on the $GABA_A$ receptor, leading to an increase of chloride flux, hyperpolarization of the neuron, and resultant inhibition of neuronal activity. The actions of ethanol on the $GABA_A$ receptor may require, at least in many instances, phosphorylation of the receptor by protein kinase C (PKC). In addition to its interaction with the $GABA_A$ receptor, ethanol may potentiate the actions of glycine on glycine-activated chloride channels (Mascia et al. 1996). The combined actions of ethanol on $GABA_A$ and glycine receptors may contribute to the inhibitory effects of ethanol on neurons. Ethanol also may inhibit neuronal function by facilitating the presynaptic release of GABA (Lovinger and Roberto 2013). This effect may occur in several key brain structures, including the amygdala, hippocampus, and cerebellum (Criswell et al. 2008; Lovinger and Roberto 2013). Ethanol may activate inositol 1,4,5-trisphosphate receptors in the cerebellum, leading to activation of PKC (Kelm et al. 2010). Protein kinase A has been implicated in the regulation of ethanol-induced GABA release (Kelm et al. 2008). A final mechanism through which ethanol may act to inhibit brain neuronal function is by increasing local levels of neuroactive steroids that potentiate the effects of GABA on the $GABA_A$ receptor (Helms et al. 2012).

$GABA_A$ receptors are pentameric ligand-gated ion channels generally composed of two α subunits, two β subunits, and either a γ or a δ subunit. Subtypes of these subunits have been identified, and the nature of the effects produced by the interaction of ethanol with $GABA_A$ receptors may be determined by the subunit composition of the receptor and its cellular location. The α_1 subunit is commonly located in synaptic $GABA_A$ receptors that control phasic activity (i.e., short duration synaptic transmission) of the neuron, whereas the α_4 subunit occurs with greater frequency in extrasynaptic areas and is more often involved in the regulation of neuronal tonic activity (i.e., sustained modulation of neuronal potential levels). Most of the findings concerning the role of $GABA_A$ receptor subtypes in mediating the effects of ethanol are from experiments involving selective gene alteration in mice. The clinical significance of these findings, therefore, requires empirical evaluation in humans. The α_1 subunit is linked to regulation of the locomotor stimulant effects of alcohol (Kumar et al. 2009). The α_1, α_4, and δ subunits may be involved in facilitating the reinforcing effects of ethanol (Kumar et al. 2009; Nie et al. 2011).

Controversial evidence indicates that $GABA_A$ receptors containing a combination of the α_4 and δ subunits may be highly sensitive to the effects of ethanol (Wallner et al. 2003). $GABA_A$ receptors that contain clones of human $\alpha_4\beta_3\delta$ receptors expressed in human cell lines were highly sensitive to alcohol, suggesting that this combination of $GABA_A$ subunits may play a major role in mediating the effects of low doses of ethanol in humans (Meera et al. 2010).

Variation in the genes encoding a few $GABA_A$ receptor subunits has been associated with alcohol dependence and related phenotypes (see Enoch 2008 for a review). We focus here on the gene encoding the α_2 subunit of the $GABA_A$ receptor (*GABRA2*), for which the largest number of studies and the most consistent findings exist. Edenberg et al. (2004) fine mapped the region identified by Porjesz et al. (2002) that implicated a cluster of GABA subunit genes on chromosome 4 and found association to alleles and haplotypes of *GABRA2*. Others (e.g., Covault et al. 2004; Enoch et al. 2006; Fehr et al. 2006; Lappalainen et al. 2005; Soyka et al. 2008) also found an association of alcohol dependence to *GABRA2*, but the risk haplotype, the nature of the association, or the specific variants that were associated with the phenotype differed from the findings of Edenberg et al. (2004). Nonreplications of the association (Drgon et al. 2006; Matthews et al. 2007) also have been reported. Zintzaras (2012), in a meta-analysis examining 14 variants in eight studies, found that 4 variants were significantly associated with alcohol dependence, but all yielded small effects on risk (i.e., all odds ratios < 1.50).

Although no specific causative variant in *GABRA2* has been identified, human laboratory and longitudinal studies support a role of *GABRA2* variation in alcohol dependence risk. Pierucci-Lagha et al. (2005) found that a *GABRA2* allele that was associated with alcohol dependence risk (Covault et al. 2004) moderated the subjective response to oral alcohol in a sample of healthy subjects. Haughey et al. (2008), in two studies of hazardous drinkers, found that three *GABRA2* single nucleotide polymorphisms (SNPs) were associated with sensitivity to the effects of oral alcohol, including its hedonic value. Reanalysis of an intravenous alcohol administration study confirmed the results of the oral alcohol challenge study. Roh et al. (2011) administered alcohol intravenously to 110 healthy social drinkers in Japan. Three SNPs showed significant associations with the subjective effects of alcohol, with individuals homozygous for the alcohol dependence–associated allele showing fewer subjective effects compared with carriers of the nonrisk allele. Uhart et al. (2012) used a cumulative oral dosing procedure to study 69 healthy subjects in a laboratory-based study. They genotyped SNPs across *GABRA2* and analyzed the effect of genotype and haplotypes on subjective responses to alcohol. SNP analysis determined that carriers of the minor alleles for six SNPs—many of which had previously been associated with alcohol dependence—had lower negative alcohol effects scores than did individuals homozygous for the common allele. One of the haplotype blocks showed concordant results with SNPs in the block.

In a follow-up of participants from a psychotherapy trial of patients with alcohol use disorder, Bauer et al. (2007) found that individuals with a *GABRA2* allele associated with risk for alcohol dependence in the Covault et al. (2004) study had higher daily probabilities of drinking and heavy drinking. The polymorphism also moderated the response to the three psychotherapies examined in the study.

Subsequent work has shown that markers in the 3′ region of *GABRA2* (the region for which the association data are most consistent) are in linkage disequilibrium with markers at the adjacent locus, *GABRG1* (Covault et al. 2008; Enoch et al. 2009; Ittiwut et al. 2008). This raises the possibility that the *GABRA2* association is at least partly attributable to variants in *GABRG1*, with risk loci in both genes (Covault et al. 2008; Enoch et al. 2009; Ittiwut et al. 2012).

Individuals at high risk for alcohol dependence challenged with benzodiazepine agonists appeared to show smaller electroencephalogram responses, less body sway, and decreased saccadic eye movements than did control subjects (Cowley et al. 1994). Reinforcing effects were inconsistent: studies that used a modified Addiction Research Center Inventory–Morphine Benzedrine Group (ARCI-MBG) scale often showed greater reinforcing effects in high-risk subjects and abstinent alcoholic persons than in healthy control subjects (Ciraulo et al. 2001; Cowley 1992; Cowley et al. 1994), whereas studies that used other scales did not find greater mood enhancement (Volkow et al. 1995). In one study, individuals receiving the $GABA_A$ receptor agonist lorazepam for alcohol withdrawal were more likely to relapse than were those receiving the anticonvulsant carbamazepine, which suggests that positive modulators of the $GABA_A$ receptor increase alcohol consumption in humans (Malcolm et al. 2002).

Together, these findings clearly implicate the $GABA_A$ receptor in the subjective effects of alcohol. The specific mechanism whereby these effects may influence alcohol dependence risk remains to be explicated. One possibility is that genetically predisposed individuals may experience lower responses to alcohol's positive effects and thereby ingest more alcohol to experience these effects. Greater alcohol consumption chronically thus could lead to the development of alcohol dependence.

NMDA, AMPA, and Kainate Receptors and Ethanol

Glutamate is the major excitatory neurotransmitter in the CNS, activating two types of receptors: ligand-gated ion channels and metabotropic receptors linked to G proteins. The ion channel receptors are classified into NMDA, α-amino-3-hydroxy-5-methylisoxazole-4-propionate (AMPA), and kainate subtypes. Ethanol inhibits the function of all three of the ionotropic glutamate receptors (Lovinger and Roberto 2013). The sensitivity of NMDA receptors to ethanol is determined by the subunit composition of the receptors. NMDA receptors consist of an NR1 subunit that combines with NR2 and NR3 subunits to form the functional receptors.

The clinical implications of the antagonism of NMDA receptors by alcohol have been discussed by Krystal and colleagues (2003a, 2003b), who have suggested that the glutamate system is closely linked to both the risk of alcoholism and the reinforcing effects of ethanol. According to their view, vulnerability to alcoholism is related to an altered NMDA response to ethanol that leads to a reduction in the negative effects of heavy drinking.

Viewing the glutamate system as central to the effects of ethanol, a therapeutic approach to the treatment of alcoholism could involve NMDA antagonists that either block the rewarding effects of ethanol or promote its dysphoric effects (Krystal et al. 2003b). Two agents that may exert their effects via inhibition of glutamate receptor activity, acamprosate and topiramate, have been shown to be efficacious in the treatment of alcohol use disorders.

Calcium Channels and Ethanol

Ethanol inhibits the influx of calcium through L-type voltage-gated calcium channels in cell culture preparations (Mullikin-Kilpatrick et al. 1995). Chronic administration of ethanol can upregulate L-type and N-type voltage-gated calcium channels (Katsura et al. 2005; Newton et al. 2005). This upregulation may contribute to ethanol withdrawal symptoms (Kahkonen and Bondarenko 2004; McMahon et al. 2000), possibly through involvement of NMDA receptors and other neural circuitry (Calton et al. 1999). The administration of L-type calcium channel blockers reduces the locomotor stimulant effect of ethanol (Balino et al. 2010). An agent that blocks both N- and T-type voltage-gated calcium channels was shown to block ethanol-induced intoxication and alcohol-seeking behaviors in animals (Newton et al. 2008). Thus, the modulation of calcium channel activity may be a useful approach to regulating alcohol consumption.

Monoamines, Acetylcholine, and Adenosine and Ethanol

Monoamines. The administration of ethanol enhances dopamine release within the nucleus accumbens (Gonzales and Weiss 1998), which contributes to its reinforcing actions. Ethanol may excite dopaminergic neurons within the VTA by inhibiting GABA interneurons that otherwise would release GABA, thereby disinhibiting dopaminergic cell bodies within this structure (Xiao and Ye 2008). This action may account, at least in part, for ethanol-induced release of dopamine within the nucleus accumbens. Nicotinic receptors located within the VTA also may mediate ethanol-induced release of dopamine within the nucleus accumbens (Larsson et al. 2002).

Ethanol also reduces the activity of the noradrenergic system in the locus coeruleus, and alterations in norepinephrine activity may account for some aspects of intoxication and the abstinence syndrome. The α_2 antagonist clonidine and the β receptor antagonist propranolol reduce some symptoms of alcohol withdrawal (Bailly et al. 1992; Carlsson and Fasth 1976; Dobrydnjov et al. 2004; Kahkonen 2003; Petty et al. 1997; Wong et al. 2003). The intravenous sedative dexmedetomidine acts more selectively on the α_2-noradrenergic receptor than does clonidine and may be useful in treating alcohol withdrawal in an intensive care unit setting (Muzyk et al. 2011).

Alterations in CNS serotonin function have been attributed to both a predisposition to alcoholism and the consequences of chronic drinking (Pierucci-Lagha et al. 2004). The behavioral effects of ethanol are altered in the presence of decreased serotonin (e.g., by parachlorophenylalanine or 5,6-dihydroxytryptamine), and this deficiency leads to increased alcohol consumption in animal models (Kranzler and Anton 1994). Human studies also suggest that serotonergic function is reduced in alcoholic patients, as evidenced by low cerebrospinal fluid levels of 5-hydroxyindoleacetic acid (5-HIAA, a metabolite of serotonin). However, interpretation of this finding is complicated by the fact that ethanol shifts serotonin metabolism from pathways leading to 5-HIAA to those producing 5-hydroxyindoleacetaldehyde and 5-hydroxytryptophol.

Other evidence supporting altered serotonin function in alcoholic patients includes blunted responses to drugs that are serotonin agonists. Fenfluramine challenge, for example, induces a smaller prolactin response in abstinent alcoholic persons than in nonalcoholic control subjects (Farren et al. 1995). Rapid tryptophan depletion, which induces a transient reduction in brain serotonin concentration, has generally produced no effects on ethanol consumption (Petrakis et al. 2001, 2002). On the other hand, a rapid tryptophan depletion study in subjects with co-occurring alcoholism and major depressive disorder found that depletion of serotonin increased depressive symptoms and the urge to drink (Pierucci-Lagha et al. 2004).

Stimulation of the serotonin type 2A (5-HT$_{2A}$) receptor may enhance ethanol-induced excitation of dopamine neurons within the VTA. Administration of a selective 5-HT$_{2A}$ antagonist into the VTA attenuated the self-administration of alcohol by animals (Ding et al. 2009b). Thus, the 5-HT$_{2A}$ receptor may be a potential target for blocking the reinforcing effects of ethanol.

Ethanol administration may facilitate the release of serotonin within the nucleus accumbens (Selim and Bradberry 1996). This and other mechanisms may be involved in the enhancement of the function of the 5-HT$_{3A}$ receptor produced by exposure to ethanol (Dopico and Lovinger 2009). The 5-HT$_{3A}$ receptor is a ligand-gated ion channel receptor that, when activated, facilitates the release of dopamine in the mesolimbic system (McBride et al. 2004). The administration of 5-HT$_{3A}$ receptor antagonists may inhibit ethanol-induced dopamine release in the VTA and the nucleus accumbens. The clinical importance of these findings was shown in treatment studies of ondansetron, a 5-HT$_{3A}$ antagonist that was efficacious in early-onset alcoholism (Johnson et al. 2000; Kranzler et al. 2003b).

Acetylcholine. Ethanol potentiates the actions of acetylcholine at nicotinic receptors containing $\alpha_4\beta_2$ subunits (Zuo et al. 2001) and may increase nicotinic receptor activity within the VTA (Ericson et al. 2008). Ethanol-induced release of dopamine within the nucleus accumbens is blocked by the administration of the nicotine receptor antagonist mecamylamine (Larsson et al. 2002). Administration of the $\alpha_4\beta_2$ partial nicotinic receptor agonist varenicline reduced ethanol consumption in both preclinical (Kamens et al. 2010) and clinical (McKee et al. 2009) studies, implicating nicotinic $\alpha_4\beta_2$ receptors in the regulation of the reinforcing effects of alcohol. One study, however, indicated that nicotinic receptors containing $\alpha_3\beta_4$ subunits may also regulate ethanol consumption, and these receptors have not been localized in the mesolimbic system (Chatterjee et al. 2011), suggesting that non-$\alpha_4\beta_2$-containing nicotinic receptors may also influence drinking behavior.

Adenosine. Limited evidence suggests that the effects of ethanol may, in part, be mediated by adenosine in the brain. Adenosine is synthesized from the purine nucleotide adenosine $5'$-triphosphate (ATP). Ethanol may increase extracellular concentrations of adenosine in the basal brain (Asatryan et al. 2011). Adenosine acts on presynaptic adenosine A_1 receptors that function to inhibit glutamate release in the nucleus accumbens. The administration of a selective adenosine A_1 receptor antagonist blocked the sleep-inducing effects of ethanol (Asatryan et al. 2011). Other evidence of the involvement of adenosine systems in regulating the effects of ethanol include the finding that administration of an adenosine A_{2A} receptor antagonist in combination with a glutamate mGluR5 receptor antagonist blocks ethanol self-administration (Adams et al. 2008).

Neuropeptides and Ethanol

Opioid peptides, such as β-endorphin, have been linked both to the rewarding effects of ethanol and to the increased risk for alcoholism (Cowen et al. 2004; Gianoulakis et al. 1989, 1996). Alcohol-preferring rats and humans with a family history of alcoholism show greater increases in β-endorphin after an ethanol challenge than do control subjects (de Waele et al. 1992, 1994). Enkephalins may also play a role in the reinforcing effects of ethanol (Ryabinin et al. 1997, 2001). As discussed later in this chapter in detail, the efficacy of opioid antagonists (e.g., naltrexone, nalmefene) in the treatment of alcoholism provides further support for the relation between the rewarding properties of ethanol and the opioid system (Mason et al. 1994, 1999).

Findings from animal studies suggest that neuropeptide Y (NPY) may modulate ethanol consumption. NPY-deficient mice consume more alcohol than do wild-type mice (Thiele et al. 1998), an effect that is mediated by the Y1 and Y2 receptors (Pandey et al. 2003; Thiele et al. 2000, 2002). By acting on Y2 receptors within the amygdala, NPY may reduce ethanol-induced GABA release, thereby blocking the actions of ethanol (Gilpin et al. 2011). NPY Y1 agonists and Y2 antagonists may have promise in the treatment of alcoholism (Cowen et al. 2004). This approach is supported by the observation that in animals, chronic treatment with NPY blocks excess responding for ethanol (Gilpin et al. 2011).

Orexins (hypocretins) (i.e., neuropeptides that regulate feeding behavior) also have been implicated in the regulation of ethanol-seeking behavior (Plaza-Zabala et al. 2012). Both cue- and context-induced alcohol-seeking behaviors occur in association with the activation of hypothalamic orexin-containing neurons. Blockade of the orexin-1 and orexin-2 receptors attenuates alcohol self-administration by animals. In alcohol-dependent subjects, orexin plasma levels were positively correlated with levels of distress during detoxification (von der Goltz et al. 2011).

Ghrelin, a stomach-derived neuropeptide that regulates appetite, also has been implicated in the regulation of alcohol-seeking behaviors. This peptide enhances dopamine release and promotes alcohol-seeking behaviors in animals (Jerlhag et al. 2009). Circulating levels of ghrelin are elevated in individuals with alcohol use disorders, and significant associations have been reported between variation in ghrelin genes and alcohol dependence in women (Landgren et al. 2008; Leggio et al. 2011). These findings support further investigation into the role of ghrelin in the development of alcohol use disorders.

Release of the peptide corticotropin-releasing factor (CRF) is increased in the amygdala during alcohol withdrawal (Merlo Pich et al. 1995). Within the amygdala of alcohol-dependent animals, ethanol-induced GABA release is potentiated by CRF (Roberto et al. 2010). CRF has been postulated to drive ethanol consumption by enhancing anxiety and other dysphoric effects of ethanol withdrawal. These actions may be counteracted by the blockade of CRF_1 receptors (Overstreet et al. 2004).

In summary, evidence indicates that neuropeptides, including CRF, ghrelin, NPY, the opioids, and the orexins, regulate ethanol-seeking behaviors and thus are targets for medications to treat alcoholism. In addition to these neuropeptides, other peptides that have been linked to the actions of ethanol include urocortin, cholecystokinin, melanocortins, and galanin (for reviews, see Cowen et al. 2004; Egli 2003; Thiele et al. 2003), which may also be targets for medications to treat alcohol dependence.

Dependence, Tolerance, Withdrawal, and Abstinence

Following chronic exposure to alcohol, tolerance develops to many of its $GABA_A$-mediated effects. This includes tolerance to the antianxiety, motor-impairing, sedative-hypnotic, and reinforcing effects of alcohol (Kumar et al. 2009). Decreased sensitivity to the effects of ethanol may be related, at least in part, to increases in the relative densities of $GABA_A$ receptors that contain α_4 subunits, with a change in the expression of these subunits from extrasynaptic to synaptic areas and enhanced expression of γ_2 subunits. The alcohol-induced increases in cortical α_4 subunits have been linked to the γ-isoform of PKC (Werner et al. 2011). Whether tolerance develops from increased association of α_4 with γ_2 subunits remains to be determined.

Prolonged exposure to ethanol can lead to dependence that becomes evident during periods of withdrawal, symptoms of which include tremor and hyperexcitability, which can lead to seizures. Levels of mRNA for both cortical α_1 and α_2 subunits are reduced by chronic alcohol exposure (Sheela Rani and Ticku 2006). In animals, such exposure may lead to the internalization of α_1-containing $GABA_A$ receptors into neurons in several brain regions, including the hippocampus and the hypothalamus. Alcohol-induced internalization of $GABA_A$ receptors that contain the α_1 subunit may result from the actions of the γ-isoform of PKC (Kumar et al. 2010).

The functional activity of NMDA receptors is increased by prolonged exposure to ethanol (Hendricson et al. 2007). Although in most brain regions (e.g., the hippocampus [Grover et al. 1994]), chronic exposure results in tolerance to ethanol's inhibitory effects on NMDA receptor function, in some brain regions (e.g., the basolateral amygdala [Floyd et al. 2003]), such tolerance to chronic ethanol's inhibitory effects does not occur. The development of tolerance to ethanol in the hippocampus may be related to alterations in protein tyrosine phosphorylation of NMDA receptor subunits (Wu et al. 2010).

The mechanism by which NMDA receptor function is increased by prolonged ethanol exposure remains to be fully characterized. Expression of mRNA involved in the formation of the NR1 subunit is increased in several brain regions as a result of chronic exposure to alcohol. Prolonged exposure to alcohol has also been found to increase the expression of NR1, NR2A, and NR2B subunits in hippocampal neurons, but only with high concentrations of ethanol (Hendricson et al. 2007). It has also been shown that ethanol-related phosphorylation by Fyn-like kinase may enhance the activity of NMDA receptors that contain NR2B subunits (Wang et al. 2007).

Given the importance of the mesolimbic system in regulating ethanol-seeking behaviors, any ethanol-induced changes in this system could have significant implications for drinking behavior and risk of alcohol use disorders. When ethanol is administered on a short-term basis (a week or less), the VTA becomes sensitized to its stimulating effect on dopamine neurons (Ding et al. 2009a). In rodents, sustained exposure to ethanol may result in an increase in the rate of reuptake of dopamine (Budygin et al. 2007) and increases in dopamine transporter levels in the nucleus accumbens (Jiao et al. 2006; Rothblat et al. 2001). In one study, no differences were found for striatal dopamine transporter binding sites between alcoholic and nonalcoholic subjects (Volkow et al. 1996). Striatal dopamine D_2 receptor availability was lower in alcoholic than in control subjects in this study. D_2 receptor levels in the ventral striatum also were lower in alcoholic individuals as compared with healthy subjects in another study (Heinz et al. 2004). In abstinent alcoholic individuals, negative correlations have been found between levels of craving for ethanol and both D_2 receptor levels and dopamine synthetic capacity. These results point to functional dopamine deficits within the striatum as neural correlates of motivation to consume alcohol.

Summary

The pharmacodynamic effects of ethanol are complex. A complicated neural network involved in the actions of ethanol accounts for its reinforcing, intoxicating, and abstinence effects. Thus, any attempt to link alcohol's actions to specific neurotransmitters or isolated brain regions is unlikely to account for many of its effects. At present, testing medications that target neurotransmitters and neuromodulators affected by ethanol is a reasonable strategy for the development of medications that reduce the reinforcing effects of alcohol and ameliorate the craving and withdrawal symptoms that commonly occur in the context of alcohol dependence. Ultimately, however, multiple medications administered together or in series may be required to treat most alcohol use disorders.

Pharmacotherapy for Heavy Drinking and Alcohol Use Disorders

The two main settings in which medications are used for alcohol treatment are to control alcohol withdrawal symptoms (i.e., detoxification) and to reduce or prevent alcohol consumption (i.e., secondary prevention or relapse prevention). In the subsections that follow, we first discuss pharmacological approaches to detoxification from alcohol. We then discuss the two major approaches to the use of pharmacotherapy in alcohol treatment: 1) the reduction or cessation of drinking, which involves direct efforts to reduce either the positive or the negative reinforcing effects of alcohol, and 2) the treatment of co-occurring psychiatric symptoms, which may be understood as the effort to reduce the mood or anxiety symptoms that commonly occur among alcoholic patients and may impede the recovery process. In discussing all of these applications, we focus on medications that are of current interest to the clinician or that are likely to yield important clinical advances in the near future. Johnson (2008) and Edwards et al. (2011) have previously published comprehensive reviews of medications to treat alcohol use disorders.

Treatment of Alcohol Withdrawal

An important initial intervention for a minority of alcohol-dependent patients (i.e., those who are most severely dependent) is the management of alcohol withdrawal through detoxification. The objectives in treating alcohol withdrawal are the relief of discomfort, prevention or treatment of complications, and preparation for rehabilitation. Effective management of the alcohol withdrawal syndrome is generally necessary for subsequent efforts at rehabilitation to be successful; treatment of withdrawal alone is usually not sufficient, because relapse occurs commonly.

The identification of co-occurring medical problems is an important element in detoxification (Naranjo and Sellers 1986). The administration of thiamine (50–100 mg po or im) and multivitamins is a low-cost, low-risk intervention for the prophylaxis and treatment of alcohol-related neurological disturbances. Good supportive care and treatment of concurrent illness, including fluid and electrolyte repletion, are essential (Naranjo and Sellers 1986).

Social detoxification, which involves the nonpharmacological treatment of alcohol withdrawal, is effective in managing mild-to-moderate alcohol withdrawal (Naranjo et al. 1983). It consists of frequent reassurance, reality orientation, monitoring of vital signs, personal attention, and general nursing care (Naranjo and Sellers 1986). The medical problems commonly associated with alcoholism (Sullivan and O'Connor 2004) may substantially complicate therapy, so care must be taken to refer patients whose condition requires medical management.

Control of early withdrawal symptoms, which prevents their progression to more serious symptoms, is the indication for which medications are most widely prescribed in the treatment of alcohol dependence (Table 1–1). The most commonly used agents to treat alcohol withdrawal are the benzodiazepines, which, by virtue of their positive modulation of activity at the $GABA_A$ receptor complex, suppress the hyperexcitability associated with alcohol withdrawal. Anticonvulsant medications, which can also decrease the CNS hyperexcitability associated with alcohol withdrawal, are increasingly being used for alcohol detoxification.

Detoxification is now frequently done on an ambulatory basis, in part because it is much less costly than inpatient detoxification (Hayashida et al. 1989). Inpatient detoxification is indicated for serious medical or surgical illness and for individuals with a history of adverse withdrawal reactions or with current evidence of more serious withdrawal (e.g., delirium tremens) (Feldman et al. 1975).

Because of their favorable side-effect profile, the benzodiazepines have supplanted older drugs such as paraldehyde and chloral hydrate (Naranjo and Sellers 1986). Although any benzodiazepine will suppress alcohol withdrawal symptoms, diazepam and chlordiazepoxide have often been used because they

Table 1–1. Management of the alcohol withdrawal syndrome

Symptom-triggered approach

Patients are monitored for withdrawal symptoms with the CIWA-Ar.

CIWA-Ar scores >10 indicate that medication is required.

Preferred medications are benzodiazepines.

Advantages of lorazepam, 2–4 mg orally: not metabolized by liver, and intravenous dose is available for rapid treatment of evolving delirium.

Oxazepam, 30–60 mg; diazepam, 10–20 mg; or chlordiazepoxide, 50–100 mg, is commonly used instead of lorazepam.

CIWA-Ar is administered hourly and dose is repeated if CIWA-Ar scores remain >10.

Goal is light sedation and CIWA-Ar scores of ≤7.

Benzodiazepine taper can be accomplished rapidly once withdrawal symptoms are stabilized.

Benzodiazepines with long-acting metabolites have the advantage of a smooth self-taper but the disadvantages of drug accumulation (if hepatic function impaired) and oversedation.

As the dose of benzodiazepine is increased, it may be difficult to distinguish alcohol withdrawal and benzodiazepine (iatrogenic) delirium.

Fixed-dose schedules

Chlordiazepoxide, 50 mg every 6 hours, followed by 25 mg every 6 hours for eight doses **or**

Diazepam, 10 mg to 5 mg, or lorazepam, 2 mg to 1 mg, at same schedule as outlined for chlordiazepoxide.

Fixed-dose schedules are most often used in patients for whom even mild symptoms may present medical risk.

CIWA-Ar monitoring should be done as needed. Despite a fixed-dose schedule, patients' withdrawal symptoms may not be adequately controlled, necessitating the use of additional doses of chlordiazepoxide or diazepam.

Delirium

Most common regimen is lorazepam, 2 mg, with haloperidol, 5 mg, intravenously.

Risk of torsades de pointes with haloperidol.

Treatment of delirium should be done on a medical unit with telemetry.

Note.   CIWA-Ar = Revised Clinical Institute Withdrawal Assessment for Alcohol.

are metabolized to long-acting compounds, which in effect are self-tapering. However, because the metabolism of these drugs is hepatic, impaired liver function may complicate their use. Oxazepam and lorazepam are not oxidized to long-acting metabolites and thus carry less risk of accumulation.

The anticonvulsant carbamazepine appears useful as a primary treatment of alcohol withdrawal (Eyer et al. 2011; Malcolm et al. 1989, 2002). Although equal to lorazepam in decreasing the symptoms of alcohol withdrawal, carbamazepine was superior to lorazepam in preventing rebound withdrawal symptoms and reducing posttreatment drinking, especially among patients with a history of multiple episodes of treated withdrawal (Malcolm et al. 2002). Other anticonvulsants also have been examined as adjuncts to standard detoxification treatment. Reoux et al. (2001) compared divalproex at a dosage of 500 mg three times daily for 7 days with matched placebo in patients receiving treatment with oxazepam in a symptom-triggered detoxification protocol. Treatment with divalproex resulted in significantly less use of oxazepam and a significantly slower progression of withdrawal symptoms. In a retrospective study, valproate was superior to carbamazepine with respect to withdrawal-related complications and adverse reactions (Eyer et al. 2011). Although carbamazepine and valproate appear to be of value in the treatment of alcohol withdrawal, the liver dysfunction that is common in alcoholic patients may reduce the metabolism of carbamazepine or increase the risk of hepatotoxicity associated with valproate, so that careful blood-level monitoring of these medications in this context is warranted.

The anticonvulsant agent gabapentin has been studied as a treatment for alcohol withdrawal. At a dosage of 1,200 mg/day, gabapentin reduced withdrawal symptom scores more than did lorazepam at 6 mg/day (Myrick et al. 2009). Zonisamide is another anticonvulsant that may have efficacy in the treatment of alcohol withdrawal (Rubio et al. 2010); more studies, however, are needed to fully establish its utility in this role. Pregabalin does not appear to have a role in the treatment of alcohol withdrawal at this time (Forg et al. 2012).

Antipsychotics are not indicated for the treatment of withdrawal except when hallucinations or severe agitation is present (Naranjo and Sellers 1986), in which case they should be added to a benzodiazepine. In addition to their potential to produce extrapyramidal side effects, antipsychotics lower seizure threshold, which increases the risk of seizure during alcohol withdrawal.

Medications to Reduce or Stop Drinking Behavior

The two major approaches to the use of medications in the secondary prevention or rehabilitation of alcoholism are 1) direct efforts to reduce or stop drinking behavior by producing adverse effects when alcohol is consumed or by modifying the neurotransmitter systems that mediate alcohol reinforcement, and 2) the treatment of persistent psychiatric symptoms, in which the aim is to reduce the risk of relapse by reducing the motivation to drink to "self-medicate" such symptoms.

Alcohol-Sensitizing Agents

In the United States, the only alcohol-sensitizing medication approved to treat alcoholism is disulfiram (Antabuse), which inhibits ALDH. The consumption of alcohol following the ingestion of disulfiram substantially elevates the plasma concentration of acetaldehyde, resulting in the signs and symptoms characteristic of the disulfiram-ethanol reaction (DER). The intensity of the DER varies with both the dose of disulfiram and the volume of alcohol ingested.

The DER includes warmness and flushing of the skin, especially that of the upper chest and face; increased heart rate; palpitations; and decreased blood pressure. It may also include nausea, vomiting, shortness of breath, sweating, dizziness, blurred vision, and confusion. Although the DER generally lasts about 30 minutes and is self-limited, occasionally it may include marked tachycardia, hypotension, or bradycardia. Rarely, cardiovascular collapse and convulsions have occurred as part of the DER.

Pharmacology of disulfiram. Disulfiram is almost completely absorbed after oral administration. Because it binds irreversibly to ALDH, renewed enzyme activity is dependent on the synthesis of new enzyme. Thus, the risk of a DER can last for at least 2 weeks from the last ingestion of disulfiram, during which time alcohol should be avoided.

Disulfiram produces a variety of adverse effects independent of the DER, which commonly include drowsiness, lethargy, and fatigue (Chick 1999). Other more serious adverse effects, such as optic neuritis, peripheral neuropathy, and hepatotoxicity, are rare. Psychiatric effects of disulfiram are also uncommon and probably occur only at higher dosages of the drug. They may result from the inhibition by disulfiram of a variety of enzymes in addition to ALDH, including dopamine β-hydroxylase. Inhibition of dopamine β-hydroxylase increases dopamine levels, which can exacerbate psychotic symptoms in schizo-phrenia and occasionally may result in psychotic or depressive symptoms among nonschizophrenic individuals.

Disulfiram is administered orally. Because of the increased risk of side ef-fects and toxic hazards as the dosage is increased, the dosage prescribed in the United States has been limited to 250–500 mg/day. However, efforts to titrate the dosage of disulfiram in relation to a challenge dose of ethanol indicate that some patients require in excess of 1 g/day of disulfiram to achieve blood con-centrations sufficient to produce a DER (Brewer 1984).

Clinical use of disulfiram.   Disulfiram has long been used in the rehabilita-tion of alcoholic patients (Favazza and Martin 1974), despite a lack of meth-odologically sound evaluations confirming its clinical efficacy. Its approval by the U.S. Food and Drug Administration (FDA) preceded the implementation of rigorous requirements for efficacy that now must be satisfied for a drug to be marketed in the United States. In the controlled studies that were con-ducted following approval, the difference in outcome between subjects receiv-ing disulfiram and those given placebo has generally been minimal.

The largest and most methodologically rigorous study of disulfiram was a multicenter trial conducted by the Veterans Administration Cooperative Studies Group, in which more than 600 male alcoholic patients were ran-domly assigned to receive 1 mg/day or 250 mg/day of disulfiram or an inactive placebo (Fuller et al. 1986). Patients assigned to the two disulfiram groups were told that they were being given the drug, but neither patients nor staff knew the dosage. Results showed a direct relation between compliance with the medication regimen (in all three groups) and complete abstinence. In a planned secondary analysis of patients who resumed drinking, those receiving 250 mg of disulfiram had significantly fewer drinking days than did patients in either of the other two groups. However, no significant differences were seen among the three groups on a variety of other outcome measures. On the basis of these findings, disulfiram may be helpful in reducing the frequency of drinking in men who cannot remain abstinent, although given the large num-ber of statistical analyses, it is possible that this finding arose by chance (Fuller et al. 1986).

In addition, disulfiram may be useful among selected groups of alcoholic patients who require special efforts to ensure compliance. Specific behavioral efforts that may enhance compliance with disulfiram (as well as other medications in the treatment of alcoholism) include providing incentives to the patient, contracting with the patient and a significant other to work together to ensure compliance, providing regular reminders and other information to the patient, and providing behavioral training and social support (Allen and Litten 1992). Azrin et al. (1982) found that a trial program of stimulus control training, role-playing, communication skills training, and recreational and vocational counseling improved outcome in disulfiram-treated patients compared with those receiving placebo. Evidence indicates that supervision of patients taking disulfiram may be essential to ensure compliance and enhance the beneficial effects of the medication (Brewer et al. 2000). Chick et al. (1992) randomly assigned patients to receive disulfiram, 200 mg/day, or placebo as an adjunct to outpatient alcoholism treatment. Medication was ingested under the supervision of an individual nominated by the patient. In this 6-month study, disulfiram treatment significantly increased abstinent days and decreased total drinks consumed, effects that were confirmed by parallel changes in levels of the hepatic enzyme γ-glutamyltransferase (GGT).

In deciding with the patient whether disulfiram should be used in alcoholism rehabilitation, the hazards of the medication should be discussed, including the need to avoid over-the-counter preparations with alcohol, foods prepared with alcohol, and drugs that can interact with disulfiram. The administration of disulfiram to anyone who does not agree to its use, does not seek to be abstinent from alcohol, or has any psychological or medical contraindications is not recommended.

Drugs That Directly Reduce Alcohol Consumption by Diminishing Its Reinforcing Effects

As reviewed earlier, several neurotransmitter systems influence the reinforcing or discriminative stimulus effects of ethanol. Although these systems function interactively in influencing drinking behavior, most of the medications that have been used to treat alcohol dependence affect neurotransmitter systems relatively selectively. Consequently, we discuss these systems individually here.

Opioidergic agents. Naltrexone and nalmefene are both opioid antagonists with no or limited intrinsic agonist properties. Naltrexone has been studied more extensively than nalmefene as a treatment for alcohol dependence. The

FDA approved oral naltrexone to treat opioid dependence in 1984 and to treat alcohol dependence in 1994. Naltrexone was approved as a long-acting injectable formulation to treat alcohol dependence in 2006 and to treat opioid dependence in 2010. Nalmefene is approved in the United States as a parenteral formulation to reverse the acute effects of opioids (e.g., following opioid overdose or analgesia) and is being developed in the European Union to reduce heavy drinking on an as-needed basis.

Naltrexone. Naltrexone is a μ opioid receptor antagonist with possible κ receptor partial agonist activity (Gastfriend 2011). The drug is converted in the liver into the metabolite 6β-naltrexol. The half-life of naltrexone is approximately 9 hours and that of 6β-naltrexol is about 8 hours (Wall et al. 1981).

Approval of naltrexone for alcohol dependence was based on the results of two single-site studies, in which it was shown to be efficacious in the prevention of relapse to heavy drinking (O'Malley et al. 1992; Volpicelli et al. 1992). In a 12-week study, Volpicelli et al. (1992) compared naltrexone with placebo in a sample of alcohol-dependent veterans, initially as an adjunct to an intensive day treatment program. In this study, naltrexone was well tolerated and resulted in significantly less craving for alcohol and fewer drinking days than did placebo. Naltrexone also limited the progression of drinking from initial sampling of alcohol to a relapse to heavy drinking. Study subjects who drank while taking the medication reported less euphoria, suggesting that naltrexone blocked the endogenous opioid system's contribution to alcohol's "priming effect" (Volpicelli et al. 1995).

Many, but not all, subsequent studies of naltrexone have provided support for its use in alcohol treatment. A series of meta-analyses have consistently shown an advantage for naltrexone over placebo, principally in reducing the risk of heavy drinking (Bouza et al. 2004; Kranzler and Van Kirk 2001; Rösner et al. 2010; Srisurapanont and Jarusuraisin 2005). The most recent meta-analysis (Rösner et al. 2010) included a total of 50 randomized controlled trials (RCTs) with 7,793 participants. It showed that naltrexone reduced the risk of heavy drinking by about 17% relative to the placebo group, a modest but significant effect. Naltrexone also decreased drinking days by about 4%, which was not statistically significant. Treatment with naltrexone also reduced the number of heavy drinking days, the amount of alcohol consumed, and GGT levels significantly more than placebo did. Differences from placebo in the therapeutic effects of the long-acting injectable formulation of naltrexone and of nalmefene were not statistically significant, but the meta-analysis included too few studies of either of these to draw meaningful conclusions.

Few naltrexone studies have exceeded 3 months in duration. One 6-month study (Landabaso et al. 1999), which was randomized but open-label, showed an advantage for naltrexone on the rate of both relapse and total abstinence. The Veterans Affairs Naltrexone Cooperative Study (Krystal et al. 2001) included both 12-week and 52-week treatment durations, neither of which showed an advantage for naltrexone over placebo on any of the outcomes examined. Treatment in the pivotal study of long-acting naltrexone for alcohol dependence (Garbutt et al. 2005) was 6 months in duration; it is discussed later in this chapter in detail.

Follow-up studies of patients taking naltrexone or placebo for 12 weeks (Anton et al. 2000; O'Malley et al. 1996) showed that among naltrexone-treated patients, the relapse rate, the number of drinking days, and the number of heavy drinking days all increased gradually following the cessation of therapy. These findings suggest that treatment with naltrexone is warranted for longer than 12 weeks, although the optimal duration of treatment remains to be determined.

An approach to the use of naltrexone based on its efficacy in reducing the risk of heavy drinking is to "target" the medication to high-risk drinking situations (Kranzler et al. 1997). Kranzler et al. (2003a) compared the effects of naltrexone, 50 mg, with those of placebo in an 8-week study of problem drinkers. Patients were randomly assigned to receive study medication either daily or targeted to situations identified by the patients as being high risk for heavy drinking. The number of tablets available for use by patients in the targeted conditions began with daily treatment, declining by one tablet each week, with no study medication available to them in the last week of the trial. Irrespective of whether they received naltrexone or placebo, patients in the targeted condition showed a reduced likelihood of any drinking. Overall, naltrexone treatment resulted in a 19% reduction in the likelihood of heavy drinking. Because of the large number of nondrinking days in the study, a secondary analysis of these data compared treatment conditions and gender effects on average drinks per day with a zero-inflated Poisson regression model (Hernandez-Avila et al. 2006).

Targeted naltrexone, and to a lesser extent targeted placebo, yielded a greater reduction in daily drinking than did daily placebo, an effect that did not differ by gender and that was greater than that seen for daily naltrexone treatment. Relative to daily placebo, daily naltrexone reduced the number of drinks per day among only men, at the level of a nonsignificant trend.

Although targeted treatments appeared to reduce the volume of drinking in both men and women, active treatment with targeted naltrexone was somewhat better than placebo. In contrast, heavy-drinking women showed no additional benefit from daily naltrexone treatment. Further evaluation of the efficacy of targeted treatments and of daily naltrexone and the relation of these treatments with gender is warranted.

In a subsequent study, Kranzler et al. (2009b) compared 12 weeks of daily or targeted naltrexone or placebo in a sample of 163 problem drinkers whose goal was to reduce their drinking to safe limits. On the primary outcome measure of mean drinks per day, men in the targeted naltrexone group drank significantly less at week 12 than did those in the other groups. On a secondary outcome measure, drinks per drinking day, the targeted naltrexone group drank significantly less than the other groups did during week 12, with no moderating gender effect. These results suggest that naltrexone may be useful for the reduction of heavy drinking, even among patients who may not meet criteria for alcohol dependence.

Heinala et al. (2001) compared naltrexone, 50 mg/day, with placebo, paired with either coping skills or supportive therapy. During the first 12 weeks of treatment, naltrexone was superior to placebo in preventing relapse to heavy drinking, but only in combination with coping skills therapy. During a subsequent 20-week period, subjects were told to use their medication only when they craved alcohol (i.e., targeted treatment). A lower risk of relapse in the naltrexone group was generally sustained during the targeted treatment. Together, findings with targeted naltrexone support its use for the initial treatment of problem drinking and to maintain the beneficial effects of an initial period of daily naltrexone.

Using a primary care model of treatment, O'Malley et al. (2003) initially prescribed open-label naltrexone to alcohol-dependent patients for 10 weeks, in combination with either cognitive-behavioral therapy (CBT) or primary care management (a less intensive, supportive approach). They found no effect of psychosocial treatment on response to treatment, although CBT was associated with a lower risk of drinking. Treatment responders from this study were then randomly assigned to one of two placebo-controlled 24-week continuation studies, in which patients received concomitant treatment with either CBT or primary care management. Although there was no advantage observed for naltrexone in combination with CBT, among patients receiving primary care management, naltrexone treatment was superior to placebo on both response rate and drinking frequency. These findings suggest that the initial treatment effects of naltrexone can be maintained during an extended period through the use of either a more intensive, skills-oriented treatment (i.e., CBT) or a less intensive, supportive treatment when combined with continued naltrexone administration.

The COMBINE Study, a large placebo-controlled trial, compared naltrexone, acamprosate, and their combination, together with either medical management or an intensive psychotherapy (Anton et al. 2006). The combination of naltrexone with medical management, compared with medical management alone, produced a modest reduction in risk of days of heavy drinking and a modest increase in the percentage of days abstinent. The efficacy of naltrexone was not enhanced by the addition of an intensive cognitive-behavioral intervention. A later analysis of the COMBINE data indicated that the effects of naltrexone treatment on heavy drinking were limited to type A alcoholic individuals (i.e., those with late-onset drinking and few childhood risk factors for drinking) (Bogenschutz et al. 2009).

Because poor compliance with oral naltrexone may reduce the potential benefits of the medication, long-acting injectable formulations have been developed. In a small pilot study, alcoholic patients receiving subcutaneous treatment with a depot formulation of naltrexone had detectable plasma concentrations of the drug for more than 30 days following the injection (Kranzler et al. 1998). The active formulation was superior to placebo in reducing the frequency of heavy drinking in these patients. Two long-acting naltrexone formulations developed for intramuscular injection also have been tested for safety and efficacy in alcoholic patients. A depot naltrexone formulation was evaluated in a 12-week, placebo-controlled trial in 315 patients who also received motivational enhancement therapy (Kranzler et al. 2004). In that study, the active formulation was well tolerated. Although it did not reduce the risk of heavy drinking, it delayed the onset of any drinking, increased the total number of days of abstinence, and doubled the likelihood of subjects remaining abstinent throughout the study period (Kranzler et al. 2004). A more definitive RCT was conducted with a different long-acting formulation (Garbutt et al. 2005), which ultimately led to the approval of that formulation by the FDA for the treatment of alcohol dependence. More than 600 alcohol-dependent adults were randomly assigned to receive six monthly long-acting injections of naltrexone, 380 mg; naltrexone, 190 mg; or matching volumes of placebo. The medication and the injections were well tolerated. Compared with placebo treatment, long-acting naltrexone, 380 mg, resulted in a 25% reduction in the rate of heavy drinking. There was a strong effect in men (48% reduction) but no advantage over placebo in women. The long-acting naltrexone at a dosage of 190 mg resulted in a 17% reduction in heavy drinking, but it was not significantly better than placebo.

Although there are no head-to-head comparisons of the long-acting formulation to oral naltrexone, adherence with the long-acting release formulation appears to be better (Gastfriend 2011). Six months of treatment with the long-acting formulation has been shown to lead to significant improvements in measures of quality of life, including those for mental health, social functioning, general health, and physical functioning. Adverse effects associated with the long-acting naltrexone formulations are similar to those associated with the oral formulation, including nausea, headache, and fatigue. Long-acting formulations are also associated with local reactions at the injection site.

Carriers of a variant (118G or Asp40 allele) of *OPRM1,* the gene encoding the μ opioid receptor, may have a better clinical response to naltrexone than do individuals homozygous for the more common A118 (or Asn40) allele (Oslin et al. 2003). A recent meta-analysis of the moderating effects of the Asp40 allele from six published studies showed that naltrexone-treated patients carrying the Asp40 allele were more than twice as likely not to relapse as Asn40 allele homozygotes. The polymorphism had no effect on abstinence rates. Identifying individuals who carry the Asp40 allele could help to differentiate a subgroup of the population that is more likely to respond to naltrexone treatment. However, the prevalence of the Asp40 allele varies widely in different populations (58% in Asians, 20% in whites of European descent, and 5% in individuals of African descent have one or two copies of the allele), so the effects of naltrexone would be predicted to vary substantially by population (Ray and Oslin 2009).

Another approach to improving the response to treatment with naltrexone has been to combine it with other medications. Kiefer et al. (2003) randomly assigned 160 detoxified alcoholic patients to receive naltrexone, acamprosate, naltrexone plus acamprosate, or placebo for 12 weeks under double-blind conditions. They found that naltrexone, acamprosate, and the two medications combined were significantly more efficacious than placebo. In addition, the naltrexone group showed a tendency to have a longer time to the first drink and time to relapse than did the acamprosate group. The combined medication group had a significantly lower relapse rate than either the placebo group or the acamprosate group, but the combined medication was not statistically superior to naltrexone. A single-blind study by Rubio et al. (2001) compared naltrexone, 50 mg/day, with acamprosate (up to 1,998 mg/day) over a 12-month treatment period. These investigators found a significant advantage for naltrexone over placebo on the following outcomes: rates of abstinence and relapse, cumulative abstinence, time to relapse, number of drinks per drinking day, severity of craving, and retention rate.

Nalmefene.   Nalmefene also has been evaluated for the treatment of alcohol dependence. A pilot study (Mason et al. 1994) showed that nalmefene, 40 mg/day, was superior either to 10 mg/day of the drug or to placebo in the prevention of relapse to heavy drinking in a small sample of alcoholic patients. A subsequent study showed no difference between 20 mg/day and 80 mg/day of nalmefene, although the combined group of nalmefene-treated subjects had significantly better outcomes on measures of heavy drinking than did the placebo group (Mason et al. 1999). A 12-week multisite, dose-ranging study comparing placebo with 5, 20, or 40 mg of nalmefene was conducted in recently abstinent alcoholic outpatients (Anton et al. 2004). During the study, all subjects showed a reduction in self-reported heavy drinking days and on biological measures of drinking, but there was no difference between the active medication and placebo groups on these measures.

After three multicenter trials of up to 12 months' duration were conducted in Europe, an application was submitted to the European Medicines Agency (EMA) to approve nalmefene, 18 mg, for use on an as-needed basis to reduce heavy drinking in alcohol-dependent individuals. The first of these studies (Mann et al. 2012) enrolled 598 patients, randomly assigning them to either nalmefene or placebo treatment for 6 months. Nalmefene was statistically superior to placebo, reducing heavy drinking days by 2.3 more days per month and total alcohol consumption by about one standard drink (i.e., 11 g) per day. The second study (Gual et al. 2012) randomly assigned 718 alcohol-dependent patients to nalmefene or placebo treatment for 6 months. This study showed a statistically significant effect of nalmefene, which reduced the number of heavy drinking days by 1.7 days per month more than placebo. Nalmefene also had a greater, but not statistically significant, effect in reducing the total alcohol consumption by about one-half of a standard drink (i.e., 5 g) per day. The third study (van den Brink et al. 2012) randomly assigned 665 patients to nalmefene or placebo for a total of 52 weeks of treatment. Nalmefene was efficacious in reducing the number of heavy drinking days and total alcohol consumption beginning in the first month and persisting throughout the treatment period. There was a statistically significant advantage for nalmefene at most time points, including at the end of treatment, but not at the midpoint of the study. In addition to the effects on self-reported drinking, nalmefene significantly reduced GGT serum concentrations in two of the three studies and alanine aminotransferase serum concentrations in all three studies.

Summary of the use of opioid antagonists to treat alcohol dependence. Abundant evidence supports the use of naltrexone to treat alcohol dependence. Although this medication has only a small effect size in unselected samples of patients (Rösner et al. 2010), there is growing evidence that naltrexone may be of particular utility in subgroups of patients. The ready identification of these individuals is of great clinical interest, as is the potential utility of combining naltrexone with other medications and with specific kinds of psychotherapy. The optimal dosage and duration of treatment are two important clinical questions that remain to be adequately addressed. New approaches to the use of naltrexone, including targeted administration and long-acting injectable formulations, promise to enhance the clinical utility of the medication. The literature supporting the use of nalmefene now includes three large multicenter trials that support its efficacy. Approval for its use in Europe appears likely.

Acamprosate.   Acamprosate (calcium acetylhomotaurinate) is an amino acid derivative with a mechanism of action that is yet to be clearly defined. It may act as a weak antagonist of NMDA receptor activity and may also inhibit the activity of the metabotropic glutamate receptor 5 (mGluR5) (Blednov and Harris

2008; Mann et al. 2008). These actions may cause acamprosate to reduce the excitability of glutamatergic systems during withdrawal from alcohol. The finding that acamprosate administration reduces anxiety in animals during ethanol withdrawal is consistent with this hypothesis (Kotlinska and Bochenski 2008). In treatment-seeking alcoholic patients, acamprosate administration reduced craving produced by alcohol priming (Hammarberg et al. 2009). This effect may involve acamprosate-induced modulation of dopamine release within the nucleus accumbens. However, evidence indicates that in alcohol-dependent individuals with high levels of craving, naltrexone is more effective than acamprosate in reducing drinking (Richardson et al. 2008).

Initially evaluated in a single-center trial in France, acamprosate was shown to be twice as effective as placebo in reducing the rate at which alcoholic individuals returned to drinking (Lhuintre et al. 1985). The safety and efficacy of the medication have been studied most widely in Europe, and three of these studies provided the basis for the approval of acamprosate by the FDA for clinical use in the United States. As with naltrexone, several meta-analytic studies provide consistent evidence of acamprosate's efficacy in the treatment of alcohol dependence.

There have been a series of meta-analyses of the effects of acamprosate (Bouza et al. 2004; Chick et al. 2003; Kranzler and Van Kirk 2001; Mann 2004; Rösner et al. 2010). The most recent of these reviewed 24 RCTs with 6,915 participants. The analysis showed that acamprosate significantly reduced the risk of any drinking and increased the cumulative abstinence duration. The likelihood of beneficial effects in industry-sponsored trials did not differ significantly from that of publicly funded trials. The authors concluded that acamprosate appeared to be a safe and effective treatment to support continuous abstinence after detoxification in patients with alcohol dependence, although the size of the treatment effects was modest (Rösner et al. 2010).

Two large multicenter trials in the United States (Anton et al. 2006; Mason et al. 2006), a large European study (Mann et al. 2009), and a large Australian study (Morley et al. 2006) failed to detect beneficial effects of acamprosate compared with placebo in the treatment of alcohol dependence. In the COMBINE Study, the administration of acamprosate did not significantly alter measures of alcohol consumption irrespective of the intensity of the concomitant psychosocial treatment provided. Furthermore, the combination of acamprosate and naltrexone did not significantly decrease measures of drinking.

Substantial differences in the results of the published studies have been attributed to the greater severity of alcohol dependence in the studies showing efficacy and the high prevalence of co-occurring drug abuse in the studies failing to show superiority of acamprosate to placebo. The small therapeutic effect of acamprosate can be difficult to detect in heterogeneous samples that are typically examined in multicenter studies.

One study had implications for the use of acamprosate in combination with disulfiram. Besson et al. (1998) randomly assigned patients to receive acamprosate or placebo. Because some of the participants were taking disulfiram when they entered the study, they were randomly assigned separately from those not taking disulfiram. Acamprosate was superior to placebo on measures of total abstinence and on cumulative abstinent days. Interestingly, the group receiving both acamprosate and disulfiram showed a significantly greater percentage of abstinent days than did any of the other three groups. However, because the design was not fully randomized, one cannot conclude that the combination would be more efficacious if initiated together or in an otherwise unselected patient group.

In summary, studies in nearly 7,000 patients provide evidence of a beneficial effect of acamprosate in relapse prevention. It must be noted, however, that acamprosate failed to show superior efficacy to placebo in several large clinical trials. Additional research is needed to identify the patient characteristics and therapeutic approaches that contribute to an optimal response to acamprosate.

Anticonvulsants.   The potential utility of anticonvulsants for the treatment of alcohol dependence was reported initially in placebo-controlled studies of carbamazepine (Mueller et al. 1997), the valproic acid derivative valproate (Salloum et al. 2005), and topiramate (Johnson et al. 2003, 2007; Miranda et al. 2008). In a 12-month pilot study, despite limited medication compliance and study completion, Mueller et al. (1997) found an early advantage to carbamazepine on drinks per drinking day, time to first heavy drinking day, and consecutive days of heavy drinking. Although Salloum et al. reported a significant decrease in alcohol consumption in bipolar patients with alcohol dependence taking valproate, Brady et al. (2002) failed to find similar differences in a 12-week double-blind, placebo-controlled pilot study of divalproex in alcohol-dependent individuals without bipolar disorder.

In both single-site and multisite placebo-controlled clinical trials, Johnson et al. (2003, 2007) found that topiramate at a target dosage of 300 mg/day resulted in large, significant reductions in drinks per day, drinks per drinking day, drinking days, heavy drinking days, and GGT concentration. The treatment of alcohol dependence with topiramate was associated with decreased compulsive thoughts about drinking, increased psychosocial well-being, and improvements in measures of quality of life, including performance of household duties and participation in leisure activities (Johnson et al. 2008). Miranda et al. (2008) conducted a double-blind study of heavy drinkers who were randomly assigned to receive treatment with topiramate, 200 mg/day; topiramate, 300 mg/day; or placebo. The medication was titrated to the target dosage over a 32-day period and then maintained at that dosage for 1 week prior to a human laboratory study. During the titration period, the frequency of heavy drinking was significantly lower in both topiramate groups than with placebo, but no significant difference was seen between the two dosages of topiramate on this measure. A larger proportion of subjects receiving 300 mg of topiramate (19%) than 200 mg of topiramate or placebo (each 5%) discontinued treatment prematurely.

Topiramate treatment is associated with a variety of adverse events, the most frequent of which are paresthesia, anorexia (with weight loss), difficulty with memory or concentration, and taste disturbances. These events are generally mild to moderate in severity. Uncommonly, topiramate causes visual adverse events including myopia, angle-closure glaucoma, and increased intraocular pressure, which require discontinuation of the medication. To minimize topiramate's adverse effects, a slow titration to the maximal dosage (e.g., 300 mg/day over a period of 8 weeks) is recommended. The optimal dosage of topiramate for alcohol dependence treatment remains to be determined; the challenge is to find a dosage that is efficacious while minimizing the likelihood of treatment discontinuation because of adverse effects. Although the report by Miranda et al. (2008) suggests that topiramate, 200 mg/day, may be equally efficacious but better tolerated than topiramate, 300 mg/day, larger prospective studies comparing different dosages are needed to test this hypothesis.

A pilot study showed that the severity of topiramate-related adverse effects in heavy drinkers was moderated by a polymorphism in *GRIK1*, the gene encoding the kainate receptor GluR5 subunit (Ray et al. 2009). The study was based on the finding that the polymorphism was associated with alcohol dependence (Kranzler et al. 2009a) and is of particular interest because the GluR5 subunit binds topiramate specifically (Gryder and Rogawski 2003). Independent validation of these findings is needed before genotyping can be recommended to identify individuals who are best able to tolerate topiramate treatment.

The anticonvulsant zonisamide has structural similarities to topiramate and has similar effects on behavior, most notably in promoting weight loss. Zonisamide has shown some promise in the treatment of alcohol use disorders in a laboratory-based study (Sarid-Segal et al. 2009) and in small open-label and placebo-controlled clinical trials (Arias et al. 2010; Knapp et al. 2010; Rubio et al. 2010).

Baclofen.   Baclofen is a $GABA_B$ agonist widely used for its antispasmodic effects. Over the past decade, it has been evaluated as a treatment for alcohol dependence. In a 30-day placebo-controlled RCT of baclofen at a maximal dosage of 10 mg three times daily in 39 patients with alcohol dependence, Addolorato et al. (2002) found that 70% of the baclofen-treated patients remained abstinent, compared with 21% of the placebo group. Baclofen also reduced anxiety symptoms and craving. Subsequently, these investigators (Addolorato et al. 2007) randomly assigned 84 patients with hepatic cirrhosis to either oral baclofen (10 mg three times daily) or placebo for 12 weeks. Consistent with their earlier finding, 71% of the baclofen-treated patients achieved and maintained abstinence compared with 29% of those assigned to placebo, with the cumulative abstinence duration in baclofen-treated patients more than double that in the placebo group. In contrast, Garbutt et al. (2010) conducted a double-blind, placebo-controlled RCT of 30 mg/day of baclofen in 80 alcohol-dependent subjects. Although baclofen significantly reduced anxiety, it had no effect on a variety of drinking outcomes.

The optimal dosage of baclofen in alcohol dependence treatment remains to be determined. Although two of three published studies showed baclofen to be efficacious at a dosage of 30 mg/day, some investigators reported that in individual cases, high-dosage baclofen therapy (>90 mg/day) has been efficacious in patients unresponsive to other treatments (Muzyk et al. 2012). Secondary analysis of an incomplete 12-week RCT comparing baclofen 30 and 60 mg/day in 42 patients (Addolorato et al. 2011) showed both dosages of the active medication to be superior to placebo regarding the number of drinks per day. Furthermore, there was evidence of a dose-effect relationship, with significantly better outcomes in the higher-dosage group.

In reviewing these studies, Muzyk et al. (2012) concluded that although baclofen appeared to be safe and well tolerated even in the setting of moderate-to-severe cirrhosis, evidence to support the use of baclofen as a first-line treatment was inadequate, except in patients with cirrhosis for whom other pharmacological treatments are not safe or practical.

Serotonergic medications.   A variety of serotonin reuptake inhibitors (SRIs) have been tested in humans to determine their effects on alcohol consumption (see Pettinati et al. 2003 for a review). Study findings on the effects of these medications for alcohol dependence treatment are inconsistent. Naranjo et al. (1990) first reported that fluoxetine, 60 mg/day, reduced average daily alcohol consumption by approximately 17% from baseline levels, whereas treatment with fluoxetine, 40 mg/day, or placebo had no effect. When alcoholic inpatients were given access to alcohol, fluoxetine pretreatment initially reduced alcohol consumption, but the effect was transient (Gorelick and Paredes 1992). Using a crossover design, Gerra et al. (1992) compared the effects of fluoxetine, acamprosate, and placebo in family-history-positive and family-history-negative alcoholic patients. Although both active medications were superior to placebo in reducing the number of drinks consumed, the effect of fluoxetine was significant only in the family-history-positive patients, whereas acamprosate produced a significant reduction only in the family-history-negative patients. Subsequent studies showed no advantage for fluoxetine over placebo in effects on drinking behavior among severe alcoholic patients recruited from an alcoholism treatment program at a Veterans Affairs Medical Center (Kabel and Petty 1996) and no advantage for fluoxetine in combination with coping skills psychotherapy in a 12-week placebo-controlled trial (Kranzler et al. 1995).

Naranjo et al. (1987) found that citalopram at 40 mg/day, but not at 20 mg/day, reduced the number of drinks per day and increased the number of abstinent days from baseline in nondepressed, early-stage problem drinkers, a finding that was subsequently replicated (Naranjo et al. 1992). In another study, however, in which citalopram, 40 mg/day, was combined with a brief psychosocial intervention in a 12-week treatment trial, the active drug show an advantage over placebo only during the first week of treatment (Naranjo et al. 1995). Balldin et al. (1994) found no overall advantage to citalopram compared with placebo; however, when the data were reanalyzed on the basis of the pretreatment level of alcohol consumption, subjects in the lighter-drinking subgroup had lower daily alcohol intake with citalopram. Tiihonen et al. (1996) found a significant advantage for citalopram over placebo in effects on study retention and on collateral informants' reports of the patient's condition, with a trend for decreased alcohol consumption and GGT levels in the active treatment group.

In a secondary analysis of their fluoxetine trial, Kranzler et al. (1996) found that individuals with high-risk or high-severity (i.e., type B) alcoholism—characterized by an earlier age at alcoholism onset—showed a poorer response to the active medication than to placebo. Pettinati et al. (2000) found that individuals with low-risk or low-severity (i.e., type A) alcoholism—characterized by a later age at alcoholism onset—drank on fewer days and were more likely to be abstinent in the 12-week treatment trial when receiving sertraline than when receiving placebo. In a 6-month posttreatment follow-up of these patients (Dundon et al. 2004), the type A subgroup taking sertraline maintained the beneficial effects that were observed during treatment. In contrast, subjects with type B alcoholism initially treated with sertraline were more likely to increase their heavy drinking during the follow-up period than were those given placebo. A recent study of sertraline (Kranzler et al. 2011) showed that its effects on drinking and heavy drinking in alcohol-dependent individuals were moderated by both age at onset of alcohol dependence and the serotonin transporter–linked polymorphic region (5-HTTLPR) polymorphism in the serotonin transporter gene. Specifically, sertraline decreased drinking significantly in patients with late-onset alcoholism with the L'/L' genotype (an effect that persisted during a 3-month follow-up period; Kranzler et al. 2012), whereas early-onset alcoholic patients with this genotype had fewer drinking and heavy drinking days when taking placebo. These results are based on small subsamples and require replication in larger studies.

The 5-HT$_3$ antagonist ondansetron was shown by Johnson et al. (2000) to reduce drinking behavior only among patients with early-onset alcoholism (onset of problem drinking before age 25). At a dosage of 4 μg/kg twice daily—substantially lower than the dosage used for its antiemetic effects—ondansetron was superior to placebo in its effects on the proportion of days abstinent and on the intensity of alcohol intake. In contrast, in late-onset alcoholism, the effects of ondansetron on drinking behavior were in nearly all respects comparable to those of placebo.

Subsequently, Johnson et al. (2011) showed that ondansetron reduced drinking only in alcoholic patients with the 5-HTTLPR L/L genotype. Furthermore, an SNP in the 3′ untranslated region (3′UTR) of the serotonin transporter gene (Seneviratne et al. 2009) interacted with the 5-HTTLPR polymorphism in the same gene to moderate the response to ondansetron. Thus, drinking was reduced by ondansetron most in individuals with the L/L genotype at 5-HTTLPR and the T/T genotype of the 3′UTR SNP.

Antipsychotic agents.   Although several studies have indicated that the atypical antipsychotic agent quetiapine may be efficacious in the treatment of alcohol dependence, a recent placebo-controlled multisite trial failed to support this effect (Litten et al. 2012).

Aripiprazole is an atypical antipsychotic agent that acts as a partial agonist at D_2 and 5-HT_{1A} receptors. A human laboratory study in healthy subjects showed that aripiprazole significantly and dose-dependently increased the sedative effects of alcohol and, to a lesser degree, decreased the euphoric effects of alcohol (Kranzler et al. 2008). The administration of aripiprazole over a 6-day period reduced drinking by alcohol-dependent subjects both prior to and during a human laboratory session (Voronin et al. 2008). Alcohol-dependent subjects who received pretreatment with aripiprazole showed less activation in the ventral striatum, which contains the nucleus accumbens, following exposure to alcohol-related cues than did those who received placebo (Myrick et al. 2010). Although these results suggest that aripiprazole has value in the treatment of alcohol dependence, a multicenter clinical trial failed to support its efficacy. In a 12-week multisite, placebo-controlled clinical trial (Anton et al. 2008), the rate of study discontinuations and treatment-related adverse events was higher in the aripiprazole group than in the placebo group. The treatment groups were similar on the primary outcome measure, the percentage of days abstinent, as well as the percentage of subjects without a heavy drinking day and the time to first drinking day, although the aripiprazole group had fewer drinks per drinking day than did the placebo group.

Partial nicotinic receptor agonists.   Varenicline, a partial nicotinic receptor agonist, is approved for the treatment of nicotine dependence. Seven days of pretreatment with this medication reduced the self-administration of alcohol in a laboratory setting and decreased alcohol craving and positive subjective responses, such as liking, to a priming drink (McKee et al. 2009). Craving for alcohol was decreased in smokers during their first weeks of treatment with varenicline (Fucito et al. 2011). The administration of varenicline to heavy-drinking smokers in a double-blind clinical trial was associated with a significant decrease in alcohol consumption (Mitchell et al. 2012), supporting the idea that partial nicotinic agonists may be of value in treating alcohol dependence.

Summary of Medications to Reduce or Stop Drinking

Currently, the most promising agents that directly reduce alcohol consumption are the opioid antagonists and topiramate. Further research is required to determine which patient groups, dosage schedules, route and duration of therapy, and concomitant psychosocial treatments are optimal for use with these medications. There is a growing literature on genetic factors that appear to moderate the response to naltrexone and serotonergic drugs in the treatment of alcohol dependence. These results suggest that a pharmacogenetic approach is one avenue by which the treatment of alcohol dependence can be enhanced. The identification of the mechanism of action (e.g., of topiramate), which would enhance the development of novel compounds that exert moderate-to-large effects on drinking behavior, is also needed to ensure widespread use of medications to treat alcohol dependence.

Drugs to Treat Co-Occurring Psychiatric Symptoms or Disorders in Alcoholic Patients

Although many alcoholic patients report substantially fewer mood or anxiety symptoms once they have completed acute withdrawal, for many others, anxiety, insomnia, and depressed mood may persist for weeks or months. Even among patients without substantial symptoms of alcohol withdrawal, persistent, low-level symptoms may develop, a condition that has been called *subacute withdrawal*. Other symptoms may reflect diagnosable psychiatric disorders. Although medications (e.g., SRIs) are often used during the postwithdrawal period to relieve these symptoms, their use in the treatment of persistent or subacute withdrawal symptoms that do not meet diagnostic criteria for a co-occurring psychiatric disorder has not been proved to result in a generally better outcome in alcoholic patients.

Many of the early studies of the efficacy of medications to treat mood disturbances were directed at symptoms of depression and anxiety in unselected groups of detoxified alcoholic patients. This approach, combined with other methodological limitations of these studies, led to a failure to show greater reductions in either psychiatric symptoms or drinking behavior than those seen with control treatments (Ciraulo and Jaffe 1981). Over the past two decades, there has been renewed interest in the incidence and prevalence of co-occurring psychiatric disturbances among individuals with alcohol use disorders. Community studies have shown high rates of co-occurrence of drug dependence and psychiatric disorders in alcohol-dependent individuals in the community (Grant and Harford 1995; Grant et al. 2004b; Kessler et al. 1994, 1997; Regier et al. 1990). It is also evident that most alcoholic patients who seek treatment meet lifetime criteria for one or more psychiatric disorders in addition to alcoholism. Most common among these co-occurring disorders are mood disorders, drug dependence, antisocial personality disorder, and anxiety disorders (Hesselbrock et al. 1985; Powell et al. 1982; Ross et al. 1988).

Medications that have been used to treat anxiety and depression in the postwithdrawal state are antidepressants, benzodiazepines and other anxiolytics, antipsychotics, and lithium. In general, the indications for use of these medications in alcoholic patients are similar to those for nonalcoholic patients with psychiatric illness. However, following careful differential diagnosis, the choice of medications should take into account the increased potential for adverse effects in alcoholic patients. For example, adverse effects can result from pharmacodynamic interactions with medical disorders commonly present among alcoholic patients, as well as from pharmacokinetic interactions with medications prescribed to treat the medical disorders (Sullivan and O'Connor 2004).

Several studies indicate that symptoms of depression in subjects with alcohol use disorders may be responsive to pharmacotherapy, including treatment with high doses of tricyclic antidepressants (Mason et al. 1996; McGrath et al. 1996) and SRIs (Cornelius et al. 1997; Roy 1998). Nunes and Levin (2004) conducted a meta-analysis of 14 RCTs of antidepressants in patients with a co-occurring substance use disorder (8 of which focused on alcohol dependence) and unipolar depression. Eight of the studies (6 of which involved alcohol-dependent patients) showed a significant or near-significant advantage for the active medication over placebo. The principal measure of effect size was the standardized difference between mean scores on a depression rating scale. The pooled effect size on this measure was in the small-to-moderate range of effect sizes. There was a trend for the medication effect to be larger in studies of alcohol dependence than in studies of dependence on other substances. The most consistent predictor of medication response was the magnitude of the placebo response: studies with a placebo response rate greater than 25% showed no advantage for the active medication, whereas those with a placebo response rate lower than 25% yielded effects in the moderate-to-large range. Moderator analysis also showed that a diagnosis of depression after a week of abstinence was associated with a better antidepressant response, whereas the presence of a larger proportion of women in the study sample, the use of SRIs (vs. tricyclic or other antidepressants), and a concurrent psychosocial intervention were associated with a poorer medication response. Studies that showed a moderate effect size for the treatment of depression yielded a substance use effect size that was also moderate, whereas those with smaller depression effects showed no beneficial effects on substance use behavior. Nunes and Levin (2004) concluded that antidepressants exert a modest beneficial effect for patients with combined depression and substance use disorders and that both disorders must be treated.

Thus, the use of combination pharmacotherapy to treat co-occurring alcohol dependence and depression is of considerable interest. In a 12-week open-label study, 14 depressed alcoholic patients who had continued to drink despite receiving antidepressants and chemical dependence counseling were prescribed naltrexone, 50 mg/day (Salloum et al. 1998). The addition of naltrexone was associated with a substantial decrease in alcohol consumption and in the urge to drink alcohol in the presence of the usual triggers. There was also a trend toward decreased depressive symptoms and improved overall functioning. In a 14-week placebo-controlled trial (Pettinati et al. 2010), 170 depressed alcohol-dependent patients were randomly assigned to receive treatment with sertraline, 200 mg/day; naltrexone, 100 mg/day; sertraline plus naltrexone; or double placebo ($N=39$). All subjects also received weekly CBT. The group receiving sertraline plus naltrexone had a higher alcohol abstinence rate (53.7%) and a longer median time to relapse to heavy drinking (98 days) than did the groups receiving naltrexone (21.3% and 29 days), sertraline (27.5% and 23 days), or placebo (23.1% and 26 days). Most patients (83.3%) in the combined medication group were not depressed at the end of treatment, with this difference from the rates in the other treatment groups approaching significance. The serious adverse event rate in the combined treatment group was about half that in the other treatment groups. Although this study requires replication, it provides the clearest support to date of the efficacy of combined medication therapy for co-occurring alcohol dependence and depression (or, for that matter, any co-occurring disorder).

A much less intensively studied group of patients are those with psychotic disorders and alcohol use disorders. A small study (Petrakis et al. 2004) showed that the addition of naltrexone to antipsychotic treatment in patients with schizophrenia and co-occurring alcohol abuse or dependence reduced the number of drinking days and heavy drinking days. Larger studies that examine this combination strategy are warranted.

In summary, despite evidence that most instances of postwithdrawal depression will spontaneously remit within a few days to several weeks of abstinence from alcohol (Brown and Schuckit 1988; Schuckit 1983), persistent depression requires treatment. SRIs have become the first-line treatment of depression because they have a more favorable side-effect profile than many other antidepressants. SRIs do not have the anticholinergic, hypotensive, or sedative effects of the tricyclic antidepressants, nor do they have the adverse cardiovascular effects of the tricyclics, which in overdose can be lethal, thereby limiting the potential for deliberate self-poisoning (Lynskey 1998). However, SRIs can exacerbate the tremor, anxiety, and insomnia often experienced by recently detoxified alcoholic patients. Although the findings of Nunes and Levin (2004) show that SRIs may be less efficacious than other antidepressants for the treatment of depression among patients with a substance use disorder, combining an SRI with naltrexone is a promising strategy for treatment of co-occurring depression and alcohol dependence.

Serotonin Reuptake Inhibitors, Benzodiazepines, and Other Anxiolytics

The effects of SRIs on co-occurring alcohol use and anxiety disorders have been examined in a few studies. In two studies, anxiety symptoms were significantly decreased in subjects taking the SRI paroxetine, but alcohol consumption was not markedly altered (Book et al. 2008; Thomas et al. 2008). In abstinent subjects, adding the SRI fluvoxamine to CBT and an intensive psychosocial relapse prevention program did not lead to greater reductions in either alcohol intake or the severity of anxiety symptoms (Schade et al. 2005).

Benzodiazepines are widely used in the treatment of acute alcohol withdrawal and to treat the anxiety, depression, and sleep disturbances that can persist for months afterward. Most nonmedical personnel, however, involved in the treatment of alcoholism are opposed to the use of any medication that can induce any level of dependence. The use of benzodiazepines in alcoholic and other substance abuse patients during the postwithdrawal period for the management of anxiety or insomnia remains controversial (Ciraulo and Nace 2000; Posternak and Mueller 2001).

The use of benzodiazepines beyond the period of acute alcohol withdrawal involves the risks of dependence and overdose, yet there may be a role for the judicious use of benzodiazepines in alcoholic patients. To the degree that early relapse, which commonly disrupts alcoholism treatment, is a result of continued withdrawal-related symptoms (e.g., anxiety, depression, insomnia) that can be suppressed by low doses of benzodiazepines, retention in treatment could be enhanced by the use of benzodiazepines (Kissin 1977). Moreover, for some patients, benzodiazepine dependence, if it does occur, may be more benign than alcoholism.

The potential benefits of benzodiazepines must be weighed against the risks of overdose and physical dependence. Although benzodiazepines alone are comparatively safe, even in overdose, their combination with other brain depressants (including alcohol) can be lethal. Although there is little doubt that alcoholic patients are more vulnerable to develop dependence on benzodiazepines than are individuals without alcoholism, the probability of abuse and dependence may be lower than was previously believed (Bliding 1978; Ciraulo et al. 1990; Marks 1978). However, dependence on both alcohol and benzodiazepines may increase depressive symptoms (Schuckit 1983), and co-occurring alcohol and benzodiazepine dependence may be more difficult to treat than alcoholism alone (Sokolow et al. 1981).

The abuse potential of benzodiazepines appears to differ widely. Benzodiazepines currently available for clinical use vary substantially in their pharmacokinetics, acute euphoriant effects, and frequency of reported dependence. Diazepam, lorazepam, and alprazolam may have greater abuse potential than chlordiazepoxide and clorazepate (Wolf et al. 1990). Similarly, oxazepam has been reported to produce low levels of abuse (Bliding 1978). Jaffe et al. (1983) found that in recently detoxified alcoholic patients, halazepam produced minimal euphoria even at a supratherapeutic dosage. The development of partial agonist and mixed agonist/antagonist compounds at the benzodiazepine receptor complex may offer an advantage over approved benzodiazepines for use in alcoholic patients.

Buspirone, a nonbenzodiazepine anxiolytic, may exert its anxiolytic effects largely via its partial agonist activity at serotonergic autoreceptors. It is comparable in efficacy to diazepam in the relief of anxiety and associated depression in outpatients with moderate-to-severe anxiety (Goldberg and Finnerty 1979; Jacobson et al. 1985). However, buspirone is less sedating than diazepam or clorazepate, does not interact with alcohol to impair psychomotor skills, and does not appear to have abuse liability (Griffith et al. 1986; Mattila et al. 1982; Seppala et al. 1982), making it more suitable than benzodiazepines to treat anxiety symptoms among alcoholic patients. In contrast to benzodiazepines, however, buspirone does not have acute anxiolytic effects nor is it useful in the treatment of alcohol withdrawal.

Four placebo-controlled, double-blind trials of buspirone to treat anxiety symptoms among alcoholic patients have been reported. An early double-blind, placebo-controlled trial of buspirone in alcoholic patients (Bruno 1989) showed significantly greater retention in treatment and greater decreases in alcohol craving, anxiety, and depression scores in buspirone-treated patients. Both buspirone and placebo groups showed significant declines in alcohol consumption during the study, with no greater effect among buspirone-treated patients. In a placebo-controlled trial in abstinent alcoholic patients with co-occurring generalized anxiety disorder, Tollefson et al. (1992) found that buspirone resulted in greater treatment retention and greater reductions in anxiety. Although buspirone-treated patients also showed greater improvement on a subjective, global measure of drinking outcome, measures of alcohol consumption were not reported in this study. Kranzler et al. (1994) also found that buspirone was more effective than placebo in retaining anxious alcoholic patients in treatment. Buspirone also delayed relapse to heavy drinking and reduced the number of drinking days during a 6-month post-treatment follow-up period. The beneficial effects of buspirone on both anxiety and drinking were most evident among patients with the highest baseline anxiety scores. In contrast, in a sample of anxious, severely alcohol-dependent patients, Malcolm et al. (1992) found that buspirone was no better than placebo in reducing either anxiety or drinking. Although there appears to be a role for buspirone in the treatment of anxiety symptoms in alcoholic patients, clinical features that can be used to identify individuals for whom buspirone may be most efficacious have not been identified.

Lithium

Although early studies of lithium, including some that used placebo controls (Kline et al. 1974; Merry et al. 1976), showed that patients receiving lithium experienced fewer days of pathological drinking, the rates of attrition in these studies were high. In a subsequent placebo-controlled study of alcoholic patients who were not selected for co-occurring depression (Fawcett et al. 1987), adherence to the medication regimen, irrespective of medication group, was associated with abstinence. Furthermore, compliant patients taking active medication who had therapeutic serum levels (0.4 mEq/L or greater) were abstinent more often than were compliant subjects with subtherapeutic lithium levels. After the first 6 months, however, even those subjects who were compliant early in the study tended to stop taking their medication. Nevertheless, the association between early compliance and sobriety persisted, suggesting that the beneficial effects of lithium are greatest in the early months after detoxification. The beneficial effect of lithium did not appear to be mediated by an antidepressant effect, because it did not affect mood in those patients who were depressed.

Dorus and colleagues (1989) conducted a multicenter, double-blind, placebo-controlled trial in depressed and nondepressed alcoholic veterans. A total of 457 male alcoholic patients, of whom approximately one-third were depressed, were randomly assigned to receive either lithium, 600–1,200 mg/day, or a comparable amount of placebo. No significant differences between lithium-treated and placebo-treated patients were found on any of a variety of outcome measures, including number of drinking days, alcohol-related hospitalizations, and severity of depression. The lack of efficacy was observed for both the depressed and the nondepressed groups. This large, carefully conducted trial suggests that lithium should be reserved for the treatment of alcoholism with co-occurring bipolar disorder. A subsequent study, in which there was no advantage to lithium over placebo in alcoholic patients who were not selected for a co-occurring psychiatric disorder (Fawcett et al. 2000), yielded results consistent with this conclusion.

Conclusion

In general, with the exception of the central role that benzodiazepines play in the treatment of alcohol withdrawal, the use of medications that have been approved for alcoholism treatment remains limited. A survey of nearly 1,400 addiction physicians (Mark et al. 2003) showed that they prescribed disulfiram to only 9% of their alcoholic patients and naltrexone to only slightly more (13%). These results contrast with findings for antidepressants, which were prescribed to 44% of alcoholic patients. Although nearly all of these physicians had heard of disulfiram and naltrexone, their self-reported level of knowledge of these medications was much lower than that of antidepressants.

Many questions must be addressed before medications are likely to be widely used for drinking reduction or relapse prevention. In addition to the issues discussed earlier in regard to specific agents (e.g., What is the optimal duration of treatment with naltrexone?), the safety and efficacy of medications to treat alcohol dependence must be examined with adequate statistical power in women, in different ethnic/racial groups, and in adolescent and geriatric samples. In addition, studies of cost-effectiveness and cost-benefit must support the routine coverage of pharmacological treatments for alcoholism under standard medical insurance plans.

The relation between substance use and psychiatric symptomatology is complex (Kranzler and Tinsley 2004; Meyer 1986). Despite ameliorating persistent mood and anxiety symptoms, medications that are prescribed to alcoholic patients with such co-occurring symptoms will not necessarily reduce alcohol consumption once a significant degree of alcohol dependence has developed, even if pathological mood states were important in the initiation of heavy drinking. The neuroadaptive changes and the complex learning that constitute the dependence syndrome (Edwards and Gross 1976) do not resolve simply because one major contributing factor is brought under control. Antidepressants with benign side-effect profiles that may also reduce alcohol intake directly warrant careful evaluation in the treatment of anxiety and depression in patients with alcoholism, particularly in combination with medications such as naltrexone (Pettinati et al. 2010). An additional challenge for those treating alcoholism is to combine efficacious medications with empirically based psychological interventions and, when feasible, self-help group participation.

The medications that have been most widely studied in alcohol rehabilitation are naltrexone and acamprosate. The effect size of these medications to treat alcohol use disorders ranges from small to moderate. Topiramate appears to have a moderate effect size, but because it is now available as a generic, there is no financial incentive for the company that owns the patent to seek approval for the treatment of alcohol dependence in the United States. As the research literature on the use of medications to treat alcohol dependence grows, it will be possible to assess the utility of different medication combinations and a variety of psychotherapies. Ongoing efforts to match medications with specific subgroups of alcoholic patients, based on clinical or genetic characteristics, remain a promising strategy.

Combining medications with self-help group participation may represent a particular challenge. Abstinence-oriented groups such as Alcoholics Anonymous may be willing to work with physicians around the issue of proper dosage, compliance, and early detection of side effects of disulfiram, the use of which is supportive of their goal of total abstinence. However, these groups may be less supportive of pharmacotherapies that focus on harm reduction through reduced heavy drinking rather than abstinence as a primary goal.

As evidence accumulates that several medications are efficacious for the treatment of co-occurring psychopathology and/or the prevention of relapse in alcoholic patients, the therapeutic options available to physicians for these patients will increase. As these developments unfold, it is crucial that efforts be directed to enhancing the acceptability of pharmacotherapy to the alcoholism treatment community as a standard part of alcoholism rehabilitation.

References

Adams CL, Cowen MS, Short JL, et al: Combined antagonism of glutamate mGlu5 and adenosine A2A receptors interact to regulate alcohol-seeking in rats. Int J Neuropsychopharmacol 11:229–241, 2008

Addolorato G, Caputo F, Capristo E, et al: Baclofen efficacy in reducing alcohol craving and intake: a preliminary double-blind randomized controlled study. Alcohol Alcohol 37:504–508, 2002

Addolorato G, Leggio L, Ferrulli A, et al: Effectiveness and safety of baclofen for maintenance of alcohol abstinence in alcohol-dependent patients with liver cirrhosis: randomised, double-blind controlled study. Lancet 370:1915–1922, 2007

Addolorato G, Leggio L, Ferrulli A, et al: Dose-response effect of baclofen in reducing daily alcohol intake in alcohol dependence: secondary analysis of a randomized, double-blind, placebo-controlled trial. Alcohol Alcohol 46:312–317, 2011

Allen JP, Litten RZ: Techniques to enhance compliance with disulfiram. Alcohol Clin Exp Res 16:1035–1041, 1992

American Psychiatric Association: Diagnostic and Statistical Manual of Mental Disorders, 3rd Edition, Revised. Washington, DC, American Psychiatric Association, 1987

American Psychiatric Association: Diagnostic and Statistical Manual of Mental Disorders, 4th Edition. Washington, DC, American Psychiatric Association, 1994

American Psychiatric Association: Diagnostic and Statistical Manual of Mental Disorders, 5th Edition. Arlington, VA, American Psychiatric Association, 2013

Anton RF, Moak DH, Lathan PK et al: Posttreatment results of combining naltrexone and cognitive-behavior therapy for the treatment of alcoholism. J Clin Psychopharmacol 21:72–77, 2000

Anton RF, Pettinati H, Zweben A, et al: A multi-site dose ranging study of nalmefene in the treatment of alcohol dependence. J Clin Psychopharmacol 24:421–428, 2004

Anton RF, O'Malley SS, Ciraulo DA, et al: Combined pharmacotherapies and behavioral interventions for alcohol dependence: the COMBINE study: a randomized controlled trial. JAMA 295:2003–2017, 2006

Anton RF, Kranzler H, Breder C, et al: A randomized, multicenter, double-blind, placebo-controlled study of the efficacy and safety of aripiprazole for the treatment of alcohol dependence. J Clin Psychopharmacol 28:5–12, 2008

Arias AJ, Feinn R, Oncken C, et al: Placebo-controlled trial of zonisamide for the treatment of alcohol dependence. J Clin Psychopharmacol 30:318–322, 2010

Asatryan L, Nam HW, Lee MR, et al: Implication of the purinergic system in alcohol use disorders. Alcohol Clin Exp Res 35:584–594, 2011

Azrin NH, Sisson RW, Meyers R, et al: Alcoholism treatment by disulfiram and community reinforcement therapy. J Behav Ther Exp Psychiatry 13:105–112, 1982

Babor TF, Kranzler HR, Lauerman RL: Social drinking as a health and psychosocial risk factor: Anstie's limit revisited, in Recent Developments in Alcoholism, Vol 5. Edited by Galanter M. New York, Plenum, 1987, pp 373–402

Bailly D, Servant D, Blandin N, et al: Effects of beta-blocking drugs in alcohol withdrawal: a double-blind comparative study with propranolol and diazepam. Biomed Pharmacother 46:419–424, 1992

Balino P, Pastor R, Aragon CM: Participation of L-type calcium channels in ethanol-induced behavioral stimulation and motor incoordination: effects of diltiazem and verapamil. Behav Brain Res 209:196–204, 2010

Balldin J, Berggren U, Engel J, et al: Effect of citalopram on alcohol intake in heavy drinkers. Alcohol Clin Exp Res 18:1133–1136, 1994

Bauer LO, Covault J, Harel O, et al: Variation in GABRA2 predicts drinking behavior in Project MATCH subjects. Alcohol Clin Exp Res 31:1780–1787, 2007

Besson J, Aeby F, Kasas A, et al: Combined efficacy of acamprosate and disulfiram in the treatment of alcoholism: a controlled study. Alcohol Clin Exp Res 22:573–579, 1998

Blednov YA, Harris RA: Metabotropic glutamate receptor 5 (mGluR5) regulation of ethanol sedation, dependence and consumption: relationship to acamprosate actions. Int J Neuropsychopharmacol 11:775–793, 2008

Bliding A: The abuse potential of benzodiazepines with special reference to oxazepam. Acta Psychiatr Scand Suppl 274:111–116, 1978

Bogenschutz MP, Tonigan JS, Pettinati HM: Effects of alcoholism typology on response to naltrexone in the COMBINE study. Alcohol Clin Exp Res 33:10–18, 2009

Book SW, Thomas SE, Randall PK, et al: Paroxetine reduces social anxiety in individuals with a co-occurring alcohol use disorder. J Anxiety Disord 22:310–318, 2008

Bouza C, Angeles M, Munoz A, et al: Efficacy and safety of naltrexone and acamprosate in the treatment of alcohol dependence: a systematic review. Addiction 99:811–828, 2004

Brady KT, Myrick H, Henderson S, et al: The use of divalproex in alcohol relapse prevention: a pilot study. Drug Alcohol Depend 67:323–330, 2002

Brewer C: How effective is the standard dose of disulfiram? A review of the alcohol-disulfiram reaction in practice. Br J Psychiatry 144:200–202, 1984

Brewer C, Meyers R, Johnsen J: Does disulfiram help to prevent relapse in alcohol abuse? CNS Drugs 14:329–341, 2000

Brown SA, Schuckit MA: Changes in depression among abstinent alcoholics. J Stud Alcohol 49:412–417, 1988

Bruno F: Buspirone in the treatment of alcoholic patients. Psychopathology 22 (suppl 1):49–59, 1989

Budygin EA, Oleson EB, Mathews TA, et al: Effects of chronic alcohol exposure on dopamine uptake in rat nucleus accumbens and caudate putamen. Psychopharmacology (Berl) 193:495–501, 2007

Calton JL, Wilson WA, Moore SD: Reduction of voltage-dependent currents by ethanol contributes to inhibition of NMDA receptor-mediated excitatory synaptic transmission. Brain Res 816:142–148, 1999

Carlsson C, Fasth BG: A comparison of the effects of propranolol and diazepam in alcoholics. Br J Addict Alcohol Other Drugs 71:321–326, 1976

Chatterjee S, Steensland P, Simms JA, et al: Partial agonists of the alpha3beta4* neuronal nicotinic acetylcholine receptor reduce ethanol consumption and seeking in rats. Neuropsychopharmacology 36:603–615, 2011

Chen S, Huang X, Zeng XJ, et al: Benzodiazepine-mediated regulation of alpha1, alpha2, beta1–3 and gamma2 GABA(A) receptor subunit proteins in the rat brain hippocampus and cortex. Neuroscience 93:33–44, 1999

Chen YC, Peng GS, Wang MF, et al: Polymorphism of ethanol-metabolism genes and alcoholism: correlation of allelic variations with the pharmacokinetic and pharmacodynamic consequences. Chem Biol Interact 178:2–7, 2009

Chick J: Safety issues concerning the use of disulfiram in treating alcohol dependence. Drug Saf 20:427–435, 1999

Chick J, Gough K, Falkowski W, et al: Disulfiram treatment of alcoholism. Br J Psychiatry 161:84–89, 1992

Chick J, Lehert P, Landron F: Does acamprosate improve reduction of drinking as well as aiding abstinence? J Psychopharmacol (Oxf) 17:397–402, 2003

Chrostek L, Jelski W, Szmitkowski M, et al: Gender-related differences in hepatic activity of alcohol dehydrogenase isoenzymes and aldehyde dehydrogenase in humans. J Clin Lab Anal 17:93–96, 2003

Ciraulo DA, Jaffe JH: Tricyclic antidepressants in the treatment of depression associated with alcoholism. J Clin Psychopharmacol 1:146–150, 1981

Ciraulo D, Nace E: Benzodiazepine treatment of anxiety or insomnia in substance abuse patients. Am J Addict 9:276–279, 2000

Ciraulo DA, Barnhill JG, Jaffe JH, et al: Intravenous pharmacokinetics of 2-hydroxyimipramine in alcoholics and normal controls. J Stud Alcohol 51:366–372, 1990

Ciraulo DA, Knapp CM, LoCastro J, et al: A benzodiazepine mood effect scale: reliability and validity determined for alcohol-dependent subjects and adults with a parental history of alcoholism. Am J Drug Alcohol Abuse 27:339–347, 2001

Cornelius JR, Salloum IM, Ehler JG, et al: Fluoxetine in depressed alcoholics: a double-blind, placebo-controlled trial. Arch Gen Psychiatry 54:700–705, 1997

Covault J, Gelernter J, Hesselbrock V, et al: Allelic and haplotypic association of GABRA2 with alcohol dependence. Am J Med Genet B Neuropsychiatr Genet 129:104–109, 2004

Covault J, Gelernter J, Jensen K, et al: Markers in the 5′-region of GABRG1 associate to alcohol dependence and are in linkage disequilibrium with markers in the adjacent GABRA2 gene. Neuropsychopharmacology 33:837–848, 2008

Cowen MS, Chen F, Lawrence AJ: Neuropeptides: implications for alcoholism. J Neurochem 89:273–285, 2004

Cowley DS: Alcohol abuse, substance abuse, and panic disorder. Am J Med 92(suppl):41S–48S, 1992

Cowley DS, Roy-Byrne PP, Radant A, et al: Eye movement effects of diazepam in sons of alcoholic fathers and male control subjects. Alcohol Clin Exp Res 18:324–332, 1994

Criswell HE, Ming Z, Kelm MK, et al: Brain regional differences in the effect of ethanol on GABA release from presynaptic terminals. J Pharmacol Exp Ther 326:596–603, 2008

de Waele JP, Papachristou DN, Gianoulakis C: The alcohol-preferring C57BL/6 mice present an enhanced sensitivity of the hypothalamic beta-endorphin system to ethanol than the alcohol-avoiding DBA/2 mice. J Pharmacol Exp Ther 261:788–794, 1992

de Waele JP, Kiianmaa K, Gianoulakis C: Spontaneous and ethanol-stimulated in vitro release of beta-endorphin by the hypothalamus of AA and ANA rats. Alcohol Clin Exp Res 18:1468–1473, 1994

Dettling A, Fischer F, Böhler S, et al: Ethanol elimination rates in men and women in consideration of the calculated liver weight. Alcohol 41:415–420, 2007

Diana M, Peana AT, Sirca D, et al: Crucial role of acetaldehyde in alcohol activation of the mesolimbic dopamine system. Ann N Y Acad Sci 1139:307–317, 2008

Ding ZM, Rodd ZA, Engleman EA, et al: Sensitization of ventral tegmental area dopamine neurons to the stimulating effects of ethanol. Alcohol Clin Exp Res 33:1571–1581, 2009a

Ding ZM, Toalston JE, Oster SM, et al: Involvement of local serotonin-2A but not serotonin-1B receptors in the reinforcing effects of ethanol within the posterior ventral tegmental area of female Wistar rats. Psychopharmacology (Berl) 204:381–390, 2009b

Dobrydnjov I, Axelsson K, Berggren L, et al: Intrathecal and oral clonidine as prophylaxis for postoperative alcohol withdrawal syndrome: a randomized double-blinded study. Anesth Analg 98:738–744, 2004

Dopico AM, Lovinger DM: Acute alcohol action and desensitization of ligand-gated ion channels. Pharmacol Rev 61:98–114, 2009

Dorus W, Ostrow DG, Anton R, et al: Lithium treatment of depressed and nondepressed alcoholics. JAMA 262:1646–1652, 1989

Drgon T, D'Addario C, Uhl GR: Linkage disequilibrium, haplotype and association studies of a chromosome 4 GABA receptor gene cluster: candidate gene variants for addictions. Am J Med Genet B Neuropsychiatr Genet 141B:854–860, 2006

Dundon W, Lynch KG, Pettinati HM, et al: Treatment outcomes in type A and B alcohol dependence 6 months after serotonergic pharmacotherapy. Alcohol Clin Exp Res 28:1065–1073, 2004

Edenberg HJ, Dick DM, Xuei X, et al: Variations in GABRA2, encoding the alpha 2 subunit of the GABA(A) receptor, are associated with alcohol dependence and with brain oscillations. Am J Hum Genet 74:705–714, 2004

Edwards G, Gross MM: Alcohol dependence: provisional description of a clinical syndrome. Br Med J 1:1058–1061, 1976

Edwards S, Kenna GA, Swift RM, et al: Current and promising pharmacotherapies, and novel research target areas in the treatment of alcohol dependence: a review. Curr Pharm Des 17:1323–1332, 2011

Egli M: Peptides: their role in excess alcohol drinking and their promise as a therapeutic tool. Physiol Behav 79:89–93, 2003

Enoch MA: The role of GABA(A) receptors in the development of alcoholism. Pharmacol Biochem Behav 90:95–104, 2008

Enoch MA, Schwartz L, Albaugh B, et al: Dimensional anxiety mediates linkage of GABRA2 haplotypes with alcoholism. Am J Med Genet B Neuropsychiatr Genet 141B:599–607, 2006

Enoch MA, Hodgkinson CA, Yuan Q, et al: GABRG1 and GABRA2 as independent predictors for alcoholism in two populations. Neuropsychopharmacology 34:1245–1254, 2009

Ericson M, Lof E, Stomberg R, et al: Nicotinic acetylcholine receptors in the anterior, but not posterior, ventral tegmental area mediate ethanol-induced elevation of accumbal dopamine levels. J Pharmacol Exp Ther 326:76–82, 2008

Eyer F, Schreckenberg M, Hecht D, et al: Carbamazepine and valproate as adjuncts in the treatment of alcohol withdrawal syndrome: a retrospective cohort study. Alcohol Alcohol 46:177–184, 2011

Farren CK, Ziedonis D, Clare AW, et al: D-fenfluramine-induced prolactin responses in postwithdrawal alcoholics and controls. Alcohol Clin Exp Res 19:1578–1582, 1995

Favazza AR, Martin P: Chemotherapy of delirium tremens: a survey of physicians' preferences. Am J Psychiatry 131:1031–1033, 1974

Fawcett J, Clark DC, Aagesen CA, et al: A double-blind, placebo-controlled trial of lithium carbonate therapy for alcoholism. Arch Gen Psychiatry 44:248–256, 1987

Fawcett J, Kravitz HM, McGuire M, et al: Pharmacological treatments for alcoholism: revisiting lithium and considering buspirone. Alcohol Clin Exp Res 24:666–674, 2000

Fehr C, Sander T, Tadic A, et al: Confirmation of association of the GABRA2 gene with alcohol dependence by subtype-specific analysis. Psychiatr Genet 16:9–17, 2006

Feldman DJ, Pattison EM, Sobell LC, et al: Outpatient alcohol detoxification: initial findings on 564 patients. Am J Psychiatry 132:407–412, 1975

Floyd DW, Jung KY, McCool BA: Chronic ethanol ingestion facilitates N-methyl-D-aspartate receptor function and expression in rat lateral/basolateral amygdala neurons. J Pharmacol Exp Ther 307:1020–1029, 2003

Forg A, Hein J, Volkmar K, et al: Efficacy and safety of pregabalin in the treatment of alcohol withdrawal syndrome: a randomized placebo-controlled trial. Alcohol Alcohol 47:149–155, 2012

Frezza M, di Padova C, Pozzato G, et al: High blood alcohol levels in women: the role of decreased gastric alcohol dehydrogenase activity and first-pass metabolism. N Engl J Med 322:95–99, 1990

Fucito LM, Toll BA, Wu R, et al: A preliminary investigation of varenicline for heavy drinking smokers. Psychopharmacology (Berl) 215:655–663, 2011

Fuller RK, Branchey L, Brightwell DR, et al: Disulfiram treatment of alcoholism: a Veterans Administration cooperative study. JAMA 256:1449–1455, 1986

Garbutt JC, Kranzler HR, O'Malley SS, et al: Efficacy and tolerability of long-acting injectable naltrexone for alcohol dependence. JAMA 293:1617–1625, 2005

Garbutt JC, Kampov-Polevoy AB, Gallop R, et al: Efficacy and safety of baclofen for alcohol dependence: a randomized, double-blind, placebo-controlled trial. Alcohol Clin Exp Res 34:1849–1857, 2010

Gastfriend DR: Intramuscular extended-release naltrexone: current evidence. Ann N Y Acad Sci 1216:144–166, 2011

Gerra G, Caccavari R, Delsignore R, et al: Effects of fluoxetine and ca-acetyl-homotaurinate on alcohol intake in familial and non familial alcoholic patients. Curr Ther Res 52:291–295, 1992

Gianoulakis C, Beliveau D, Angelogianni P, et al: Different pituitary beta-endorphin and adrenal cortisol response to ethanol in individuals with high and low risk for future development of alcoholism. Life Sci 45:1097–1109, 1989

Gianoulakis C, Krishnan B, Thavundayil J: Enhanced sensitivity of pituitary beta-endorphin to ethanol in subjects at high risk of alcoholism. Arch Gen Psychiatry 53:250–257, 1996

Gilpin NW, Misra K, Herman MA, et al: Neuropeptide Y opposes alcohol effects on gamma-aminobutyric acid release in amygdala and blocks the transition to alcohol dependence. Biol Psychiatry 69:1091–1099, 2011

Goldberg HL, Finnerty RJ: The comparative efficacy of buspirone and diazepam in the treatment of anxiety. Am J Psychiatry 136:1184–1187, 1979

Goldman D: Recent developments in alcoholism: genetic transmission. Recent Dev Alcohol 11:231–248, 1993

Gonzales RA, Weiss F: Suppression of ethanol-reinforced behavior by naltrexone is associated with attenuation of the ethanol-induced increase in dialysate dopamine levels in the nucleus accumbens. J Neurosci 18:10663–10671, 1998

Gorelick DA, Paredes A: Effect of fluoxetine on alcohol consumption in male alcoholics. Alcohol Clin Exp Res 16:261–265, 1992

Grant BF: Alcohol consumption, alcohol abuse and alcohol dependence. the United States as an example. Addiction 89:1357–1365, 1994

Grant BF: Theoretical and observed subtypes of DSM-IV alcohol abuse and dependence in a general population sample. Drug Alcohol Depend 60:287–293, 2000

Grant BF, Harford TC: Comorbidity between DSM-IV alcohol use disorders and major depression: results of a national survey. Drug Alcohol Depend 39:197–206, 1995

Grant BF, Dawson DA, Stinson FS, et al: The 12-month prevalence and trends in DSM-IV alcohol abuse and dependence: United States, 1991–1992 and 2001–2002. Drug Alcohol Depend 74:223–234, 2004a

Grant BF, Stinson FS, Dawson DA, et al: Prevalence and co-occurrence of substance use disorders and independent mood and anxiety disorders: results from the National Epidemiologic Survey on Alcohol and Related Conditions. Arch Gen Psychiatry 61:807–816, 2004b

Griffith JD, Jasinski DR, Casten GP, et al: Investigation of the abuse liability of buspirone in alcohol-dependent patients. Am J Med 80 (suppl 3B):30–35, 1986

Grobin AC, Matthews DB, Devaud LL, et al: The role of GABA(A) receptors in the acute and chronic effects of ethanol. Psychopharmacology (Berl) 139:2–19, 1998

Grover CA, Frye GD, Griffith WH: Acute tolerance to ethanol inhibition of NMDA-mediated EPSPs in the CA1 region of the rat hippocampus. Brain Res 642:70–76, 1994

Gryder DS, Rogawski MA: Selective antagonism of GluR5 kainate-receptor-mediated synaptic currents by topiramate in rat basolateral amygdala neurons. J Neurosci 23:7069–7074, 2003

Gual A, He Y, Torup L, van den Brink W, et al: ESENSE 2: a randomized, double-blind, placebo-controlled study of nalmefene, as-needed use in alcohol dependent patients. Alcohol Clin Exp Res 36 (suppl 1):246A, 2012

Hammarberg A, Jayaram-Lindstrom N, Beck O, et al: The effects of acamprosate on alcohol-cue reactivity and alcohol priming in dependent patients: a randomized controlled trial. Psychopharmacology (Berl) 205:53–62, 2009

Haughey HM, Ray LA, Finan P, et al: Human gamma-aminobutyric acid A receptor alpha2 gene moderates the acute effects of alcohol and brain mRNA expression. Genes Brain Behav 7:447–454, 2008

Hayashida M, Alterman AI, McLellan AT, et al: Comparative effectiveness and costs of inpatient and outpatient detoxification of patients with mild-to-moderate alcohol withdrawal syndrome. N Engl J Med 320:358–365, 1989

Heinala P, Alho H, Kiianmaa K, et al: Targeted use of naltrexone without prior detoxification in the treatment of alcohol dependence: a factorial double-blind, placebo-controlled trial. J Clin Psychopharmacol 21:287–292, 2001

Heinz A, Goldman D, Gallinat J, et al: Pharmacogenetic insights to monoaminergic
dysfunction in alcohol dependence. Psychopharmacology (Berl) 174:561–570,
2004

Helms CM, Rossi DJ, Grant KA: Neurosteroid influences on sensitivity to ethanol.
Front Endocrinol (Lausanne) 3:10, 2012

Hendricson AW, Maldve RE, Salinas AG, et al: Aberrant synaptic activation of N-
methyl-D-aspartate receptors underlies ethanol withdrawal hyperexcitability. J
Pharmacol Exp Ther 321:60–72, 2007

Hernandez-Avila CA, Song C, Kuo L, et al: Targeted versus daily naltrexone: secondary analysis of effects on average daily drinking. Alcohol Clin Exp Res 30:860–
865, 2006

Hesselbrock MN, Meyer RE, Keener JJ: Psychopathology in hospitalized alcoholics.
Arch Gen Psychiatry 42:1050–1055, 1985

Ittiwut C, Listman J, Mutirangura A, et al: Inter-population linkage disequilibrium
(LD) patterns of GABRA2 and GABRG1 genes at the GABA cluster locus on human chromosome 4. Genomics 91:61–69, 2008

Ittiwut C, Yang, BZ, Kranzler HR, et al: GABRG1 and GABRA2 variation associated
with alcohol dependence in African Americans. Alcohol Clin Exp Res 36:588–
593, 2012

Jacobson AF, Dominguez RA, Goldstein BJ, et al: Comparison of buspirone and diazepam in generalized anxiety disorder. Pharmacotherapy 5:290–296, 1985

Jaffe JH, Ciraulo DA, Nies A, et al: Abuse potential of halazepam and of diazepam in
patients recently treated for acute alcohol withdrawal. Clin Pharmacol Ther
34:623–630, 1983

Jerlhag E, Egecioglu E, Landgren S, et al: Requirement of central ghrelin signaling for
alcohol reward. Proc Natl Acad Sci U S A 106:11318–11323, 2009

Jiao X, Pare WP, Tejani-Butt SM: Alcohol consumption alters dopamine transporter
sites in Wistar-Kyoto rat brain. Brain Res 1073–1074:175–182, 2006

Johnson BA: Update on neuropharmacological treatments for alcoholism: scientific
basis and clinical findings. Biochem Pharmacol 75:34–56, 2008

Johnson BA, Roache JD, Javors MA, et al: Ondansetron for reduction of drinking
among biologically predisposed alcoholic patients: a randomized controlled trial.
JAMA 284:963–971, 2000

Johnson BA, Ait-Daoud N, Bowden CL, et al: Oral topiramate for treatment of alcohol dependence: a randomised controlled trial. Lancet 361:1677–1685, 2003

Johnson BA, Rosenthal N, Capece JA, et al: Topiramate for treating alcohol dependence: a randomized controlled trial. JAMA 298:1641–1651, 2007

Johnson BA, Rosenthal N, Capece JA, et al: Improvement of physical health and quality of life of alcohol-dependent individuals with topiramate treatment: US multisite randomized controlled trial. Arch Intern Med 168:1188–1199, 2008

Johnson BA, Ait-Daoud N, Seneviratne C, et al: Pharmacogenetic approach at the serotonin transporter gene as a method of reducing the severity of alcohol drinking. Am J Psychiatry 168:265–275, 2011

Kabel DI, Petty F: A placebo-controlled double-blind study of fluoxetine in severe alcohol dependence: adjunctive pharmacotherapy during and after inpatient treatment. Alcohol Clin Exp Res 20:780–784, 1996

Kahkonen S: Alcohol withdrawal changes cardiovascular responses to propranolol challenge. Neuropsychobiology 47:192–197, 2003

Kahkonen S, Bondarenko BB: L-type Ca2+ channels mediate cardiovascular symptoms of alcohol withdrawal in humans. Prog Neuropsychopharmacol Biol Psychiatry 28:45–48, 2004

Kamens HM, Andersen J, Picciotto MR: Modulation of ethanol consumption by genetic and pharmacological manipulation of nicotinic acetylcholine receptors in mice. Psychopharmacology (Berl) 208:613–626, 2010

Karahanian E, Quintanilla ME, Tampier L, et al: Ethanol as a prodrug: brain metabolism of ethanol mediates its reinforcing effects. Alcohol Clin Exp Res 35:606–612, 2011

Katsura M, Torigoe F, Hayashida S, et al: Ethanol physical dependence is accompanied by up-regulated expression of L-type high voltage-gated calcium channel alpha1 subunits in mouse brain. Brain Res 1039:211–215, 2005

Kelm MK, Criswell HE, Breese GR: The role of protein kinase A in the ethanol-induced increase in spontaneous GABA release onto cerebellar Purkinje neurons. J Neurophysiol 100:3417–3428, 2008

Kelm MK, Weinberg RJ, Criswell HE, et al: The PLC/IP 3 R/PKC pathway is required for ethanol-enhanced GABA release. Neuropharmacology 58:1179–1186, 2010

Kessler RC, McGonagle KA, Zhao S, et al: Lifetime and 12-month prevalence of DSM-III-R psychiatric disorders in the United States: results from the National Comorbidity Survey. Arch Gen Psychiatry 51:8–19, 1994

Kessler RC, Crum RM, Warner LA, et al: Lifetime co-occurrence of DSM-III-R alcohol abuse and dependence with other psychiatric disorders in the National Comorbidity Survey. Arch Gen Psychiatry 54:313–321, 1997

Kiefer F, Jahn H, Tarnaske T, et al: Comparing and combining naltrexone and acamprosate in relapse prevention of alcoholism: a double-blind, placebo-controlled study. Arch Gen Psychiatry 60:92–99, 2003

Kissin B: Medical management of the alcoholic patient, in The Biology of Alcoholism, Vol 5: Treatment and Rehabilitation of the Chronic Alcoholic. Edited by Kissin B, Begleiter H. New York, Plenum, 1977, pp 55–103

Kline NS, Wren JC, Cooper TB, et al: Evaluation of lithium therapy in chronic and periodic alcoholism. Am J Med Sci 268:15–22, 1974

Knapp CM, Sarid-Segal O, Richardson MA, et al: Open label trial of the tolerability and efficacy of zonisamide in the treatment of alcohol dependence. Am J Drug Alcohol Abuse 36:102–105, 2010

Kotlinska J, Bochenski M: The influence of various glutamate receptors antagonists on anxiety-like effect of ethanol withdrawal in a plus-maze test in rats. Eur J Pharmacol 598:57–63, 2008

Kranzler HR, Anton RF: Implications of recent neuropsychopharmacologic research for understanding the etiology and development of alcoholism. J Consult Clin Psychol 62:1116–1126, 1994

Kranzler HR, Tinsley JA (eds): Dual Diagnosis: Substance Abuse and Comorbid Medical and Psychiatric Treatment, 2nd Edition. New York, Marcel Dekker, 2004

Kranzler HR, Van Kirk J: Efficacy of naltrexone and acamprosate for alcoholism treatment: a meta-analysis. Alcohol Clin Exp Res 25:1335–1341, 2001

Kranzler HR, Babor TF, Lauerman RJ: Problems associated with average alcohol consumption and frequency of intoxication in a medical population. Alcohol Clin Exp Res 14:119–126, 1990

Kranzler HR, Burleson JA, Del Boca FK, et al: Buspirone treatment of anxious alcoholics: a placebo-controlled trial. Arch Gen Psychiatry 51:720–731, 1994

Kranzler HR, Burleson JA, Korner P, et al: Placebo-controlled trial of fluoxetine as an adjunct to relapse prevention in alcoholics. Am J Psychiatry 152:391–397, 1995

Kranzler HR, Burleson JA, Brown J, et al: Fluoxetine treatment seems to reduce the beneficial effects of cognitive-behavioral therapy in type B alcoholics. Alcohol Clin Exp Res 20:1534–1541, 1996

Kranzler HR, Tennen H, Penta C, et al: Targeted naltrexone treatment of early problem drinkers. Addict Behav 22:431–436, 1997

Kranzler HR, Modesto-Lowe V, Nuwayser ES: Sustained-release naltrexone for alcoholism treatment: a preliminary study. Alcohol Clin Exp Res 22:1074–1079, 1998

Kranzler HR, Armeli S, Tennen H, et al: Targeted naltrexone for early problem drinkers. J Clin Psychopharmacol 23:294–304, 2003a

Kranzler HR, Pierucci-Lagha A, Feinn R, et al: Effects of ondansetron in early versus late-onset alcoholics: a prospective, open-label study. Alcohol Clin Exp Res 27:1150–1155, 2003b

Kranzler HR, Wesson DR, Billot L: Naltrexone depot for treatment of alcohol dependence: a multicenter, randomized, placebo-controlled clinical trial. Alcohol Clin Exp Res 28:1051–1059, 2004

Kranzler HR, Covault J, Pierucci-Lagha A, et al: Effects of aripiprazole on subjective and physiological responses to alcohol. Alcohol Clin Exp Res 32:573–579, 2008

Kranzler HR, Gelernter J, Anton RF, et al: Association of markers in the 3' region of the GluR5 kainate receptor subunit gene (GRIK1) to alcohol dependence. Alcohol Clin Exp Res 33:1–6, 2009a

Kranzler HR, Tennen H, Armeli S, et al: Targeted naltrexone for problem drinkers. J Clin Psychopharmacol 29:350–357, 2009b

Kranzler HR, Armeli S, Tennen H, et al: A double-blind, randomized trial of sertraline for alcohol dependence: moderation by age of onset and 5-hydroxytryptamine transporter-linked promoter region genotype. J Clin Psychopharmacol 31:22–30, 2011

Kranzler HR, Armeli S, Tennen H: Post-treatment outcomes in a double-blind, randomized trial of sertraline for alcohol dependence. Alcohol Clin Exp Res 36:739–744, 2012

Krystal JH, Cramer JA, Krol WF, et al: Naltrexone in the treatment of alcohol dependence. N Engl J Med 345:1734–1739, 2001

Krystal JH, Petrakis IL, Limoncelli D, et al: Altered NMDA glutamate receptor antagonist response in recovering ethanol-dependent patients. Neuropsychopharmacology 28:2020–2028, 2003a

Krystal JH, Petrakis IL, Mason G, et al: N-methyl-D-aspartate glutamate receptors and alcoholism: reward, dependence, treatment, and vulnerability. Pharmacol Ther 99:79–94, 2003b

Kumar S, Porcu P, Werner DF, et al: The role of GABA(A) receptors in the acute and chronic effects of ethanol: a decade of progress. Psychopharmacology (Berl) 205:529–564, 2009

Kumar S, Suryanarayanan A, Boyd KN, et al: Ethanol reduces GABAA alpha1 subunit receptor surface expression by a protein kinase C gamma-dependent mechanism in cultured cerebral cortical neurons. Mol Pharmacol 77:793–803, 2010

Lai CL, Chao YC, Chen YC, et al: No sex and age influence on the expression pattern and activities of human gastric alcohol and aldehyde dehydrogenases. Alcohol Clin Exp Res 24:1625–1632, 2000

Landabaso M, Iraurgi I, Sanz J, et al: Naltrexone in the treatment of alcoholism: two years follow-up results. Eur Psychiatry 13:97–105, 1999

Landgren S, Jerlhag E, Zetterberg H, et al: Association of pro-ghrelin and GHS-R1A gene polymorphisms and haplotypes with heavy alcohol use and body mass. Alcohol Clin Exp Res 32:2054–2061, 2008

Lappalainen J, Krupitsky E, Remizov M, et al: Association between alcoholism and gamma-amino butyric acid alpha2 receptor subtype in a Russian population. Alcohol Clin Exp Res 29:493–498, 2005

Larsson A, Svensson L, Soderpalm B, et al: Role of different nicotinic acetylcholine receptors in mediating behavioral and neurochemical effects of ethanol in mice. Alcohol 28:157–167, 2002

Leggio L, Addolorato G, Cippitelli A, et al: Role of feeding-related pathways in alcohol dependence: a focus on sweet preference, NPY, and ghrelin. Alcohol Clin Exp Res 35:194–202, 2011

Lhuintre JP, Daoust M, Moore ND, et al: Ability of calcium bis acetyl homotaurine, a GABA agonist, to prevent relapse in weaned alcoholics. Lancet 1:1014–1016, 1985

Litten RZ, Fertig JB, Falk DE, et al: A double-blind, placebo-controlled trial to assess the efficacy of quetiapine fumarate XR in very heavy-drinking alcohol-dependent patients. Alcohol Clin Exp Res 36:406–416, 2012

Lovinger DM, Roberto M: Synaptic effects induced by alcohol. Curr Top Behav Neurosci 13:31–86, 2013

Lynskey MT: The comorbidity of alcohol dependence and affective disorders: treatment implications. Drug Alcohol Depend 52:201–209, 1998

Malcolm R, Ballenger JC, Sturgis ET, et al: Double-blind controlled trial comparing carbamazepine to oxazepam treatment of alcohol withdrawal. Am J Psychiatry 146:617–621, 1989

Malcolm R, Anton RF, Randall CL, et al: A placebo-controlled trial of buspirone in anxious inpatient alcoholics. Alcohol Clin Exp Res 16:1007–1013, 1992

Malcolm R, Myrick H, Roberts J, et al: The effects of carbamazepine and lorazepam on single versus multiple previous alcohol withdrawals in an outpatient randomized trial. J Gen Intern Med 17:349–355, 2002

Mann K: Pharmacotherapy of alcohol dependence: a review of the clinical data. CNS Drugs 18:485–504, 2004

Mann K, Kiefer F, Spanagel R, et al: Acamprosate: recent findings and future research directions. Alcohol Clin Exp Res 32:1105–1110, 2008

Mann K, Kiefer F, Smolka M, et al: Searching for responders to acamprosate and naltrexone in alcoholism treatment: rationale and design of the PREDICT study. Alcohol Clin Exp Res 33:674–683, 2009

Mann K, Bladstrom A, Torup L, et al: Shifting the paradigm: ESENSE1—a randomised, double-blind, placebo controlled study of nalmefene, as-needed use in alcohol dependent patients Alcohol Clin Exp Res 36 (suppl 1):246A, 2012

Mark TL, Kranzler HR, Song X, et al: Physicians' opinions about medications to treat alcoholism. Addiction 98:617–626, 2003

Marks J: The Benzodiazepines: Use, Misuse, Abuse. Lancaster, UK, MTP Press, 1978

Mascia MP, Mihic SJ, Valenzuela CF, et al: A single amino acid determines differences in ethanol actions on strychnine-sensitive glycine receptors. Mol Pharmacol 50:402–406, 1996

Mason BJ, Ritvo EC, Morgan RO, et al: A double-blind, placebo-controlled pilot study to evaluate the efficacy and safety of oral nalmefene HCl for alcohol dependence. Alcohol Clin Exp Res 18:1162–1167, 1994

Mason BJ, Kocsis JH, Ritvo EC, et al: A double-blind, placebo-controlled trial of desipramine for primary alcohol dependence stratified on the presence or absence of major depression. JAMA 275:761–767, 1996

Mason BJ, Salvato FR, Williams LD, et al: A double-blind, placebo-controlled study of oral nalmefene for alcohol dependence. Arch Gen Psychiatry 56:719–724, 1999

Mason BJ, Goodman AM, Chabac S, et al: Effect of oral acamprosate on abstinence in patients with alcohol dependence in a double-blind, placebo-controlled trial: the role of patient motivation. J Psychiatr Res 40:383–393, 2006

Matthews AG, Hoffman EK, Zezza N, et al: The role of the GABRA2 polymorphism in multiplex alcohol dependence families with minimal comorbidity: within-family association and linkage analyses. J Stud Alcohol Drugs 68:625–633, 2007

Mattila MJ, Aranko K, Seppala T: Acute effects of buspirone and alcohol on psychomotor skills. J Clin Psychiatry 43:56–61, 1982

McBride WJ, Lovinger DM, Machu T, et al: Serotonin-3 receptors in the actions of alcohol, alcohol reinforcement, and alcoholism. Alcohol Clin Exp Res 28:257–267, 2004

McGrath PJ, Nunes EV, Stewart JW, et al: Imipramine treatment of alcoholics with primary depression: a placebo-controlled clinical trial. Arch Gen Psychiatry 53:232–240, 1996

McKee SA, Harrison EL, O'Malley SS, et al: Varenicline reduces alcohol self-administration in heavy-drinking smokers. Biol Psychiatry 66:185–190, 2009

McMahon T, Andersen R, Metten P, et al: Protein kinase C epsilon mediates up-regulation of N-type calcium channels by ethanol. Mol Pharmacol 57:53–58, 2000

Meera P, Olsen RW, Otis TS, et al: Alcohol- and alcohol antagonist-sensitive human GABAA receptors: tracking delta subunit incorporation into functional receptors. Mol Pharmacol 78:918–924, 2010

Merlo Pich E, Lorang M, Yeganeh M, et al: Increase of extracellular corticotropin-releasing factor-like immunoreactivity levels in the amygdala of awake rats during restraint stress and ethanol withdrawal as measured by microdialysis. J Neurosci 15:5439–5447, 1995

Merry J, Reynolds CM, Bailey J, et al: Prophylactic treatment of alcoholism by lithium carbonate: a controlled study. Lancet 1:481–482, 1976

Meyer RE: How to understand the relationship between psychopathology and addictive disorders: another example of the chicken and the egg, in Psychopathology and Addictive Disorders. Edited by Meyer RE. New York, Guilford, 1986, pp 3–16

Miranda R Jr, MacKillop J, Monti PM, et al: Effects of topiramate on urge to drink and the subjective effects of alcohol: a preliminary laboratory study. Alcohol Clin Exp Res 32:489–497, 2008

Mitchell JM, Teague CH, Kayser AS, et al: Varenicline decreases alcohol consumption in heavy-drinking smokers. Psychopharmacology (Berl) 223:299–306, 2012

Morley KC, Teesson M, Reid SC, et al: Naltrexone versus acamprosate in the treatment of alcohol dependence: a multi-centre, randomized, double-blind, placebo-controlled trial. Addiction 101:1451–1462, 2006

Mueller TI, Stout RL, Rudden S, et al: A double-blind, placebo-controlled pilot study of carbamazepine for the treatment of alcohol dependence. Alcohol Clin Exp Res 21:86–92, 1997

Mullikin-Kilpatrick D, Mehta ND, Hildebrandt JD, et al: Gi is involved in ethanol inhibition of L-type calcium channels in undifferentiated but not differentiated PC-12 cells. Mol Pharmacol 47:997–1005, 1995

Muzyk AJ, Fowler JA, Norwood DK, et al: Role of alpha2-agonists in the treatment of acute alcohol withdrawal. Ann Pharmacother 45:649–657, 2011

Muzyk AJ, Rivelli S, Gagliardi J: Defining the role of baclofen for the treatment of alcohol dependence. CNS Drugs 26:69–78, 2012

Myrick H, Malcolm R, Randall PK, et al: A double-blind trial of gabapentin versus lorazepam in the treatment of alcohol withdrawal. Alcohol Clin Exp Res 33:1582–1588, 2009

Myrick H, Li X, Randall PK, et al: The effect of aripiprazole on cue-induced brain activation and drinking parameters in alcoholics. J Clin Psychopharmacol 30:365–372, 2010

Naranjo CA, Sellers EM: Clinical assessment and pharmacotherapy of the alcohol withdrawal syndrome. Recent Dev Alcohol 4:265–281, 1986

Naranjo CA, Sellers EM, Chater K, et al: Nonpharmacologic intervention in acute alcohol withdrawal. Clin Pharmacol Ther 34:214–219, 1983

Naranjo CA, Sellers EM, Sullivan JT, et al: The serotonin uptake inhibitor citalopram attenuates ethanol intake. Clin Pharmacol Ther 41:266–274, 1987

Naranjo CA, Kadlec KE, Sanhueza P, et al: Fluoxetine differentially alters alcohol intake and other consummatory behaviors in problem drinkers. Clin Pharmacol Ther 47:490–498, 1990

Naranjo CA, Poulos CX, Bremner KE, et al: Citalopram decreases desirability, liking, and consumption of alcohol in alcohol-dependent drinkers. Clin Pharmacol Ther 51:729–739, 1992

Naranjo CA, Bremner KE, Lanctot KL: Effects of citalopram and a brief psycho-social intervention on alcohol intake, dependence and problems. Addiction 90:87–99, 1995

Newton PM, Tully K, McMahon T, et al: Chronic ethanol exposure induces an N-type calcium channel splice variant with altered channel kinetics. FEBS Lett 579:671–676, 2005

Newton PM, Zeng L, Wang V, et al: A blocker of N- and T-type voltage-gated calcium channels attenuates ethanol-induced intoxication, place preference, self-administration, and reinstatement. J Neurosci 28:11712–11719, 2008

Nie H, Rewal M, Gill TM, et al: Extrasynaptic delta-containing GABAA receptors in the nucleus accumbens dorsomedial shell contribute to alcohol intake. Proc Natl Acad Sci USA 108:4459–4464, 2011

Nunes EV, Levin FR: Treatment of depression in patients with alcohol or other drug dependence: a meta-analysis. JAMA 291:1887–1896, 2004

O'Malley SS, Jaffe AJ, Chang G, et al: Naltrexone and coping skills therapy for alcohol dependence: a controlled study. Arch Gen Psychiatry 49:881–887, 1992

O'Malley SS, Jaffe AJ, Chang G, et al: Six-month follow-up of naltrexone and psycho-therapy for alcohol dependence. Arch Gen Psychiatry 53:217–224, 1996

O'Malley SS, Rounsaville BJ, Farren C, et al: Initial and maintenance naltrexone treatment for alcohol dependence using primary care vs specialty care: a nested sequence of 3 randomized trials. Arch Intern Med 163:1695–1704, 2003

Oslin DW, Berrettini W, Kranzler HR, et al: A functional polymorphism of the mu-opioid receptor gene is associated with naltrexone response in alcohol-dependent patients. Neuropsychopharmacology 28:1546–1552, 2003

Overstreet DH, Knapp DJ, Breese GR: Modulation of multiple ethanol withdrawal-induced anxiety-like behavior by CRF and CRF1 receptors. Pharmacol Biochem Behav 77:405–13, 2004

Pandey SC, Carr LG, Heilig M, et al: Neuropeptide Y and alcoholism: genetic, molecular, and pharmacological evidence. Alcohol Clin Exp Res 27:149–154, 2003

Peer K, Rennert L, Lynch K, et al: Prevalence of DSM-IV and DSM-5 alcohol, cocaine, opioid, and cannabis use disorders in a largely substance dependent sample. Drug Alcohol Depend Aug 9, 2012 [Epub ahead of print]

Petrakis IL, Trevisan L, Boutros NN, et al: Effect of tryptophan depletion on alcohol cue-induced craving in abstinent alcoholic patients. Alcohol Clin Exp Res 25:1151–1155, 2001

Petrakis IL, Buonopane A, O'Malley S, et al: The effect of tryptophan depletion on alcohol self-administration in non-treatment-seeking alcoholic individuals. Alcohol Clin Exp Res 26:969–975, 2002

Petrakis IL, O'Malley S, Rounsaville B, et al: Naltrexone augmentation of neuroleptic treatment in alcohol abusing patients with schizophrenia. Psychopharmacology (Berl) 172:291–297, 2004

Pettinati HM, Volpicelli JR, Kranzler HR, et al: Sertraline treatment for alcohol dependence: interactive effects of medication and alcoholic subtype. Alcohol Clin Exp Res 24:1041–1049, 2000

Pettinati HM, Kranzler HR, Madaras J: The status of serotonin-selective pharmacotherapy in the treatment of alcohol dependence. Recent Dev Alcohol 16:247–262, 2003

Pettinati HM, Oslin DW, Kampman KM, et al: A double-blind, placebo-controlled trial combining sertraline and naltrexone for treating co-occurring depression and alcohol dependence. Am J Psychiatry 167:668–675, 2010

Petty F, Kramer GL, Davis LL, et al: Plasma gamma-aminobutyric acid (GABA) predicts outcome in patients with alcohol dependence. Prog Neuropsychopharmacol Biol Psychiatry 21:809–816, 1997

Pierucci-Lagha A, Feinn R, Modesto-Lowe V, et al: Effects of rapid tryptophan depletion on mood and urge to drink in patients with co-morbid major depression and alcohol dependence. Psychopharmacology (Berl) 171:340–348, 2004

Pierucci-Lagha A, Covault J, Feinn R, et al: GABRA2 alleles moderate the subjective effects of alcohol, which are attenuated by finasteride. Neuropsychopharmacology 30:1193–1203, 2005

Plaza-Zabala A, Maldonado R, Berrendero F: The hypocretin/orexin system: implications for drug reward and relapse. Mol Neurobiol 45:424–439, 2012

Porjesz B, Begleiter H, Wang K, et al: Linkage and linkage disequilibrium mapping of ERP and EEG phenotypes. Biol Psychol 61:229–248, 2002

Posternak MA, Mueller TI: Assessing the risks and benefits of benzodiazepines for anxiety disorders in patients with a history of substance abuse or dependence. Am J Addict 10:48–68, 2001

Powell BJ, Penick EC, Othmer E, et al: Prevalence of additional psychiatric syndromes among male alcoholics. J Clin Psychiatry 43:404–407, 1982

Quertemont E, Eriksson CJ, Zimatkin SM, et al: Is ethanol a pro-drug? Acetaldehyde contribution to brain ethanol effects. Alcohol Clin Exp Res 29:1514–1521, 2005

Radel M, Goldman D: Pharmacogenetics of alcohol response and alcoholism: the interplay of genes and environmental factors in thresholds for alcoholism. Drug Metab Dispos 29:489–494, 2001

Ray LA, Oslin DW: Naltrexone for the treatment of alcohol dependence among African Americans: results from the COMBINE Study. Drug Alcohol Depend 105:256–258, 2009

Ray LA, Miranda R Jr, MacKillop J, et al: A preliminary pharmacogenetic investigation of adverse events from topiramate in heavy drinkers. Exp Clin Psychopharmacol 17:122–129, 2009

Regier DA, Farmer ME, Rae DS, et al: Comorbidity of mental disorders with alcohol and other drug abuse: results from the Epidemiologic Catchment Area (ECA) Study. JAMA 264:2511–2518, 1990

Reoux JP, Saxon AJ, Malte CA, et al: Divalproex sodium in alcohol withdrawal: a randomized double-blind placebo-controlled clinical trial. Alcohol Clin Exp Res 25:1324–1329, 2001

Richardson K, Baillie A, Reid S, et al: Do acamprosate or naltrexone have an effect on daily drinking by reducing craving for alcohol? Addiction 103:953–959, 2008

Roberto M, Cruz MT, Gilpin NW, et al: Corticotropin releasing factor-induced amygdala gamma-aminobutyric acid release plays a key role in alcohol dependence. Biol Psychiatry 67:831–839, 2010

Roh S, Matsushita S, Hara S, et al: Role of GABRA2 in moderating subjective responses to alcohol. Alcohol Clin Exp Res 35:400–407, 2011

Rösner S, Hackl-Herrwerth A, Leucht S, et al: Acamprosate for alcohol dependence. Cochrane Database of Systematic Reviews 2010, Issue 9. Art. No.: CD004332. DOI: 10.1002/14651858.CD004332.pub2.

Ross HE, Frederick B, Glaser MD, et al: The prevalence of psychiatric disorders in patients with alcohol and other drug problems. Arch Gen Psychiatry 45:1023–1031, 1988

Rothblat DS, Rubin E, Schneider JS: Effects of chronic alcohol ingestion on the mesostriatal dopamine system in the rat. Neurosci Lett 300:63–66, 2001

Roy A: Placebo-controlled study of sertraline in depressed recently abstinent alcoholics. Biol Psychiatry 44:633–637, 1998

Rubio G, Jimenez-Arriero MA, Ponce G, et al: Naltrexone versus acamprosate: one year follow-up of alcohol dependence treatment. Alcohol Alcohol 36:419–425, 2001

Rubio G, Lopez-Munoz F, Ponce G, et al: Zonisamide versus diazepam in the treatment of alcohol withdrawal syndrome. Pharmacopsychiatry 43:257–262, 2010

Ryabinin AE, Criado JR, Henriksen SJ, et al: Differential sensitivity of c-Fos expression in hippocampus and other brain regions to moderate and low doses of alcohol. Mol Psychiatry 2:32–43, 1997

Ryabinin AE, Bachtell RK, Freeman P, et al: ITF expression in mouse brain during acquisition of alcohol self-administration. Brain Res 890:192–195, 2001

Salloum IM, Cornelius JR, Thase ME, et al: Naltrexone utility in depressed alcoholics. Psychopharmacol Bull 34:111–115, 1998

Salloum IM, Cornelius JR, Daley DC, et al: Efficacy of valproate maintenance in patients with bipolar disorder and alcoholism: a double-blind placebo-controlled study. Arch Gen Psychiatry 62:37–45, 2005

Sarid-Segal O, Knapp CM, Burch W, et al: The anticonvulsant zonisamide reduces ethanol self-administration by risky drinkers. Am J Drug Alcohol Abuse 35:316–319, 2009

Schade A, Marquenie LA, van Balkom AJ, et al: The effectiveness of anxiety treatment on alcohol-dependent patients with a comorbid phobic disorder: a randomized controlled trial. Alcohol Clin Exp Res 29:794–800, 2005

Schuckit M: Alcoholic patients with secondary depression. Am J Psychiatry 140:711–714, 1983

Selim M, Bradberry CW: Effect of ethanol on extracellular 5-HT and glutamate in the nucleus accumbens and prefrontal cortex: comparison between the Lewis and Fischer 344 rat strains. Brain Res 716:157–164, 1996

Seneviratne C, Huang W, Ait-Daoud N, et al: Characterization of a functional polymorphism in the 3′ UTR of SLC6A4 and its association with drinking intensity. Alcohol Clin Exp Res 33:332–339, 2009

Seppala T, Aranko K, Mattila MJ, et al: Effects of alcohol on buspirone and lorazepam actions. Clin Pharmacol Ther 32:201–207, 1982

Sheela Rani CS, Ticku MK: Comparison of chronic ethanol and chronic intermittent ethanol treatments on the expression of GABA(A) and NMDA receptor subunits. Alcohol 38:89–97, 2006

Sokolow L, Welte J, Hynes G, et al: Multiple substance use by alcoholics. Br J Addict 76:147–158, 1981

Soyka M, Preuss UW, Hesselbrock V, et al: GABA-A2 receptor subunit gene (GABRA2) polymorphisms and risk for alcohol dependence. J Psychiatr Res 42:184–91, 2008

Srisurapanont M, Jarusuraisin N: Naltrexone for the treatment of alcoholism: a meta-analysis of randomized controlled trials. Int J Neuropsychopharmacol 8:267–280, 2005

Substance Abuse and Mental Health Services Administration: Results from the 2009 National Survey on Drug Use and Health: Volume I. Summary of National Findings (Office of Applied Studies, NSDUH Series H-38A, HHS Publ No SMA 10-4856 Findings). Rockville, MD, Substance Abuse and Mental Health Services Administration, 2010. Available at: http://www.samhsa.gov/data/NSDUH/2k9NSDUH/2k9Results.htm. Accessed November 18, 2012.

Sullivan LE, O'Connor PG: Medical disorders in substance abuse patients, in Dual Diagnosis and Psychiatric Treatment: Substance Abuse and Comorbid Disorders, 2nd Edition. Edited by Kranzler HR, Tinsley JA. New York, Marcel Dekker, 2004, pp 515–553

Sun F, Tsuritani I, Yamada Y: Contribution of genetic polymorphisms in ethanol-metabolizing enzymes to problem drinking behavior in middle-aged Japanese men. Behav Genet 32:229–236, 2002

Thiele TE, Marsh DJ, Ste Marie L, et al: Ethanol consumption and resistance are inversely related to neuropeptide Y levels. Nature 396:366–369, 1998

Thiele TE, Miura GI, Marsh DJ, et al: Neurobiological responses to ethanol in mutant mice lacking neuropeptide Y or the Y5 receptor. Pharmacol Biochem Behav 67:683–691, 2000

Thiele TE, Koh MT, Pedrazzini T: Voluntary alcohol consumption is controlled via the neuropeptide Y Y1 receptor. J Neurosci 22:RC208, 2002

Thiele TE, Navarro M, Sparta DR, et al: Alcoholism and obesity: overlapping neuropeptide pathways: Neuropeptides 37:321–337, 2003

Thomas SE, Randall PK, Book SW, et al: A complex relationship between co-occurring social anxiety and alcohol use disorders: what effect does treating social anxiety have on drinking? Alcohol Clin Exp Res 32:77–84, 2008

Thomasson HR, Crabb DW, Edenberg HJ, et al: Low frequency of the ADH2*2 allele among Atayal natives of Taiwan with alcohol use disorders. Alcohol Clin Exp Res 18:640–643, 1994

Tiihonen J, Ryynanen OP, Kauhanen J, et al: Citalopram in the treatment of alcoholism: a double-blind placebo-controlled study. Pharmacopsychiatry 29:27–29, 1996

Tollefson GD, Montague-Clouse J, Tollefson SL: Treatment of comorbid generalized anxiety in a recently detoxified alcohol population with a selective serotonergic drug (buspirone). J Clin Psychopharmacol 12:19–26, 1992

Tu GC, Israel Y: Alcohol consumption by orientals in North America is predicted largely by a single gene. Behav Genet 25:59–65, 1995

Uhart M, Weerts EM, McCaul ME, et al: GABRA2 markers moderate the subjective effects of alcohol. Addict Biol Apr 13, 2012 [Epub ahead of print]

van den Brink W, Sørensen P, Torup L, et al: Long-term efficacy, tolerability, and safety of nalmefene as-needed in alcohol dependence: a randomised, double-blind, placebo-controlled study. Alcohol Clin Exp Res 36 (suppl 1):247A, 2012

Volkow ND, Wang GJ, Begleiter H, et al: Regional brain metabolic response to lorazepam in subjects at risk for alcoholism. Alcohol Clin Exp Res 19:510–516, 1995

Volkow ND, Wang GJ, Fowler JS, et al: Decreases in dopamine receptors but not in dopamine transporters in alcoholics. Alcohol Clin Exp Res 20:1594–1598, 1996

Volpicelli JR, Alterman AI, Hayashida M, et al: Naltrexone in the treatment of alcohol dependence. Arch Gen Psychiatry 49:876–880, 1992

Volpicelli JR, Watson NT, King AC, et al: Effect of naltrexone on alcohol "high" in alcoholics. Am J Psychiatry 152:613–615, 1995

von der Goltz C, Koopmann A, Dinter C, et al: Involvement of orexin in the regulation of stress, depression and reward in alcohol dependence. Horm Behav 60:644–650, 2011

Voronin K, Randall P, Myrick H, et al: Aripiprazole effects on alcohol consumption and subjective reports in a clinical laboratory paradigm—possible influence of self-control. Alcohol Clin Exp Res 32:1954–1961, 2008

Wall ME, Brine DR, Perez-Reyes M: Metabolism and disposition of naltrexone in man after oral and intravenous administration. Drug Metab Dispos 9:369–375, 1981

Wallner M, Hanchar HJ, Olsen RW: Ethanol enhances alpha 4 beta 3 delta and alpha 6 beta 3 delta gamma-aminobutyric acid type A receptors at low concentrations known to affect humans. Proc Natl Acad Sci USA 100:15218–15223, 2003

Wang J, Carnicella S, Phamluong K, et al: Ethanol induces long-term facilitation of NR2B-NMDA receptor activity in the dorsal striatum: implications for alcohol drinking behavior. J Neurosci 27:3593–3602, 2007

Werner DF, Kumar S, Criswell HE, et al: PKCγ is required for ethanol-induced increases in GABA$_A$ receptor α4 subunit expression in cultured cerebral cortical neurons. J Neurochem 116: 554–63, 2011

Wolf B, Iguchi MY, Griffiths RR: Sedative/tranquilizer use and abuse in alcoholics currently in outpatient treatment: incidence, pattern and preference, in Problems of Drug Dependence 1989 (NIDA Research Monograph No 95. DHHS Publ No ADM-90-a663). Edited by Harris LS. Washington, DC, U.S. Government Printing Office, 1990, pp 376–377

Wong DF, Maini A, Rousset OG, et al: Positron emission tomography—a tool for identifying the effects of alcohol dependence on the brain. Alcohol Res Health 27:161–173, 2003

Wu PH, Coultrap S, Browning MD, et al: Correlated changes in NMDA receptor phosphorylation, functional activity, and sedation by chronic ethanol consumption. J Neurochem 115:1112–1122, 2010

Xiao C, Ye JH: Ethanol dually modulates GABAergic synaptic transmission onto dopaminergic neurons in ventral tegmental area: role of mu-opioid receptors. Neuroscience 153:240–248, 2008

Zimatkin SM, Buben AL: Ethanol oxidation in the living brain. Alcohol Alcohol 42:529–532, 2007

Zintzaras E: Gamma-aminobutyric acid A receptor, alpha-2 (GABRA2) variants as individual markers for alcoholism: a meta-analysis. Psychiatr Genet 22:189–196, 2012

Zuo Y, Aistrup GL, Marszalec W, et al: Dual action of n-alcohols on neuronal nicotinic acetylcholine receptors. Mol Pharmacol 60:700–711, 2001

2

Tobacco

Cheryl A. Oncken, M.D., M.P.H.

Tony P. George, M.D., F.R.C.P.C.

Comprehensive treatment of tobacco addiction is necessary because of the addictive nature of nicotine and the serious health consequences of tobacco dependence (Fiore et al. 2008). Approximately one-third of individuals who experiment with cigarettes become regular smokers (Giovino 2007). Once dependence develops, tobacco addiction can become a chronic relapsing disorder with dire medical consequences. Indeed, cigarette smoking is responsible for approximately 443,000 deaths each year in the United States (Centers for Disease Control and Prevention 2010).

Fortunately, effective smoking treatments (both behavioral and pharmacological) are available (George and O'Malley 2004; Polosa and Benowitz

The preparation of this chapter was supported in part by grant R01-HD069314 (to Dr. Oncken) and the Chair in Addiction Psychiatry at the University of Toronto and Canadian Institutes of Health Research (CIHR) grant MOP#115145 (to Dr. George).

2011). Although behavioral interventions are an integral part of tobacco treatment, our chapter includes only pharmacotherapies that aid in smoking cessation (see George and O'Malley 2004; Polosa and Benowitz 2011). Several recent publications discuss the behavioral treatment of tobacco dependence (Fiore et al. 2008). Specifically, we discuss here the phenomenology of nicotine addiction and clinical aspects of tobacco dependence and withdrawal, the first-line tobacco pharmacotherapies—nicotine replacement therapy (NRT) products, sustained-release bupropion (bupropion SR) and varenicline—and other medications that may enhance smoking cessation rates and/or reduce smoking relapse, as outlined in Table 2–1. We also briefly review nicotine dependence pharmacotherapies for persons with psychiatric and medical comorbidity and other special populations such as pregnant women.

Phenomenology of Tobacco Addiction and Clinical Aspects of Withdrawal

The primary addictive substance in cigarette smoke is nicotine. Cigarette smoking is a very efficient nicotine delivery system because nicotine is aerosolized and subsequently readily absorbed through the extensive pulmonary vasculature. Consequently, smoking produces high arterial nicotine concentrations (i.e., compared with venous concentrations) (Benowitz 2010). These high arterial concentrations deliver a bolus of 1–3 mg of nicotine rapidly to the brain (i.e., within seconds after the onset of smoking) (Benowitz 2010). Several neurotransmitters are released with nicotinic receptor activation, including dopamine, norepinephrine, serotonin, and endogenous opioids. The immediate positive reinforcing effects of smoking include a reduction in anxiety and increased alertness and concentration.

Nicotine's half-life is 60–90 minutes, so repeated administration is needed throughout the day for continued effects. Consequently, daily smokers usually smoke at frequent intervals to maintain a narrow range of nicotine levels. Paradoxically, chronic administration of nicotine results in an increase in the number of nicotinic receptors, presumably resulting from chronic nicotinic receptor desensitization and inactivation. An increased number of receptors may play a role in the cravings and nicotine withdrawal symptoms many smokers experience with prolonged cigarette abstinence (Dani and Balfour

Table 2–1. Pharmacological treatments for tobacco dependence

Nicotine replacement therapies	Mechanism of action	Efficacy rating
Nicotine gum or lozenge (OTC)[a]	Intermediate nicotine absorption, full agonist gradually reduces cravings and nicotine withdrawal	1
Transdermal nicotine (OTC)[a]	Slow nicotine absorption, full agonist gradually reduces cravings and nicotine withdrawal	1
Nicotine nasal spray (prescription)[a]	Fast nicotine absorption leads to stimulation of nAChR, which rapidly reduces craving and nicotine withdrawal	1
Nicotine inhaler (prescription)[a]	Intermediate nicotine absorption, full agonist reduces craving and nicotine withdrawal	1
Nonnicotine medications (all by prescription)		
Bupropion SR[a]	Blocks neuronal reuptake of dopamine and norepinephrine; high-affinity, noncompetitive nAChR antagonist reduces craving and nicotine withdrawal and nicotine reinforcement	1
Varenicline[a]	Partial agonist of $\alpha_4\beta_2$ nAChRs; relieves cravings and blocks reinforcing effects of nicotine	1
Nortriptyline	Noradrenergic and serotonergic reuptake blockade; reduces withdrawal symptoms and probably comorbid depressive symptoms; adverse effects limit its utility	1–2

Table 2–1.   Pharmacological treatments for tobacco dependence (*continued*)

Nicotine replacement therapies	Mechanism of action	Efficacy rating
Nonnicotine medications (all by prescription) (*continued*)		
Mecamylamine	Noncompetitive, high-affinity nAChR antagonist combined with transdermal nicotine reduces nicotine reinforcement, craving, and withdrawal	2
Clonidine	α_2-Adrenoreceptor agonist reduces cravings and nicotine withdrawal symptoms	2
Naltrexone	Endogenous μ opioid receptor antagonist reduces craving and nicotine withdrawal symptoms in combination with transdermal nicotine; may reduce alcohol use and prevent cessation-induced weight gain	3
Monoamine oxidase inhibitors	Increase monoamine levels; can reduce reinforcing effects of nicotine, craving, and withdrawal symptoms; may be useful for smokers with co-occurring mood disorders	2
Cytisine	Partial agonist of $\alpha_4\beta_2$ nAChRs; low cost, may be useful to treat smokers in low- and middle-income countries	2
Nicotine vaccine	Limited evidence of efficacy for smoking cessation in early human trials; may also have utility in relapse prevention	2

Note.   nAChRs=nicotinic acetylcholine receptors; OTC=over the counter. Efficacy rating: 1=strong evidence of efficacy, 2=moderate evidence of efficacy, 3=limited evidence of efficacy.
[a]U.S. Food and Drug Administration approved for smoking cessation.

Source.   Adapted from George 2011.

2011). Withdrawal symptoms include dysphoria or depressed mood, insomnia, irritability, anxiety, frustration, difficulty in concentration, and increased appetite and weight gain. Withdrawal symptoms typically peak within 24–36 hours after cessation and usually diminish after 1 week of abstinence, but prolonged withdrawal may occur in some individuals. Thus, some individuals may continue to smoke cigarettes to avoid the negative symptoms of withdrawal (i.e., negative reinforcement of smoking behavior) (Polosa and Benowitz 2011). It seems probable that both the primary, positively reinforcing effects of smoking and the avoidance of withdrawal symptoms sustain tobacco use in most smokers.

Pharmacological Treatments for Tobacco Dependence

Nicotine Replacement Therapies

NRTs, which are considered first-line treatment for smoking cessation, were designed to enhance efficacy rates during smoking cessation by replacing some of the nicotine usually delivered by smoking (George 2011). The U.S. Food and Drug Administration (FDA)–approved NRTs for smoking cessation include 2- and 4-mg nicotine polacrilex gum and nicotine lozenge, transdermal nicotine, nicotine nasal spray, and nicotine inhaler. All NRTs have been shown to approximately double the smoking cessation success rate seen with placebo treatment (Stead 2012). (Specific odds ratios [ORs] for individual NRTs relative to placebo therapies can be found in Fiore et al. 2008.) The choice of NRT for an individual patient depends on the patient's preference, the adverse-effect profile of the NRT, the presence of other medical conditions, and previous success or failure with a certain type of NRT.

Nicotine Gum

Nicotine polacrilex gum was the first NRT marketed for smoking cessation. It is available for over-the-counter purchase in 2- and 4-mg dose forms. Nicotine gum contains nicotine bound to an ion-exchange resin. The nicotine in nicotine gum is released slowly into the mouth and absorbed through the buccal mucosa. Nicotine gum is most beneficial with concurrent behavioral therapy and when used on a fixed schedule (i.e., chewing one piece every 1–2 hours) rather than ad libitum dosing. The usual treatment duration for nicotine gum is 6–14 weeks; however, benefits may occur with a longer duration of treatment (Fiore et al. 2008).

The gum should be chewed slowly, with intermittent "parking" of the gum at the side of the mouth, to avoid adverse effects (e.g., hiccups, heartburn, stomach upset). Only 50% of the nicotine in a piece of gum is systemically absorbed. Nicotine concentrations peak approximately 30 minutes after the onset of chewing (Benowitz 2010). The starting dose for individuals who smoke fewer than 20 cigarettes per day is 2 mg, whereas the 4-mg dose is recommended for heavier smokers (Le Foll and George 2007). This recommendation comes in part from studies that show a higher dose of gum is more beneficial for heavier smokers (Fiore et al. 2008). The gum probably should not be prescribed to persons with temporomandibular joint disease or those who have dental or oral problems that could be exacerbated by gum chewing.

Nicotine Lozenge

The nicotine lozenge contains nicotine bound to a polacrilex ion-exchange resin (similar to the nicotine gum). It is available for over-the-counter purchase in 2- and 4-mg dose forms. Because the lozenge does not require chewing, it may be preferable to the gum for patients with dental problems and for patients who find chewing gum objectionable. The lozenge formulations release 25% more nicotine than an equal dose of the gum (Shiffman et al. 2002). In a large randomized trial, low-dependence smokers (i.e., those who waited longer than 30 minutes on awakening to have their first cigarette) were randomly assigned to receive the 2-mg lozenge or a matching placebo, and highly dependent smokers (i.e., those who had their first cigarette within 30 minutes of awakening) were randomly assigned to receive the 4-mg lozenge or placebo for at least 24 weeks (Shiffman et al. 2002). Participants in the active lozenge groups had a significantly higher 28-day abstinence rate at 6 weeks, compared with the placebo group, for both the 2-mg (46.0% vs. 29.7%; $P<0.001$) and the 4-mg doses (48.7% vs. 20.8%; $P<0.001$). Efficacy of the drug was sustained through a 1-year follow-up.

Patients who use the lozenge for smoking cessation should use one lozenge every 1–2 hours for the first 2–4 weeks, decreasing the interval of use to every 2–4 hours thereafter. Adverse effects that are common with the nicotine lozenge include heartburn, hiccups, and nausea (Shiffman et al. 2002). Because the product contains phenylalanine, the lozenge should not be used for smoking cessation by individuals with phenylketonuria.

Transdermal Nicotine

Transdermal nicotine (i.e., the nicotine patch) is also available over the counter for smoking cessation. This form of nicotine delivery may be especially useful for smoking cessation because a constant delivery of nicotine may aid in patients' adherence to NRT. Eight weeks of treatment are generally sufficient for smoking cessation (Fiore et al. 2008). Compared with other NRTs, transdermal nicotine probably has the lowest abuse potential, because there are few or no withdrawal symptoms after treatment has ended, and the patient does not have control over nicotine delivery.

Transdermal nicotine is available in a variety of formulations and dosing schedules (e.g., 15 mg/16 hours; 7, 14, and 21 mg/24 hours). Peak nicotine concentrations for the various systems are reached 2–6 hours after application, and steady-state conditions occur 2–3 days after continued patch use (Benowitz 2010). The highest-dose patch (i.e., 21 or 22 mg/24 hours or 15 mg/ 16 hours) delivers approximately 0.9 mg of nicotine per hour transdermally (Benowitz 2010).

The transdermal system is applied in the morning and removed either before bedtime or the next morning. Among individuals smoking 10 or more cigarettes per day, the highest-dose patch should be used to start; a lower dose can be used if the patient smokes fewer than 10 cigarettes per day (Benowitz 2010). Although dosage reduction is usually recommended after 2–4 weeks with most formulations to taper the NRT because of clinical concerns about nicotine withdrawal from transdermal nicotine, one meta-analysis showed no benefit of dosage reduction on patch efficacy (Fiore et al. 2008). In fact, there is little evidence for a clinically significant nicotine withdrawal syndrome after transdermal nicotine discontinuation. Transdermal nicotine should not be used for patients with skin conditions that could be exacerbated by the patch.

Nicotine Nasal Spray

Nicotine nasal spray delivers nicotine through the nasal mucosa. One advantage of this formulation is that it relieves tobacco cravings quickly. In one study, the nicotine nasal spray was 2.6 times more likely to produce smoking cessation than placebo, at 1 year (Sutherland et al. 1992). The nicotine spray was most beneficial among highly dependent smokers.

The nasal spray is available only by prescription. One spray to each nostril constitutes a dose. Although one dose delivers approximately 1 mg of nicotine, only 0.5 mg of nicotine is systemically absorbed. Patients should initially use 1 or 2 doses per hour but should not exceed 5 doses per hour or 40 doses per day (Sutherland et al. 1992). The nasal spray delivers nicotine rapidly, with venous nicotine concentrations peaking at 5–10 minutes after administration (Sutherland et al. 1992). Of the nicotine delivery systems, nicotine nasal spray most closely approximates the pharmacokinetic profile of nicotine following smoking. Because this form of NRT is administered nasally, patients with rhinitis, nasal polyps, or sinusitis probably should not use nicotine nasal spray for smoking cessation. The nasal spray produces some initial irritation of the nasal mucosa at the dosage formulation (10 mg/mL) that is available commercially, but this effect subsides with repeated dosing.

Nicotine Inhaler

Nicotine inhalers, which are used by puffing through a cartridge inhaler, may be useful for smoking cessation in some patients because their use is similar to the smoking ritual (i.e., holding the device, with repeated hand-to-mouth activity, and puffing on the device replicate many of the sensory and motoric aspects of smoking), and they deliver nicotine rapidly (although not as rapidly as the nasal spray). In one placebo-controlled study, in which subjects were allowed to use an inhaler for up to 6 months, quit rates at 1 year remained higher in the nicotine inhaler group than in the placebo inhaler group (28% and 18%, respectively; $P=0.046$) (Hjalmarson et al. 1997).

This product is available only by prescription. The usual treatment period is up to 24 weeks (Fiore et al. 2008). Using the inhaler by puffing 80 deep inhalations over 20 minutes results in a systemic absorption through the buccal mucosa of 2 mg of nicotine, with maximal nicotine concentrations occurring 15 minutes after the end of inhalation (Pfizer and Pharmacia and Upjohn Company 2008). When the product is used as directed, the patient will likely use 6–16 inhalers per day. This form of NRT is contraindicated in patients with known hypersensitivity to nicotine or menthol. The inhaler should be used with caution in persons with asthma, because although most of the nicotine is absorbed through the buccal mucosa and is not delivered to the lungs, nicotine by inhalation may produce bronchial constriction.

Combined NRT Formulations

As previously discussed, currently available NRT products typically double the rate of smoking cessation, relative to placebo. One way to improve efficacy further is to combine a passive and continuous nicotine delivery system (i.e., the patch) with an active and intermittent delivery system (e.g., the gum, inhaler, or spray) (Fiore et al. 2008; Kleber et al. 2007). The rationale for combined treatment is that smokers may need a constant delivery of nicotine to alleviate withdrawal symptoms as well as an ad libitum nicotine medication that can be used to control smoking urges and further relieve withdrawal symptoms (Sweeney et al. 2001). Moreover, two nicotine replacement products may provide a higher degree of nicotine substitution than monotherapy.

Findings from one meta-analysis (Fiore et al. 2008) showed that combination regimens may increase effectiveness of the nicotine patch. In particular, three studies that evaluated the patch (> 14 weeks) plus either ad libitum nicotine gum or nasal spray (range = 26–52 weeks) found an estimated OR of 1.9 (95% confidence interval [CI], 1.3–2.7) for the combined therapy compared with the patch alone.

Nonnicotine Pharmacotherapies

Not all smokers respond well to NRT. Furthermore, many smokers have comorbid symptoms suggesting that mechanisms independent of the nicotinic receptor may increase vulnerability to nicotine dependence. Thus, there has been considerable interest in nonnicotine medications to treat nicotine dependence, either alone or in combination with NRTs. The observations that the antidepressant bupropion has potential as a treatment for smoking cessation and that other antidepressants (e.g., tricyclic antidepressants and selective serotonin reuptake inhibitors [SSRIs]) may modify smoking behaviors have catalyzed intensive research on medications that act directly on dopamine, norepinephrine, serotonin, glutamate, γ-aminobutyric acid (GABA), nicotinic, cannabinoid, or opioid receptors. We review here data on the safety and efficacy of bupropion and other nonnicotine therapies. Of the nonnicotine medications for smoking cessation, only bupropion SR and varenicline are currently considered a first-line treatment for cigarette smokers.

Sustained-Release Bupropion

The phenylaminoketone atypical antidepressant agent bupropion (amfebutamone) in the SR formulation (Zyban) is considered a first-line pharmacological treatment for smoking cessation. The mechanism of action of this antidepressant in the treatment of nicotine dependence likely involves blockade of dopamine and norepinephrine reuptake (Ascher et al. 1995), as well as antagonism of high-affinity nicotinic acetylcholine receptors (Slemmer et al. 2000). The goals of bupropion therapy for nicotine dependence are 1) cessation of smoking behavior and 2) reduction of nicotine withdrawal symptoms. In addition, bupropion SR may delay cessation-induced weight gain.

Efficacy.   A pivotal study by Hurt et al. (1997) established the efficacy and safety of bupropion SR for treatment of nicotine dependence, which led to its approval for this indication by the FDA in 1997. This study was a 7-week, double-blind, placebo-controlled, multicenter trial of three dosages of bupropion SR (100 mg/day, 150 mg/day, or 300 mg/day in twice-daily dosing). Participants comprised 615 cigarette smokers who smoked at least 15 cigarettes per day. The medication was administered in combination with weekly individual cessation counseling. End-of-trial 7-day point prevalence cessation rates were 19.0% for placebo and 28.8%, 38.6%, and 44.2% for the 100 mg/day, 150 mg/day, and 300 mg/day bupropion dosages, respectively. At 1-year follow-up, cessation rates were 12.4% for placebo and 19.6%, 22.9%, and 23.1% for the 100 mg/day, 150 mg/day, and 300 mg/day bupropion dosages, respectively. Bupropion treatment dose-dependently reduced weight gain associated with smoking cessation and significantly reduced nicotine withdrawal symptoms at the 150 mg/day and 300 mg/day dosages. In this study, the major adverse effects associated with bupropion, compared with placebo, were insomnia and dry mouth. Accordingly, the target dosage for bupropion treatment of smoking cessation that was approved was 150 mg/day for 3–4 days, with a subsequent increase to 150 mg twice daily. The "target quit date" is typically set on the eighth day of bupropion treatment, when bupropion levels are at steady-state concentrations.

The combination of bupropion SR with the nicotine transdermal patch was evaluated in a double-blind, double placebo-controlled, randomized multicenter trial (Jorenby et al. 1999). A total of 893 cigarette smokers who smoked at least 15 cigarettes per day were randomly assigned to one of four groups: 1) placebo bupropion (0 mg/day) plus placebo patch, 2) bupropion (300 mg/day) plus placebo patch, 3) placebo bupropion plus nicotine patch (21 mg/day for 4 weeks, followed by 2 weeks of 14 mg/day and 2 weeks of 7 mg/day), and 4) bupropion (300 mg/day) plus nicotine patch (21 mg/day for 4 weeks, followed by 2 weeks of 14 mg/day and 2 weeks of 7 mg/day). Treatment with bupropion was initiated 1 week before the target quit date (day 15), at which time patch treatment was added for a total of 8 weeks. All subjects received weekly individual smoking cessation counseling. Cessation rates at the 1-year follow-up assessment were 15.6% for placebo, 16.4% for active nicotine transdermal patch alone, 30.3% for bupropion alone, and 35.5% for the combination of patch and bupropion. The rates for both the group receiving bupropion plus the patch and the bupropion-only group were significantly better than those for the placebo group and the patch-only group, but the rate for the combination was not significantly better than that for bupropion only. Weight suppression after cessation was most robust in the combination therapy group. The combination was well tolerated, with adverse effects those expected from the patch and bupropion. It is noteworthy that the patch-only treatment was significantly different from placebo at the end of the trial but not at the follow-up assessments. In this trial, 6.1% of the subjects who were randomly assigned to receive combination treatment with the nicotine patch and bupropion developed hypertension. Most of the subjects who developed hypertension had preexisting hypertension; however, patients who are using NRT and bupropion together for smoking cessation should have their blood pressure monitored. The combination of the transdermal nicotine and bupropion has been FDA approved for smoking cessation. In one meta-analysis, bupropion SR and transdermal nicotine had an estimated OR of 1.3 (95% CI, 1.0–1.8) compared with nicotine patch alone (Fiore et al. 2008).

Use in smoking cessation in tobacco smokers with comorbid psychiatric or substance use disorders.   Some studies have suggested that bupropion SR may be useful for smoking cessation or reduction in psychiatric patients who smoke or in substance-misusing smokers. Hayford et al. (1999), in a secondary analysis of data from the study by Hurt et al. (1997), found that bupropion SR was efficacious for smoking cessation in smokers irrespective of a history of major depression or alcoholism. A recent study has shown the safety of bupropion SR in cigarette smokers in recovery from alcohol dependence

(Kalman et al. 2011). There are also preliminary reports of the safety and effectiveness of bupropion SR for smoking cessation in patients with major depression (Chengappa et al. 2001), bipolar disorder (Weinberger et al. 2008; George et al. 2012), and posttraumatic stress disorder (Hertzberg et al. 2001; McFall et al. 2005, 2010).

Bupropion SR has been evaluated in several trials involving patients with schizophrenia, including an open-label trial of 300 mg/day (Weiner et al. 2001) and placebo-controlled trials of 150 mg/day (Evins et al. 2001) and 300 mg/day (George et al. 2002). Similarly, in a double-blind trial of 12 weeks' duration, Evins et al. (2001) found that among 18 patients with schizophrenia who were smokers, bupropion (150 mg/day) led to a 40%–50% reduction in carbon monoxide (CO) levels, compared with placebo. One of nine subjects in the bupropion group versus none of nine in the placebo group had achieved smoking cessation by the end of the trial. During this trial, bupropion reduced both positive and negative symptoms of schizophrenia. George et al. (2002) conducted a double-blind, placebo-controlled, 10-week trial of bupropion SR (300 mg/day) in a sample of 32 nicotine-dependent smokers with schizophrenia or schizoaffective disorder. Trial endpoint cessation rates (confirmed by a CO level < 10 ppm) were 8 of 16 (50%) in the bupropion group and 2 of 16 (12.5%) in the placebo group ($P<0.05$). Positive symptoms of schizophrenia were not affected, but negative symptom scores were reduced by approximately 15% in the bupropion group. In addition, treatment with atypical antipsychotic (vs. neuroleptic) drugs strongly predicted success in smoking cessation in schizophrenia. Accordingly, results from these preliminary studies suggest that 1) smoking reduction or cessation is possible in patients with schizophrenia (with endpoint cessation rates ranging from 11% to 50%); 2) exacerbation of psychotic symptoms is unlikely, and negative symptoms of schizophrenia may be reduced; and 3) the drug's efficacy for smoking cessation may be greater at higher doses in this population. Subsequent studies from Evins et al. (2007) and George et al. (2008) have shown the safety and efficacy of NRTs in combination with bupropion SR in smokers with schizophrenia.

Adverse effects. The primary adverse effects reported with bupropion administration in cigarette smokers are headache, dry mouth, nausea and vomiting, insomnia, and activation. Although most of these adverse effects occur during the first week of treatment, insomnia can persist. Seizures occur very rarely (incidence < 0.5%) at dosages of 300 mg/day or less, but a history of seizures or a seizure disorder contraindicates its use.

Varenicline

Varenicline tartrate, an $\alpha_4\beta_2$ nicotinic acetylcholine receptor partial agonist, was FDA approved as a first-line smoking cessation medication in 2006 and by regulatory bodies in Canada and Europe in 2007. Varenicline is marketed as Chantix in the United States and as Champix in Europe and Canada. Varenicline reduces cravings and blocks some of the reinforcing effects of smoking. An initial Phase II trial of varenicline established its efficacy and safety in comparison to placebo and suggested an optimal dosage of 2 mg/day, with dose titration during the first week of use (Oncken et al. 2006). Subsequently, two identical, independent 12-week Phase III trials comparing varenicline (2 mg/day) with bupropion SR (300 mg/day) with placebo were conducted (Gonzales et al. 2006; Jorenby et al. 2006). The continuous abstinence rates for both studies were similar over the last 4 weeks (weeks 9–12) of medication treatment: in Study 1 (Jorenby et al. 2006) varenicline quit rates were 44.0%, bupropion SR quit rates were 29.5%, and placebo quit rates were 17.7%; in Study 2 (Gonzales et al. 2006) varenicline quit rates were 43.9%, bupropion SR quit rates were 29.8%, and placebo quit rates were 17.6%. The continuous abstinence rates during the last 4 weeks were significantly higher for subjects taking varenicline than for those taking bupropion SR; both varenicline and bupropion SR resulted in significantly higher continuous abstinence rates than did placebo. Continuous abstinence rates over the weeks 9–52 follow-up period were lower; however, subjects taking varenicline continued to show higher abstinence rates than did subjects taking bupropion or placebo.

Varenicline is generally well tolerated. The most common adverse events occurring in Phase II and III studies were nausea and insomnia. However, postmarketing concerns have arisen over neuropsychiatric adverse events such as agitation, mania and psychosis, and suicidal and homicidal ideation (McClure et al. 2010). These events have been reported during medication treatment and after medication discontinuation. Williams et al. (2012) found that varenicline (2 mg/day) was associated with significantly better 12-week smoking cessation outcomes than placebo, with no evidence of exacerbation of psychotic or depressive symptoms or suicidal ideation, in 127 cigarette smokers with schizophrenia or schizoaffective disorder. Nonetheless, close monitoring of smokers is advised when prescribing this medication, especially among smokers with a history of psychiatric illness. Concerns over adverse cardiovascular effects of varenicline are described later in this chapter (see section "Treatment of Smokers With Comorbid Medical Problems") in relation to medical adverse effects of nicotine dependence medications.

Other Nonnicotine Pharmacotherapies

Findings from studies of several non-FDA-approved nonnicotine pharmacotherapies for nicotine dependence are summarized in the following subsections.

Nortriptyline.   Nortriptyline, a tricyclic antidepressant, has been shown in randomized, double-blind, placebo-controlled trials to be superior to placebo for smoking cessation (Prochazka et al. 1998). Nortriptyline appears to have efficacy comparable to that of bupropion for smoking cessation (Hall et al. 2002). The efficacy of this agent may be improved with more intensive behavioral therapies (Hall et al. 1998). Nortriptyline's mechanism of action is thought to relate to its noradrenergic and serotonergic reuptake blockade, two neurotransmitters that have been implicated in the neurobiology of nicotine dependence. Adverse effects of nortriptyline are typical of tricyclic antidepressants and include dry mouth, blurred vision, constipation, and orthostatic hypotension. Although it appears to have some utility for smokers with a history of major depression and can be recommended as a second-line agent after NRTs and bupropion, more study of nortriptyline is needed.

Mecamylamine.   Mecamylamine, a noncompetitive blocker at the ion channel site of both high-affinity central nervous system and peripheral nicotinic receptors, may decrease some of the positive subjective effects of cigarette smoking (Bacher et al. 2009). Mecamylamine does not precipitate withdrawal in humans, perhaps because it is a noncompetitive antagonist of high-affinity nicotinic receptors that does not bind to the nicotine binding site (Eissenberg et al. 1996). Adverse effects of the drug included abdominal cramps, constipation, dry mouth, and headaches. On the hypothesis that combined blockade and agonist therapy might be beneficial (Rose and Levin 1991), two randomized controlled trials were conducted comparing the addition of mecamylamine or placebo to the nicotine patch (Rose et al. 1994, 1998). The rationale for the study design was that mecamylamine would reduce the rewarding effects of nicotine, and the nicotine patch would reduce nicotine withdrawal symptoms. The study provided evidence of the efficacy of the combination therapy; however, a multicenter controlled trial of the combination of transdermal mecamylamine (0, 3, and 6 mg) and transdermal nicotine (21 mg) was negative (Glover et al. 2007). Accordingly, mecamylamine lacks sufficient evidence to be recommended for smoking cessation, but it remains a promising approach.

Clonidine. Clonidine dampens sympathetic activity originating at the locus coeruleus by stimulation of presynaptic α_2-adrenergic receptors in the sympathetic chain (Covey and Glassman 1991; Hughes 1994). It appears to have some efficacy for alcohol and opioid withdrawal and thus was evaluated for the treatment of nicotine withdrawal as well (Covey and Glassman 1991; Hughes 1994). Clinical trials have used oral or transdermal clonidine at a dosage of 0.1–0.4 mg/day for 2–6 weeks, with or without behavioral therapy. Three meta-analytic reviews reported that clonidine improved quit rates (Covey and Glassman 1991; Gourlay and Benowitz 1995).

The most common adverse effects of clonidine are dry mouth, sedation, and constipation (Gourlay and Benowitz 1995). Postural hypotension, rebound hypertension, and depression were rare with use of clonidine for smoking cessation (Gourlay and Benowitz 1995). Several studies have shown that clonidine is more effective in women than in men; however, other studies have failed to find this association (Gourlay and Benowitz 1995). In general, the effects of clonidine are not as consistent as those of NRTs, but this agent should be considered as a second-line therapy for smokers for whom initial treatment with NRTs, bupropion, and varenicline failed.

Naltrexone. Naltrexone hydrochloride is an orally bioactive form of the opioid antagonist naloxone. The rationale for using naltrexone for smoking cessation is that the performance-enhancing and other positive effects of nicotine may be mediated by opioid receptors (Pomerleau and Pomerleau 1984). Most, but not all, studies have shown that naltrexone increases smoking (interpreted again as an attempt to overcome blockade) (Hughes 1994; Sutherland et al. 1995), although a trial in recovering alcoholic patients showed that naltrexone may reduce smoking by about 5 cigarettes per day, even though it appears to have little utility in smoking cessation (Rohsenow et al. 2003). The adverse effects of naltrexone include elevated liver enzyme values, nausea, and blockade of analgesia from narcotic pain relievers (Hughes 1994). Little evidence supports the efficacy of naltrexone hydrochloride alone for smoking cessation (Sutherland et al. 1995), and results are conflicting as to whether adding it to the nicotine patch enhances efficacy (Covey et al. 1999; Krishnan-Sarin et al. 2003; O'Malley et al. 2006).

SSRIs.   Little available evidence supports the use of SSRIs for smoking cessation, either alone (Niaura et al. 2002) or in combination with NRT. Placebo-controlled trials of fluoxetine combined with the nicotine inhaler (Blondal et al. 1999) and of paroxetine combined with the nicotine patch (Killen et al. 2000) failed to show that either of these combinations is superior to NRT plus placebo for smoking cessation. Thus, the use of SSRIs for smoking cessation is not recommended. However, SSRIs may be of some use in smokers with a history of depression.

Monoamine oxidase (MAO) inhibitors.   Drugs that inhibit the enzymes MAO-A and MAO-B theoretically could be helpful for smoking cessation. These drugs block the metabolism of neurotransmitters involved in the biology of nicotine dependence, including dopamine (MAO-B inhibitors) and serotonin and norepinephrine (MAO-A inhibitors), leading to increases in their synaptic levels, which are reduced during acute tobacco withdrawal. The net effect of treatment with these agents could be to reverse the effects of withdrawal, thereby ameliorating withdrawal symptoms and the risk of a relapse to smoking. In a preliminary trial of the MAO-A inhibitor moclobemide, the active medication resulted in a higher short-term rate of self-reported smoking cessation than placebo in a sample of 88 smokers (Berlin et al. 1995). Moreover, a preliminary trial by George et al. (2003) in 40 smokers provided support for the short-term efficacy of the MAO-B inhibitor selegiline hydrochloride for smoking cessation. However, larger trials of selegiline in both oral (Weinberger et al. 2010) and transdermal (Kahn et al. 2012) formulations failed to support the efficacy of this MAO-B inhibitor for smoking cessation.

Cytisine.   Cytisine, an alkaloid extracted from the seeds of the *Cytisus laburnum* plant, is a partial agonist of the $\alpha_4\beta_2$ receptor (similar to varenicline). It has been sold under the trade name Tabex for many years (in many European countries and over the Internet) and is much less expensive than other pharmacotherapies for smoking cessation. In a recent placebo-controlled study, a 25-day standard treatment course resulted in a sustained 12-month abstinence rate of 8.4% in the cytisine group and 2.4% in the placebo group ($P=0.001$). Seven-day point prevalence rates at 12 months were 13.2% in the cytisine group and 7.3% in the placebo group. Gastrointestinal adverse events were observed more frequently in the cytisine group than in the placebo group, and serious adverse events were few and similar between groups. In this study, cytisine was effective for smoking cessation, with an OR similar to that of NRT. Cytisine may be particularly useful in low- to middle-income countries, where tobacco rates are rising and the cost of standard pharmacotherapies is high (West et al. 2011).

Nicotine vaccine.   Nicotine vaccines have been developed for smoking cessation (Fagerström and Balfour 2006). They are designed to stimulate an antibody response to nicotine, which binds nicotine in the plasma and reduces brain exposure to the drug. Although nicotine is not immunogenic, it stimulates an immune response when linked to an appropriate carrier protein (e.g., cholera B toxin, Pseudomonas exotoxin) (Fagerström and Balfour 2006). A gradual reduction in the brain's exposure to nicotine could facilitate smoking cessation. Although early studies provided proof of concept for the vaccine (i.e., a greater antibody response was associated with higher cessation rates), recent large-scale Phase III trials have not shown its efficacy. Further research is needed to establish the safety and efficacy of the different vaccine formulations.

Relapse Prevention

Although numerous studies have examined the use of pharmacotherapy for smoking cessation, there are far fewer studies of its use in preventing smoking relapse over the longer term. The paucity of reports on the extended use of NRTs for the prevention of smoking relapse may be related to few studies examining the safety of long-term use (www.treatobacco.net). However, for a patient who reports prolonged urges to smoke or nicotine withdrawal symptoms, the clinician should consider extending the current approved pharmacotherapy or adding an additional pharmacotherapy (Fiore et al. 2008). If a patient is concerned that weight gain may threaten relapse, continued use of bupropion SR or nicotine gum is warranted, because these treatments have been shown to delay weight gain (Fiore et al. 2008).

Studies have extended the use of bupropion for smoking cessation to the prevention of smoking relapse. Hays et al. (2001) compared the effects of bupropion with placebo for the prevention of smoking relapse in 784 cigarette smokers who achieved smoking abstinence after a 7-week, open-label trial of bupropion (300 mg/day). Abstinent smokers were randomly assigned to receive bupropion (300 mg/day) or placebo for a total of 45 weeks. Of the smokers enrolled in the open-label phase of the trial, 58.8% quit smoking. Significantly more smokers were abstinent at the end of the 52-week treatment period in the bupropion group than in the placebo group (55.1% vs. 42.3%; $P<0.01$), but no difference was evident at the 1-year posttreatment follow-up assessment. In addition, the number of days to smoking relapse was greater in the bupropion group, compared with the placebo group (156 vs. 65 days, $P<0.05$). Weight gain was significantly less in the bupropion group, both at the end of treatment and at the 1-year follow-up. The results of this study support the efficacy of bupropion SR in preventing smoking relapse. However, the question of how long bupropion therapy can be continued as a maintenance treatment requires further study.

A large placebo-controlled trial of varenicline (2 mg/day) for 12 weeks after initial abstinence showed that this agent delays relapse to smoking compared with placebo (Tonstad et al. 2006). On the basis of that study, an additional period of 12 weeks of varenicline was approved by the FDA for tobacco relapse prevention.

Treatment of Smokers With Comorbid Medical Conditions

General precautions for each medication that has been used for smoking cessation are listed in the sections describing each medication. All FDA-approved first-line medications for smoking cessation have a relatively good safety profile. Consensus opinions on the safety of the various medications for persons with cardiovascular disease, other medical conditions, and pregnancy are beyond the scope of this chapter but can be found elsewhere (www.treatobacco.net).

Cardiovascular Disease

In general, for smokers with cardiac disease, the benefits of NRT outweigh the potential risks. In a safety and efficacy study that included veterans with cardiac disease, smoking while using the nicotine patch was not associated with an increase in adverse events (Joseph et al. 1996). Bupropion SR is generally well tolerated in smokers with cardiovascular disease (Rigotti et al. 2006). However, because rare cases of elevated blood pressure can occur with bupropion treatment (Fiore et al. 2008), it is prudent to monitor blood pressure during bupropion treatment in individuals with cardiovascular disease. A multicenter randomized, placebo-controlled study of the safety and efficacy of varenicline was conducted in 714 individuals with cardiovascular disease (Rigotti et al. 2010). Although the sample size was too small to make definitive conclusions about safety, there was approximately a 1% greater risk of nonfatal myocardial infarction and need for coronary cardiovascularization in the varenicline group compared with placebo group and a 0.5% greater risk of new diagnosis or need for a procedure for peripheral arterial disease. Consequently, the FDA required the addition of a new safety warning to the package insert for varenicline highlighting the drug's potential to increase the risk for certain cardiovascular events in persons with cardiovascular disease.

Pregnancy

Prescription NRTs are listed by the FDA as Category D medications (i.e., those for which there is evidence of fetal harm), which are to be used only if the potential benefits outweigh the risks. This classification is based mainly on animal studies showing that nicotine is a neurobehavioral teratogen. Over-the-counter NRT products advise pregnant smokers to ask their health professional before using the product for smoking cessation. With these considerations in mind, the use of NRT should be considered for smoking cessation if the pregnant woman is unable to quit without such treatment.

Because nicotine is a neurobehavioral teratogen that may contribute to sudden infant death syndrome, using the lowest dose of nicotine replacement that aids in smoking cessation seems prudent. Consequently, during pregnancy, use of intermittent NRTs (e.g., gum, lozenge, inhaler) may be preferable to the constant delivery of nicotine that results from the nicotine patch for smoking cessation, although this approach has not been adequately studied. One study of the 15 mg/16 hours nicotine patch in pregnant smokers showed no improvement in overall quit rates at 6 weeks among women randomly assigned to receive the nicotine or placebo patch. However, women randomly assigned to receive the active patch delivered infants with higher birth weights than those born to women who had received placebo (Wisborg et al. 2000). Similarly, a study of 2-mg nicotine gum compared with placebo gum showed no difference in quit rates but lower cotinine concentrations and greater birth weight and longer gestational age in the nicotine group than in the placebo group (Oncken et al. 2008).

A large clinical trial of 1,050 pregnant smokers comparing 15 mg/16 hour transdermal nicotine with placebo for 8 weeks combined with behavioral counseling similar to that observed in a clinical setting was recently reported (Coleman et al. 2012). This study found that although quit rates were higher in the nicotine group than in the placebo group after 1 month of treatment (21.3% vs. 11.7%), quit rates at the end of pregnancy were similar between groups (9.4% and 7.6%, respectively). However, compliance was poor, with most subjects not using the transdermal nicotine patch after 1 month of treatment. Because medication compliance is a known determinant of efficacy, it seems probable that low medication adherence may have contributed to lack of nicotine patch efficacy in this trial. However, because the clearance of nicotine is accelerated during pregnancy, higher doses of NRT may be needed to optimize efficacy in pregnant smokers (Coleman et al. 2012).

Although placebo-controlled studies have not shown NRTs to be efficacious, open-label studies have shown that behavioral therapy combined with NRT can increase quit rates. In one study, behavioral therapy and the choice of nicotine patch, gum, or lozenge was associated with an 18% quit rate at 7 weeks postrandomization compared with a 3% quit rate in the control group that received behavioral therapy alone ($P=0.006$) (Pollak et al. 2007). Similar significant effects favoring the nicotine group were observed at the end of pregnancy (Pollak et al. 2007). A meta-analysis of NRT pregnancy trials that included both open-label and placebo-controlled trials also showed a significant effect of NRT (Lumley et al. 2009).

Although bupropion is listed as a Category C medication in pregnancy (i.e., there may be some risk in humans), no placebo-controlled studies have examined its safety and efficacy in pregnant women. The clinical efficacy of bupropion for smoking cessation during pregnancy was supported by a prospective observational study, in which pregnant smokers receiving bupropion achieved a higher quit rate than did control subjects (10 of 22 [45%] vs. 3 of 22 [14%]; $P=0.047$) (Chan et al. 2005). Placebo-controlled studies are needed to establish the safety and efficacy of bupropion use for smoking cessation during pregnancy.

In summary, the safety and efficacy of pharmacotherapy for smoking cessation during pregnancy have not been established. In the absence of such data, no definitive recommendations can be made for the use of either NRT or bupropion SR during pregnancy. Individual decisions as to the best options to promote smoking cessation during pregnancy should be made by the clinician in collaboration with the patient.

Conclusion

Seven first-line agents are recommended for smoking cessation: transdermal nicotine, nicotine gum, nicotine lozenge, nicotine inhaler, nicotine nasal spray, bupropion SR, and varenicline. Nortriptyline is a promising second-line, nonnicotine pharmacotherapy that should be considered for the treatment of smokers with comorbid depressive symptoms, major depression, or a history of major depression. Clonidine also may have some merit as a second-line agent, possibly in female smokers, but adverse effects limit its safety and may limit patients' adherence to treatment with this medication. Cytisine is a nicotinic pharmacotherapy shown to have promise in recent studies. Other agents to be considered as third-line treatments are naltrexone, nicotine vaccines, and MAO inhibitors, but their efficacy for smoking cessation has not been clearly established.

Pharmacotherapies should be used for the treatment of tobacco dependence, with optimal results produced by the combination of medications with behavioral support. More study is needed to determine how the intensity of behavioral treatments interacts with different pharmacotherapeutic agents. Although varenicline, bupropion SR, and NRTs significantly increase smoking cessation rates, most smokers are unable to achieve long-term abstinence, and absolute 1-year quit rates remain low. Additional research is warranted to determine whether medications for smoking cessation, used as monotherapies (e.g., bupropion, varenicline) or in combination (e.g., nicotine patch plus bupropion; varenicline plus naltrexone), prevent smoking relapse. New medications should be evaluated for the treatment of tobacco dependence. Well-controlled, large-scale studies are also needed to identify specific therapies that are safe and effective for smoking cessation in patients with comorbid psychiatric, substance abuse, and medical problems.

References

Ascher JA, Cole JO, Colin JN, et al: Bupropion: a review of its mechanism of antidepressant activity. J Clin Psychiatry 56:395–401, 1995

Bacher I, Wu B, Shytle DR, et al: Mecamylamine—a nicotinic acetylcholine receptor antagonist with potential for the treatment of neuropsychiatric disorders. Expert Opin Pharmacother 10:2709–2721, 2009

Benowitz N: Nicotine addiction. N Engl J Med 17:2295–2303, 2010

Berlin I, Said S, Spreux-Varoquaux O, et al: A reversible monoamine oxidase A inhibitor (moclobemide) facilitates smoking cessation and abstinence in heavy, dependent smokers. Clin Pharmacol Ther 58:444–452, 1995

Blondal T, Gudmundsson LJ, Tomasson K, et al: The effects of fluoxetine combined with nicotine inhalers in smoking cessation—a randomized trial. Addiction 94:1007–1015, 1999

Centers for Disease Control and Prevention: Vital signs: current cigarette smoking among adults aged ≥18 years—United States, 2009. MMWR Morb Mortal Wkly Rep 59:1135–1140, 2010

Chan B, Einarson A, Koren G: Effectiveness of bupropion for smoking cessation during pregnancy. J Addict Dis 24:19–23, 2005

Chengappa KN, Kambhampati R, Perkins K, et al: Bupropion sustained release as a smoking cessation treatment in remitted depressed patients maintained on treatment with selective serotonin reuptake inhibitor antidepressants. J Clin Psychiatry 62:503–508, 2001

Coleman, T, Cooper S, Thornton JG, et al: A randomized trial of nicotine replacement therapy patches in pregnancy. N Engl J Med 366:808–818, 2012

Covey LS, Glassman AH: A meta-analysis of double-blind placebo controlled trials of clonidine for smoking cessation. Br J Addict 86:991–998, 1991

Covey LS, Glassman AH, Stetner F: Naltrexone effects on short-term and long-term smoking cessation. J Addict Dis 18:31–40, 1999

Dani JA, Balfour DM: Historical and current perspectives on tobacco use and nicotine addiction. Trends Neurosci Jun 20, 2011 [Epub ahead of print]

Eissenberg T, Griffiths RR, Stitzer ML: Mecamylamine does not precipitate withdrawal in cigarette smokers. Psychopharmacology (Berl) 127:328–336, 1996

Evins AE, Mays VK, Rigotti NA, et al: A pilot trial of bupropion added to cognitive behavioral therapy for smoking cessation in schizophrenia. Nicotine Tob Res 3:397–403, 2001

Evins AE, Cather C, Culhane MA, et al: A 12-week double-blind, placebo-controlled study of bupropion SR added to high-dose dual nicotine replacement therapy for smoking cessation or reduction in schizophrenia. J Clin Psychopharmacol 27:380–386, 2007

Fagerstrom K, Balfour DJ: Neuropharmacology and potential efficacy of new treatments for tobacco dependence. Expert Opin Investig Drugs 15:107–116, 2006

Fiore MC, Jaén RC, Baker TB, et al: Treating Tobacco Use and Dependence: 2008 Update. Clinical Practice Guideline. Rockville, MD, U.S. Department of Health and Human Services, Public Health Service, May 2008. Available at: http://www.ahrq.gov/clinic/tobacco/treating_tobacco_use08.pdf. Accessed November 29, 2012.

George TP: Nicotine and tobacco, in Cecil Textbook of Medicine, 24th Edition. Edited by Goldman L, Schacter A. New York, Elsevier Health Sciences, 2011, pp 142–145

George TP, O'Malley SS: Current pharmacological treatments for nicotine dependence. Trends Pharmacol Sci 25:42–48, 2004

George TP, Vessicchio JC, Termine A, et al: A placebo-controlled trial of bupropion for smoking cessation in schizophrenia. Biol Psychiatry 52:53–61, 2002

George TP, Vessicchio JC, Termine A, et al: A preliminary placebo-controlled trial of selegiline hydrochloride for smoking cessation. Biol Psychiatry 53:136–143, 2003

George TP, Vessicchio JC, Sacco KA, et al: A double-blind, randomized, placebo-controlled trial of sustained-release bupropion combined with transdermal nicotine patch for smoking cessation in schizophrenia. Biol Psychiatry 63:1092–1096, 2008

George TP, Wu BS, Weinberger AH: A review of smoking cessation in bipolar disorder: implications for future research. J Dual Diagnosis 8: 126–130, 2012

Giovino GA: The tobacco epidemic in the United States. Am J Prev Med 33(suppl):S318–S326, 2007

Glover ED, Laflin MT, Schuh KJ, et al: A randomized, controlled trial to assess the efficacy and safety of a transdermal delivery system of nicotine/mecamylamine in cigarette smokers. Addiction 102:795–802, 2007

Gonzales D, Rennard SI, Nides M, et al: Varenicline, an alpha4beta2 nicotinic acetylcholine receptor partial agonist, vs sustained-release bupropion and placebo for smoking cessation: a randomized controlled trial. JAMA 296:47–55, 2006

Gourlay SG, Benowitz NL: Is clonidine an effective smoking cessation therapy? Drugs 50:197–207, 1995

Hall SM, Reus VI, Munoz RF, et al: Nortriptyline and cognitive-behavioral therapy in the treatment of cigarette smoking. Arch Gen Psychiatry 55:683–690, 1998

Hall SM, Humfleet GL, Reus VI, et al: Psychological intervention and antidepressant treatment in smoking cessation. Arch Gen Psychiatry 59:930–936, 2002

Hayford KE, Patten CA, Rummans TA, et al: Efficacy of bupropion for smoking cessation in smokers with a former history of major depression or alcoholism. Br J Psychiatry 174:173–178, 1999

Hays JT, Hurt RD, Rigotti NA, et al: Sustained-release bupropion for pharmacologic relapse prevention after smoking cessation. Ann Intern Med 135:423–433, 2001

Hertzberg MA, Moore SD, Feldman ME, et al: A preliminary study of bupropion sustained-release for smoking cessation in patients with chronic posttraumatic stress disorder. J Clin Psychopharmacol 21:94–98, 2001

Hjalmarson A, Nilsson F, Sjostrom L, et al: The nicotine inhaler in smoking cessation. Arch Intern Med 157:1721–1728, 1997

Hughes JR: Non-nicotine pharmacotherapies for smoking cessation. J Drug Dev 6:197–203, 1994

Hurt RD, Sachs DP, Glover ED, et al: A comparison of sustained-release bupropion and placebo for smoking cessation. N Engl J Med 337:1195–1202, 1997

Jorenby DE, Leischow SJ, Nides MA, et al: A controlled trial of sustained-release bupropion, a nicotine patch, or both for smoking cessation. N Engl J Med 340:685–691, 1999

Jorenby DE, Hays JT, Rigotti NA, et al: Efficacy of varenicline, an alpha4beta2 nicotinic acetylcholine receptor partial agonist, vs placebo or sustained-release bupropion for smoking cessation: a randomized controlled trial. JAMA 296:56–63, 2006

Joseph AM, Norman SM, Ferry LH, et al: The safety of transdermal nicotine as an aid to smoking cessation in patients with cardiac disease. N Engl J Med 335:1792–1798, 1996

Kahn R, Gorgon L, Jones K, et al: Selegiline transdermal system (STS) as an aid for smoking cessation. Nicotine Tob Res 14:377–382, 2012

Kalman D, Herz L, Monti P, et al: Incremental efficacy of adding bupropion to the nicotine patch for smoking cessation in smokers with a recent history of alcohol dependence: results from a randomized, double-blind, placebo-controlled study. Drug Alcohol Depend 118:111–118, 2011

Killen JD, Fortmann SP, Schatzberg AF, et al: Nicotine patch and paroxetine for smoking cessation. J Consult Clin Psychol 68:883–889, 2000

Kleber HB, Weiss RD, Anton RF, et al: Practice guideline for the treatment of patients with substance use disorders. Am J Psychiatry 163(suppl):5–83, 2007

Krishnan-Sarin S, Meandzija B, O'Malley S: Naltrexone and nicotine patch smoking cessation: a preliminary study. Nicotine Tob Res 5:851–857, 2003

Le Foll B, George TP: Treatment of tobacco dependence: integrating recent progress into practice. CMAJ 177:1373–1380, 2007

Lumley J, Chamberlain C, Dowswell T, et al: Interventions for promoting smoking cessation during pregnancy. Cochrane Database of Systematic Reviews 2009, Issue 3. Art. No.: CD001055. DOI: 10.1002/14651858.CD001055.pub3.

McClure JB, Swan GE, Catz SL, et al: Smoking outcome by psychiatric history after behavioral and varenicline treatment. J Subst Abuse Treat 38:394–402, 2010

McFall M, Saxon AJ, Thompson CE, et al: Improving the rates of quitting smoking for veterans with posttraumatic stress disorder. Am J Psychiatry 162:1311–1319, 2005

McFall M, Saxon AJ, Malte CA, et al: Integrating tobacco cessation into mental health care for posttraumatic stress disorder: a randomized controlled trial. JAMA 304:2485–2493, 2010

Niaura R, Spring B, Borrelli B, et al: Multicenter trial of fluoxetine as an adjunct to behavioral smoking cessation treatment. J Consult Clin Psychol 70:887–896, 2002

O'Malley SS, Cooney JL, Krishnan-Sarin S, et al: A controlled trial of naltrexone augmentation of nicotine replacement therapy for smoking cessation. Arch Intern Med 166:667–674, 2006

Oncken C, Gonzales D, Nides M, et al: Efficacy and safety of the novel selective nicotinic acetylcholine receptor partial agonist, varenicline, for smoking cessation. Arch Intern Med 166:1571–1577, 2006

Oncken C, Dornelas E, Greene J, et al: Nicotine gum for pregnant smokers: a randomized controlled trial. Obstet Gynecol 112:859–867, 2008

Pfizer and Pharmacia and Upjohn Company: Nicotrol inhaler (nicotine inhalation system) package insert. New York, Pfizer and Pharmacia and Upjohn Company, revised December 2008

Pollak KI, Oncken CA, Lipkus IM, et al: Nicotine replacement and behavioral therapy for smoking cessation in pregnancy. Am J Prev Med 33:297–305, 2007

Polosa R, Benowitz NL: Treatment of nicotine addiction: present therapeutic options and pipeline developments. Trends Pharmacol Sci 32:281–289, 2011

Pomerleau OF, Pomerleau CS: Neuroregulators and the reinforcement of smoking: towards a biobehavioral explanation. Neurosci Biobehav Rev 8:503–513, 1984

Prochazka AV, Weaver MJ, Keller RT, et al: A randomized trial of nortriptyline for smoking cessation. Arch Intern Med 158:2035–2039, 1998

Rigotti NA, Thorndike AN, Regan S, et al: Bupropion for smokers hospitalized with acute cardiovascular disease. Am J Med 119:1080–1087, 2006

Rigotti NA, Pipe AL, Benowitz NL et al: Efficacy and safety of varenicline for smoking cessations in patients with cardiovascular disease: a randomized trial. Circulation 121:221–229, 2010

Rohsenow DJ, Monti PM, Colby SM, et al: Naltrexone treatment for alcoholics: effect on cigarette smoking rates. Nicotine Tob Res 5:231–236, 2003

Rose JE, Levin ED: Concurrent agonist-antagonist administration for the analysis and treatment of drug dependence. Pharmacol Biochem Behav 41:219–226, 1991

Rose JE, Behm FM, Westman EC, et al: Mecamylamine combined with nicotine skin patch facilitates smoking cessation beyond nicotine patch treatment alone. Clin Pharmacol Ther 56:86–99, 1994

Rose JE, Behm FM, Westman EC: Nicotine-mecamylamine treatment for smoking cessation: the role of pre-cessation therapy. Exp Clin Psychopharmacol 6:331–343, 1998

Shiffman S, Dresler CM, Hajek P, et al: Efficacy of a nicotine lozenge for smoking cessation. Arch Intern Med 162:1267–1276, 2002

Slemmer JE, Martin BR, Damaj MI: Bupropion is a nicotinic antagonist. J Pharmacol Exp Ther 295:321–327, 2000

Stead LF, Perera R, Bullen C, et al: Nicotine replacement therapy for smoking cessation. Cochrane Database of Systematic Reviews 2012, Issue 11. Art. No.: CD000146. DOI: 10.1002/14651858.CD000146.pub4.

Sutherland G, Stapleton JA, Russel MA, et al: Randomised controlled trial of nasal nicotine spray in smoking cessation. Lancet 340:324–329, 1992

Sutherland G, Stapleton JA, Russell MA, et al: Naltrexone, smoking behaviour and cigarette withdrawal. Psychopharmacology (Berl) 120:418–425, 1995

Sweeney CT, Fant RV, Fagerstrom KO, et al: Combination nicotine replacement therapy for smoking cessation. CNS Drugs 15:453–467, 2001

Tonstad S, Tønnesen P, Hajek P, et al: Effect of maintenance therapy with varenicline on smoking cessation: a randomized controlled trial. JAMA 296:64–71, 2006

Weinberger AH, Vessicchio JC, Sacco KA, et al: A preliminary study of sustained-release bupropion for smoking cessation in bipolar disorder. J Clin Psychopharmacol 28:584–587, 2008

Weinberger AH, Reutenauer EL, Jatlow PI, et al: A double-blind, placebo-controlled, randomized clinical trial of oral selegiline hydrochloride for smoking cessation in nicotine-dependent cigarette smokers. Drug Alcohol Depend 107:188–195, 2010

Weiner E, Ball MP, Summerfelt A, et al: Effects of sustained-release bupropion and supportive group therapy on cigarette consumption in patients with schizophrenia. Am J Psychiatry 158:635–637, 2001

West R, Zatonski W, Cedzynska M, et al: Placebo-controlled trial of cytisine for smoking cessation. N Engl J Med 365:1193–1200, 2011

Williams JM, Anthenelli RM, Morris C, et al: A randomized double-blind, placebo-controlled study evaluating the safety and efficacy of varenicline for smoking cessation in patients with schizophrenia or schizoaffective disorder. J Clin Psychiatry 73:654–660, 2012

Wisborg K, Henriksen TB, Jespersen LB, et al: Nicotine patches for pregnant smokers: a randomized controlled study. Obstet Gynecol 96:967–971, 2000

3

Opioids

John A. Renner Jr., M.D.

Clifford M. Knapp, Ph.D.

Domenic A. Ciraulo, M.D.

Steven Epstein, M.D.

Prevalence and Natural History

Prevalence and Patterns of Opioid Use and Dependence

Major epidemics of heroin abuse occurred in the United States following World War I, World War II, and the Vietnam conflict. However, opioid abuse patterns changed significantly in the late 1990s when the number of new nonmedical users of opioid pain relievers almost tripled, from 700,000–800,000 to almost 2.5 million (Substance Abuse and Mental Health Services Administration [SAMHSA] 2003). In 2011, there were more than 1.8 million new illicit users of pain relievers, making this class of drugs the second most common new drug of abuse, ahead of marijuana (SAMHSA 2011a, 2012). This change

began with the introduction in 1996 of OxyContin, a potent time-release formulation of oral oxycodone. When the OxyContin tablet is crushed or
chewed, a rapid release of intoxicating, and sometimes fatal, amounts of oxycodone occurs.

It is estimated that 10%–30% of individuals exposed to licit and illicit
opioids may develop substance abuse or dependence. As these findings indicate, opioid pharmaceuticals have replaced heroin as the primary opioids of
abuse in the United States (SAMHSA 2011b, 2012). As was true for heroin,
nonmedical use of opioid pharmaceuticals is predominantly a problem of young
adults (SAMHSA 2011c, 2012).

It was long thought that opioid dependence rarely results from the legitimate prescribing of opioids for the treatment of acute or chronic pain
(Portenoy and Foley 1986). However, recent experience with potent, long-
acting pain relievers suggests that they have a significant risk for abuse or dependence in individuals with a history of drug abuse or other co-occurring
psychiatric disorders (Cheatle and O'Brien 2011). The anticipated U.S. Food
and Drug Administration (FDA) approval of timed-release formulations of
hydrocodone (Zohydro and others) has raised concerns about the wisdom of
adding another potent opioid to the U.S. market. Several pharmaceutical
companies are developing products containing pure hydrocodone as alternatives to existing products, such as Vicodin, which combine hydrocodone with
acetaminophen. The effort to avoid exposing patients to the liver problems associated with high doses of acetaminophen runs the risk of making widely
available products that contain up to 10 times the amount of opioid in Vicodin. Drug abuse experts are concerned that these new products can be crushed
to release a highly abusable and potentially lethal opioid dose. Nonetheless,
concerns about the abuse potential of opioids should not preclude the appropriate use of these medications for the treatment of chronic pain that is not responsive to nonopioid therapies.

In 2011, the Institute of Medicine, in its report "Relieving Pain in America," identified untreated or poorly treated pain as a major public health problem and recommended a plan to transform prevention, care, education, and
research to provide relief for people with pain problems in America. The education of health professionals regarding patient assessment and appropriate
treatment, including the safe and effective prescription of opioids, is central to
their recommendations.

Natural History and Treatment Outcomes

Although many who experiment with opioids experience euphoria or symptom relief with the first use, some experimenters use these drugs only a few times and then avoid further use because of an awareness of the risks involved. Even for those who become dependent, the most common pattern is one of alternating periods of use and abstinence, whether voluntary or due to external pressure. Many opioid-dependent individuals recover without ever having formal treatment. Individuals addicted to opioids who recover without treatment have less psychopathology, fewer legal problems, and more adequate social functioning, but not less drug dependence (Rounsaville and Kleber 1985). For those who seek treatment, the average time from dependence to first treatment is approximately 2–3 years. Initial treatment typically involves detoxification, with little or no aftercare. Up to two-thirds of individuals who undergo only detoxification will relapse to opioid use, most within the first few months following treatment.

There have been several long-term follow-up studies of patients addicted to opioids who sought treatment from publicly supported programs. A 33-year follow-up of 581 opioid-addicted patients who had received treatment in the California Civil Addict Program between 1962 and 1964 showed a very high mortality rate of 49% (Hser et al. 2001). Of the 242 individuals interviewed at follow-up, 20.7% had positive urine test results for heroin, an additional 9.5% refused a urine test, and 14% were incarcerated. The authors concluded that for most of these subjects, heroin dependence was a lifelong condition that had a severe effect on their health and social functioning. By the end of the 33-year follow-up period, only 25% of individuals had achieved abstinence; for most of those years, less than 6% of the subjects were in treatment at any one time. A second study of this cohort examined premature mortality in terms of years of potential life lost. The addicted cohort lost 34.29 years (years of potential life lost per 1,000) because of injury and disease compared with 5.63 years (years of potential life lost per 1,000) for the overall U.S. population (Smith et al. 2007).

In another study, selected daily opioid users who entered treatment in 1969–1974 were followed up for 12 years after initial treatment. At that point, 24% of the addicted males had used opioids daily during the previous year, and 25% reported that they had never returned to daily opioid use

(Simpson and Marsh 1986; Simpson et al. 1982). Of the entire sample, 35% never relapsed after they quit. During the previous year, 13% had been arrested, and 29% had spent time in jail or prison.

A third study interviewed more than 10,000 patients addicted to drugs who entered treatment during 1979–1981; a sample of these individuals was reinterviewed 3–5 years later (Hubbard et al. 1989). Among these individuals, heroin use declined during and following treatment. For those who stayed in treatment, the rate of regular use of heroin declined from 63.5% before treatment to 17.5% 3–5 years later.

In general, physicians and other health professionals with opioid dependence have a remarkably good prognosis when their license to practice is made contingent on continued abstinence and their abstinence monitored by random urine tests. A cohort outcome study of 904 physicians treated in 16 state physician health programs documented a very positive response to treatment. At the time of a 5-year follow up, almost 78.7% were licensed and working as physicians. The authors noted the high quality of the treatment received, the importance of regular monitoring (urine testing), and that treatment of this quality, duration, and intensity is rarely available in standard treatment settings (Dupont et al. 2009; McLellan et al. 2008).

Currently, no reliable means are available to predict an opioid-addicted individual's long-term prognosis as measured by drug use, work, crime, and psychological adjustment. Although the achievement of even temporary abstinence is associated with improvement in several factors (legal problems in particular), simply achieving abstinence does not ensure an adequate psychosocial adjustment. Therefore, treatment also must address other problem areas. In general, outcome in a particular area (e.g., employment or criminal behavior) is best predicted by past behavior in that domain (Kosten et al. 1987a; Rounsaville et al. 1987).

Opioid dependence has always been associated with high mortality rates related to factors such as overdose, suicide, homicide, and infection. The authors of a study in Sweden reported a 20% mortality rate during a 1-year period in a group of patients who were addicted to opioids who served as the control group in a double-blind, placebo-controlled buprenorphine maintenance study (Kakko et al. 2003). All patients underwent buprenorphine detoxification (as the initial phase of an intended 1-year placebo arm of the maintenance trial) and were offered intensive outpatient counseling services.

These results underscore the shortcomings and risks of treatment consisting of detoxification and outpatient counseling, even for addicted individuals with a relatively short history of dependence.

Clinical Pharmacology

Three types of opioid receptors have been identified: μ, δ, and κ receptors. A nociceptin receptor/orphanin FQ receptor also has been identified that is technically classified as an opioid receptor because of its structure but does not directly mediate the effects of opioid agonists. These receptors are coupled to guanine nucleotide–binding proteins (G proteins). Opioid agonists produce intracellular effects through their actions on G proteins, which include the inhibition of adenylyl cyclase, producing a decrease in cyclic adenosine monophosphate (cAMP) levels, a reduction in the opening of voltage-gated calcium channels, an increase in potassium channel current flows, and the activation of protein kinase C. Opioids may inhibit the release of neurotransmitters—most notably, γ-aminobutyric acid (GABA) and substance P—from neurons (Williams et al. 2001).

The maximal effects that are produced by a particular opioid are determined by the nature of its interactions with receptor-coupled G proteins (Selley et al. 1998, 2003). Full opioid receptor agonists, which include methadone, can maximally activate G proteins. Partial agonists, including morphine and buprenorphine, are limited in the degree to which they produce G-protein activation. Morphine, however, can produce a sufficient degree of activation to cause severe respiratory depression. Other partial agonists, such as buprenorphine, however, stimulate G proteins to a very limited extent, showing "ceiling effects" in their respiratory depressant actions and many of their subjective effects (Ciraulo et al. 2006). Early assumptions about a ceiling effect for analgesia have been brought into question by clinical experience (Malinoff et al. 2005) and research. In 2008, a consensus group of experts reviewed recent research and concluded that although in clinical practice buprenorphine acts as a full μ opioid agonist for analgesia, with no ceiling effect, it has a ceiling effect for respiratory depression (Pergolizzi et al. 2010). Another study found that the addition of ultra-low-dose naloxone to buprenorphine results in enhanced analgesic effects in humans without significant side effects (La Vincente et al. 2008). A recent review, however, indicated that patients with chronic pain may be more likely to discontinue buprenorphine as an analgesic medication than morphine (Bekkering et al. 2011), leaving open the question of whether the analgesia produced by the two medications is equivalent.

Opioid agonists include several classes of endogenous peptides, including the endorphins, enkephalins, endomorphins, and dynorphins, and numerous exogenous opioid drugs. The exogenous opioid agonists are used to treat cough, diarrhea, and pain. They include *Papaver somniferum* (i.e., poppy) plant derivatives such as morphine and codeine; morphine-related semisynthetic drugs, including heroin and oxycodone; and synthetic agents such as fentanyl, methadone, and meperidine. The effects of the opioid agonists can be blocked by opioid antagonists, which include naloxone, naltrexone, and nalmefene. These antagonists bind to opioid receptors to block the actions of opioid agonists, but at therapeutic doses they appear to have few other pharmacological effects.

Most opioid analgesic medications in current use are thought to exert their actions primarily through the μ opioid receptor (Zhang et al. 1998). A few opioid analgesics, including butorphanol and nalbuphine, may produce analgesia by stimulating κ opioid receptors. Although the stimulation of κ opioid receptors produces analgesia, dysphoria and hallucinations also may occur in response to the activation of these receptors. Nalbuphine is also a μ opioid receptor antagonist that may induce withdrawal in opioid-dependent individuals.

Central nervous system effects of μ opioid receptor agonist medications include analgesia, sedation, "mental clouding" (apathy and difficulty concentrating), mood changes, nausea, and vomiting. Meperidine's metabolite normeperidine may also lead to delirium. In abstinent persons who were addicted to opioids, euphoria is greater and mental clouding is less pronounced than in nonaddicted subjects. Tolerance develops to these effects with chronic use. Opioids acutely inhibit gonadotropin-releasing hormone and corticotropin-releasing hormone secretion, but tolerance develops with chronic use. Therefore, male methadone patients who have been maintained for more than a year with stable doses generally have been found to have normal levels of cortisol, luteinizing hormone, and testosterone (for general references, see Gutstein and Akil 2001).

Major gastrointestinal effects that result from the administration of μ receptor agonists include decreased gut motility and changes in secretion of gastric and intestinal fluids. Morphine and most μ opioid receptor agonists cause pupillary constriction (miosis). Some tolerance to this effect may develop, but addicted individuals with high opioid levels will still have miosis. Respiratory depression is the usual cause of death from opioid overdose.

After rapid intravenous injection of an opioid, the user experiences warm skin flushing and a "rush" that lasts about 45 seconds. In one retrospective study (Seecof and Tennant 1987), the most common feelings associated with the rush were pleasure, relaxation, and satisfaction. Although at one time the rush was classically reported to be similar to a sexual orgasm, in a study of the phenomenon, such a feeling was reported in only 18% of men and 10% of women (Seecof and Tennant 1987).

Opioids are absorbed from the gastrointestinal tract, nasal mucosa (e.g., when heroin is used as snuff), and lung (e.g., when opium is smoked). The potent opioid agent fentanyl can be absorbed transdermally, and the partial opioid agonist buprenorphine can be administered sublingually. After absorption from the gastrointestinal tract, morphine undergoes a substantial first-pass effect (i.e., it is extensively metabolized in the liver) and consequently is more potent when administered by injection.

Pharmacokinetic features distinguish some of the commonly used opioids. Codeine must undergo biotransformation into morphine by the liver enzyme cytochrome P450 (CYP) 2D6 to exert its full therapeutic effects. About 90% of the excretion of morphine occurs during the first 24 hours, but traces are detectable in urine for more than 48 hours. Heroin (diacetylmorphine) is hydrolyzed to monoacetylmorphine, which is then hydrolyzed to morphine. Morphine and monoacetylmorphine are responsible for the pharmacological effects of heroin. Heroin produces effects more rapidly than morphine because it is more lipid soluble and therefore crosses the blood-brain barrier faster. In the urine, heroin is detected as free morphine and morphine glucuronide (Gutstein and Akil 2001; Jaffe et al. 2004).

Opioid Receptors

Three distinct opioid receptor genes have been identified: *OPRM1* encodes the μ opioid receptor, *OPRK1* encodes the κ opioid receptor, and *OPRD1* encodes the δ opioid receptor. These genes have extensive shared nucleic acid sequences and produce receptors with extensive amino acid sequence homologies. The structure of the opioid receptors is largely shared by the nociceptin receptor/

orphanin FQ receptor, which is not sensitive to the antagonist effects of naloxone but nevertheless is classified as an opioid receptor gene.

Pharmacological evidence suggests that there may be several subtypes of the three basic opioid agonist–sensitive receptors, but this is not supported by molecular evidence. Differences in the functioning of the different opioid receptors of the same type may occur because of single nucleotide polymorphisms in the receptors (see, e.g., Kroslak et al. 2007). The alternative splicing that occurs during the translation of opioid messenger RNA may also be a source of functional differences in opioid receptors generated from the same gene (Dietis et al. 2011). Variation in the pharmacology of opioid receptors also may result from the existence of opioid heterodimers, which arise from the interaction of the different opioid receptor types. An example of this is seen in differences in the actions of morphine and oxycodone—oxycodone exhibits features of a κ agonist in some experimental models of analgesia. This phenomenon may occur because of the interaction of this drug with a κ opioid receptor/δ opioid receptor heterodimer (Dietis et al. 2011).

High densities of μ opioid receptors in the nervous system are found in the dorsal horn of the spinal cord, brain stem, thalamus, and cortex, where they can modulate the intensity of incoming pain signals. Within the mesolimbic system, μ opioid receptors may play a role in regulating reward-motivated behaviors. The reinforcing actions of opioid agonists are produced, at least in part, by the induction of dopamine release by these agents in the nucleus accumbens, a mesolimbic structure implicated in mediating the effects of rewarding stimuli on behavior (Nestler et al. 2001).

Mechanisms of Tolerance and Dependence

The prolonged administration of opioid analgesics results in the development of tolerance to these drugs, manifested as the need to administer a larger dose of the drug to produce a given level of effect. The mechanisms that mediate the occurrence of opioid tolerance are not fully characterized and may involve changes in the intracellular regulation of opioid receptor activity and adaptations in the wider networks of neurons that mediate the physiological effects of the opioids. Discontinuation of chronic opioid agonist administration results in a distinct pattern of withdrawal symptoms, which are indicative of opioid physical dependence. At least some of the cellular mechanisms that mediate opioid withdrawal also may play a role in the development of opioid tolerance.

Much of the research on the mechanisms that mediate the development of tolerance to opioid agonists has focused on factors that directly regulate the functionality of opioid receptors. These include opioid receptor desensitization, phosphorylation, resensitization, and internalization (i.e., endocytosis). Receptor desensitization involves the acute loss of receptor function that may result from the uncoupling of a receptor from its G protein as a result of phosphorylation of the receptor protein produced by G protein–coupled receptor kinases and the subsequent enhanced binding to β-arrestins (Christie 2008). Resensitization of the receptor can occur by the recycling of the desensitized receptor through intracellular pathways. For opioid receptors, this process may involve phosphorylation of the agonist-bound receptor, followed by binding of the receptor to β-arrestin. This receptor complex then undergoes endocytosis, and receptors resensitized within the cell are then recycled to the cell surface. Other mechanisms, which have not been fully characterized, may exist that allow resensitization of opioid receptors that remain on the cell surface (Dang and Christie 2012).

It has been postulated that tolerance to morphine occurs because desensitized receptors remain on the cell surface following prolonged exposure to this drug. Chronic exposure to morphine may lead to persistence of desensitization, which may be related to changes in signaling systems that mediate the effects of the enzyme protein kinase C (Christie 2008). Tolerance to the analgesic effects of morphine, which is reliably seen after the chronic administration of this agent, is attenuated in mutant animals that have the β-arrestin-2 gene (ARRB2) deleted (Bohn et al. 2000). Although morphine does not readily interact with β-arrestin-1, fentanyl and methadone do interact with this protein (Groer et al. 2011). Agonist-related changes in the affinity of the μ opioid receptor for different forms of β-arrestin may be an important factor in the mechanisms responsible for the development of tolerance to different opioid medications.

The administration of several full opioid agonists, including fentanyl and methadone, produces μ opioid receptor resensitization by a mechanism that may involve internalization of these receptors into the interior of the neuron. In contrast to the full opioid receptor agonists, many partial opioid receptor agonists—most notably, morphine—do not produce marked or rapid endocytosis (Schulz et al. 2004). Evidence from animal studies indicates that tolerance to morphine may be more pronounced than it is in animals treated with agents that readily facilitate the internalization of opioid receptors. At present, however, no evidence in humans shows that the opioid medications that are known to readily promote endocytosis produce tolerance to a lesser degree than do drugs that are poor promoters of receptor internalization (Morgan and Christie 2011).

Another mechanism implicated in the development of tolerance to opioids involves a reduction in the inhibitory effects of morphine on cAMP pathway activity. The acute administration of opioid agonists such as morphine decreases the activity of cAMP second-messenger pathways through the inhibition of adenylyl cyclase activity. However, following chronic exposure to morphine, this inhibitory effect is lost in many brain areas, and there may be upregulation of the cAMP pathway, in at least some neurons (Cao et al. 2010; Nestler et al. 2001).

The upregulation of the cAMP pathway may play an important role in opioid withdrawal. Once morphine treatment is discontinued, rebound activity may occur in the cAMP pathway. Rebound activity may be related to an increase in the extracellular levels of the excitatory neurotransmitters glutamate and aspartate during withdrawal from opioids (Aghajanian et al. 1994). The increase in cAMP pathway activity may lead to enhanced phosphorylation of the cAMP response element binding protein (CREB), which alters transcription of some genes in brain regions associated with withdrawal (Delfs et al. 2000; Shaw-Lutchman et al. 2002). Symptoms of physical withdrawal following morphine administration are reduced in mice mutated to produce only residual levels of CREB (Maldonado et al. 1996).

Etiology of Opioid Dependence

It is difficult to delineate, even for a specific individual, the precise etiology of dependence. Each of the etiological factors discussed in this section may play different roles in initiation and maintenance of use, relapse, and recovery.

Opioids can be reinforcing by directly inducing pleasurable effects (positive reinforcement) or by reducing aversive affects or the experience of noxious stimuli (negative reinforcement). They may reduce pain or anxiety and, for some users, decrease depression or boredom, relieve the experience of intense aggression, and increase self-esteem. Social approval among peers may be a factor in initial opioid use. The rituals of injecting opioids often become associated with a "high," so that even an occasional placebo injection still may elicit pleasurable effects. Even after tolerance has developed to some of the effects of opioids, the rush may still be experienced briefly after an intravenous injection. Animal studies indicate that low doses of opioids lower the threshold to produce reinforcing (pleasurable) effects by means of self-administration of electrical currents to certain brain regions (Kornetsky 2004). Tolerance to this effect does not seem to occur. The experience of withdrawal relief also contributes to repeated opioid use. Because of heroin's brief duration of action, withdrawal occurs several times a day, and its repeated relief leads to a strongly reinforced behavior pattern.

The paraphernalia and setting associated with drug use can become cues, indicating that a high or relief of distress is possible. Craving or desire to use the drug is increased in the presence of such stimuli. Withdrawal symptoms also may become conditioned to such stimuli. The addicted person may experience conditioned withdrawal as an increase in craving or desire to use opioids (McLellan et al. 1986; Meyer and Mirin 1979; Wikler 1980). The most intense craving appears to be elicited by conditions associated with opioid use rather than those associated with withdrawal. The role that conditioned phenomena play in relapse and the perpetuation of use is currently unknown. Research findings suggest that these phenomena may be clinically important and that their extinction may be helpful in treatment (Childress et al. 1988).

Psychosocial and environmental factors play a major role in the development of and recovery from opioid dependence; however, a detailed discussion is beyond the scope of this chapter. The use of licit drugs such as nicotine and alcohol typically precedes the use of opioids (Clayton and Voss 1981; Kandel and Yamaguchi 1993). Although one cannot predict definitively which users will proceed to opioid use, those who do generally have low self-esteem, disrupted families, and difficult relationships with their parents (Farrell and White 1998). The increased availability of opioids in inner cities of major urban centers contributes to the initiation of use in naïve individuals and to relapse in experienced users. It is particularly difficult to avoid use and relapse in areas with high unemployment, poor school systems, and high crime rates. Living in such an area may contribute to the negative affects that opioid use temporarily relieves.

Brief experimentation with illicit opioids rarely leads to dependence, but persons who use opioids at least once a month for even a brief period commonly escalate to daily use. Epidemiological studies and treatment facilities report a high prevalence of anxiety, mood disorders, bipolar disorder, and alcoholism, as well as antisocial personality, among individuals with opioid dependence (Cacciola et al. 2001; Callaly et al. 2001; Hien et al. 2000; Krausz et al. 1998, 1999; Marsden et al. 2000; Milby et al. 1996; Regier et al. 1990; Roozen et al. 2003).

Dole and Nyswander (1967) postulated a biological etiology for opioid dependence. They proposed that a preexisting metabolic deficiency could lead to dependence or that changes induced by opioid use could perpetuate dependence. Dole (1988) later hypothesized that opioid receptor dysfunction is a primary etiological factor. Recent research efforts have focused on the hypothesis that individuals with a genetic vulnerability to opioid abuse have defects in the genes for the opioid peptides and receptors. Variants of the μ and δ receptors have been associated with opioid and/or alcohol addiction. However, the associations are weak, suggesting that either the opioid system plays a relatively small part in the genesis of these disorders or combinations of opioid system polymorphisms may be necessary to show a relation (Mayer and Höllt 2001). Antisocial personality and alcoholism are more common in opioid users. Because both of these disorders appear to be influenced by genetic factors, a stronger link with genetic factors in opioid abuse may someday be established.

Phenomenology of Opioid Withdrawal

Tolerance

Some degree of tolerance to the euphorigenic effects of heroin in addicted individuals may develop in 1–2 weeks (Cami and Farre 2003). Therefore, to obtain a rush or a high, the addicted individual progressively increases the dose. Although some individuals build up to extraordinarily high doses, there is always a dose capable of causing death from respiratory depression. Physical dependence and tolerance occur more rapidly in those who were formerly addicted; individuals addicted to morphine can reach a daily dose of 500 mg within 10 days of the resumption of use. Tolerance largely disappears after withdrawal; addicted persons have unwittingly taken fatal doses by returning to their previous doses after detoxification. Receptor upregulation may occur with chronic administration of opioid antagonists and may render addicted patients taking these agents more sensitive to opioids when the antagonists are discontinued.

Withdrawal

Administration of sufficient doses of an opioid antagonist after only a single therapeutic dose of morphine results in withdrawal phenomena (Bickel et al. 1987; Heishman et al. 1989; Jones 1979). Some degree of clinically detectable physical dependence develops in people who are given opioids regularly for more than a few days. However, relatively few become chronic users. Physical dependence and the presence of tolerance and withdrawal symptoms thus cannot be viewed as the only causes of continued use and relapse. However, the presence of physical dependence clearly contributes to difficulty with or fear of withdrawal and to a tendency to relapse.

The intensity of withdrawal depends on the following factors: 1) the dose of the opioid used (however, increasing beyond the equivalent of 500 mg/day of morphine does not significantly increase severity), 2) the duration of use, 3) the rate of removal of opioids from receptors, and 4) the extent of continuous use. Generally, the character of the signs and symptoms is opposite to that of the acute agonist effects. For example, constipation occurs during acute treatment, and bowel hypermotility occurs with withdrawal. Individual sensitivity also may affect the nature of the withdrawal syndrome. Generally, the shorter the duration of action of the drug, the more severe is the withdrawal syndrome, the more rapid is the onset of symptoms, and the shorter is the total duration of the symptoms. With short-acting drugs such as heroin and morphine, early symptoms may occur 8–12 hours after the last dose. Severe syndromes peak 48–72 hours after the last dose. In some individuals, subjective symptoms predominate over objective signs. Untreated, the acute phase of morphine or heroin withdrawal lasts 7–10 days. Withdrawal from κ agonists (e.g., nalorphine) is generally mild and qualitatively distinct. The onset of withdrawal with longer-acting drugs such as methadone or buprenorphine can be delayed until 1–3 days after the last dose. Peak symptoms often may not occur until days 3–5. Withdrawal from methadone includes complaints of pain, which patients state originates from muscle or bone. Meperidine withdrawal develops within 3 hours after the last dose, peaks in 5–12 hours, and generally ends in 4–5 days. With meperidine, subjective symptoms, such as craving and restlessness, may be much more severe than the autonomic changes. Codeine withdrawal is less severe than that for the more potent opioid agonists.

A protracted abstinence syndrome may follow the acute opioid withdrawal syndrome and last for many weeks (Martin et al. 1973). In one study of heroin-addicted patients detoxified with methadone, withdrawal distress peaked at day 20, the final day of methadone detoxification, and it was not until day 40 that their symptom scores reached normal levels (Gossop et al. 1987). During this phase, there may be excessive somatic concerns, decreased stress tolerance, poor self-image, and disturbed sleep. Opioid effects are especially reinforcing at this time, perhaps providing one explanation for early relapse (Cushman and Dole 1973; Martin et al. 1973).

Formerly, ratings of withdrawal severity from drugs such as heroin, morphine, and methadone were made with the Himmelsbach scale (Himmelsbach 1941), which emphasized "objective" or measurable signs over subjective reports. With such a system, the sequence of signs observed was as shown in Table 3–1. However, more recent work giving greater weight to subjective aspects of withdrawal distress has shown that drug users experience mood changes, fatigue, dysphoria, and vague discomforts many hours before signs such as lacrimation or yawning can be detected. A useful scale that combines both objective and subjective measures is the Clinical Opiate Withdrawal Scale (COWS; Wesson and Ling 2003). This instrument is particularly useful when assessing patients for induction on to buprenorphine (see the discussion of buprenorphine in the subsection "Relapse Prevention" later in this chapter).

Personality variables, state of mind at the time of withdrawal, and expectations of the severity of symptoms all may affect withdrawal severity (Kleber 1981). One study found that merely providing information about the withdrawal syndrome to the addicted individual resulted in lower levels of withdrawal symptoms (Green and Gossop 1988).

Pharmacological Treatment

Opioid Dependence

Treatment approaches include 1) short-term detoxification, usually with methadone, buprenorphine, or clonidine; 2) opioid substitution therapy, consisting of maintenance treatment with methadone or buprenorphine; and 3)

Table 3–1.   Signs and symptoms of opioid withdrawal

Early	Middle	Late
Lacrimation	Restless sleep	Increased severity of earlier symptoms
Yawning	Dilated pupils	Tachycardia
Rhinorrhea	Anorexia	Nausea
Sweating	Gooseflesh	Vomiting
	Restlessness	Diarrhea
	Irritability	Abdominal cramps
	Tremor	Increased blood pressure
		Mood lability
		Depression
		Muscle spasms
		Weakness
		Bone pain

Source.   Adapted from Ciraulo and Ciraulo 1988.

antagonist treatment with naltrexone. An addicted individual often has experience with more than one treatment modality in his or her career. It is often difficult to ascertain for such individuals exactly which was the key ingredient for recovery.

Opioid Withdrawal

Opioid Detoxification

Methadone.   In the United States, methadone has traditionally been the standard drug used to treat withdrawal symptoms. Detoxification can be accomplished over a period as long as 6 months in an ambulatory methadone maintenance program or as brief as several days in a hospital setting. The goal in brief detoxification is to make the experience less distressing, but the suppression of all withdrawal symptoms should not be expected. If the daily opioid dose is known, one can administer the pharmacologically equivalent methadone dose. The drawback to this approach is that the published equivalencies of oral methadone vary markedly. For example, one source cited reported equivalencies of oral morphine to oral methadone ranging from 4:1 to 14:1 (Gordon et al. 1999), although the equivalency may be as low as 2.5:1 (Ripamonti et al. 1998). Thus, caution should be used when dosing is guided by equivalency tables. As a consequence of methadone's longer duration of action and oral efficacy, withdrawal may be suppressed with lower doses of oral methadone than would be predicted from the published analgesic equivalency ratios.

For patients taking street heroin, the initial dose of methadone is usually 15–20 mg orally. If withdrawal symptoms or signs persist, one may repeat the dose in a few hours. Although some addicted persons with access to pure drugs (not uncommon in some U.S. cities) may require higher doses, generally a dosage of 40 mg/day of methadone is adequate. Once a stabilizing dosage has been found, methadone can be reduced by about 5 mg/day to achieve full detoxification within 5–8 days (American Psychiatric Association 2006). The rate of decrease can be more rapid if clonidine is used (see the following subsection on clonidine). To facilitate compliance in outpatient detoxification, the treatment period may need to be prolonged. Reasonable tapering schedules are 10% per week from high doses and 3% per week from dosages less than 20 mg/day (Senay et al. 1977).

Relapse rates after detoxification are very high, so strong efforts must be made to interest the detoxifying addicted patient in further treatment. Although extension of the withdrawal period for up to 6 months does not appear to improve outcome (Sees et al. 2000), patients who have received methadone maintenance and who have a good therapeutic relationship have more successful outcomes.

Clonidine.   Clonidine, an α_2 agonist used primarily as an antihypertensive, is another agent commonly used for detoxification. It has been shown to suppress many of the autonomic symptoms of the withdrawal syndrome (Gold et al. 1978; Kleber et al. 1985). Patients taking opioids can be transitioned to taking oral clonidine at dosages starting at 0.1–0.2 mg three times per day (up to 0.6 mg/day in inpatient settings). Clonidine should be given for approximately 10 days for heroin detoxification and for 14 days for individuals who are discontinuing methadone. Limiting the outpatient use of clonidine are two major side effects: hypotension, which may be marked, and sedation. For this reason, dosages greater than 1.0 mg/day are not recommended in outpatient settings. Another important limitation of clonidine is that although it suppresses autonomic signs of withdrawal, subject-reported symptoms, such as lethargy, restlessness, insomnia, and craving, are not well relieved (Charney et al. 1981; Jasinski et al. 1985). Anxiety may be alleviated with benzodiazepines, and some data suggested that low-dose propranolol may reduce restlessness (Roehrich and Gold 1987). Although not currently approved by the FDA, lofexidine, another α_2 agonist, has been used extensively in Europe for detoxification. Compared with clonidine, it is less likely to produce hypotension or sedation (Strang et al. 1999).

Detoxification is more successful when the patient is transitioned from a stable methadone dose with the support of ongoing therapy than when the patient comes directly from the street for detoxification from heroin. Clonidine has been used in combination with naltrexone to facilitate rapid withdrawal as well as to ease rapid transition to treatment with the antagonist. Patients usually begin by taking both clonidine and a very low dose of naltrexone on day 1. Clonidine is given in divided doses, adjusted for severity of withdrawal, to a dosage of up to 2.5 mg/day. The dosage of naltrexone is gradually increased to 50–150 mg/day by approximately day 5 or 6; 80%–90% of patients are able to complete the transition to naltrexone in less than 1 week (Charney et al. 1986; Kleber et al. 1987; Vining et al. 1988). In one of the few randomized trials comparing some of the newer detoxification protocols, O'Connor et al. (1997) reported that patients detoxified with a combination of clonidine and naltrexone, or with buprenorphine alone, were more likely to complete detoxification than were those taking clonidine alone. Subjects assigned to the buprenorphine group reported less severe withdrawal symptoms than did those in the other two groups.

Buprenorphine.   Since the late 1990s, buprenorphine has been recognized as an effective agent for opioid detoxification. Sublingual buprenorphine, available for the office-based treatment of opioid dependence, has become one of the standard options for detoxification treatment. However, the optimal withdrawal protocol is still under study. Currently, most clinicians follow the guidelines for buprenorphine induction outlined in Table 3–2 (described in the discussion of buprenorphine maintenance therapies in the subsection "Relapse Prevention"), followed by a 2- to 5-day medication taper (Cheskin et al. 1994; Horspool et al. 2008). Buprenorphine is clearly preferred by many addicted patients as a medication for detoxification. In one study, sublingual buprenorphine appeared to be as effective as methadone in a 7-week detoxification (Bickel et al. 1987). The buprenorphine withdrawal syndrome has been characterized as relatively mild (Fudala et al. 1990; Jasinski et al. 1978; Kosten and Kleber 1988; Mello and Mendelson 1980). However, clinical experience with patients following prolonged substitution therapy has identified a wide range of symptomatology, with some patients reporting a prolonged and significant opioid withdrawal state. After 6 weeks of treatment with 8 mg/day of buprenorphine sublingually, withdrawal was measurable by a symptom checklist and appeared to peak at about 72 hours after the last dose. No increase in withdrawal symptoms was observed with the Himmelsbach scale, which emphasizes physiological signs and symptoms (Fudala et al. 1990). The low severity of buprenorphine withdrawal seems to facilitate rapid induction of naltrexone after buprenorphine discontinuation (Kosten and Kleber 1988). In contrast to these reports, some patients undergoing gradual detoxification from long-term buprenorphine treatment have reported significant withdrawal symptoms. Protocols to manage these symptoms are still under study (Ling et al. 2009).

Ultrarapid detoxification uses general anesthesia and opioid antagonists to accomplish withdrawal more quickly and with less discomfort (Brewer and Maksoud 1997; Kleber 1998; Rabinowitz et al. 1998). However, its efficacy and safety have been questioned (Brewer et al. 1998; O'Connor and Kosten 1998; San and Arranz 1999; Shreeram et al. 2001; Stephenson 1997). Several deaths have been reported during the 16–40 hours following ultrarapid detoxification (Kleber 2007).

Relapse Prevention

Agonist Replacement/Opioid Substitution Therapy

The effectiveness of methadone maintenance and other types of opioid substitution therapy has been well documented (Ball and Ross 1991; Ling et al. 1998). Each prospective methadone maintenance patient needs to be evaluated extensively, with attention paid to several factors, including 1) motivation for a particular type of treatment, 2) presence of co-occurring psychopathology, 3) presence of other substance abuse, 4) availability and feasibility of various types of treatment, and 5) success or failure of prior treatments. Research on the efficacy of methadone maintenance suggests that counseling and/or psychotherapy plays a critical role in the success of opioid substitution

Table 3–2. Buprenorphine induction schedule

	Sublingual buprenorphine/naloxone tablets[a]		
	Day 1		Day 2
Patient type	First dose	Supplemental dose	
Not currently dependent	2/0.5 mg		4/1 mg
Dependent on heroin or pain medications	2/0.5 to 4/1 mg[b]	Redose every 1–2 hours, if withdrawal continues, up to a total of 8/2 mg	If the patient is still in withdrawal, give first-day dosage plus 2/0.5 to 4/1 mg
Dependent on methadone (≤30 mg/day)	2/0.5 mg[b]	Redose every 1–2 hours, if withdrawal continues, up to a total of 8/2 mg	If the patient is still in withdrawal, give first-day dosage plus 2/0.5 to 4/1 mg; if oversedated, give <8/2 mg

[a]Dose amounts consist of the buprenorphine dose (the number before the slash) and the naloxone dose (the number after the slash).
[b]Do not begin buprenorphine until patient shows evidence of opioid withdrawal.
Source. Adapted from McNicholas and Howell 2000.

therapy (Ball and Ross 1991; O'Brien et al. 1995; Woody et al. 1995). Two recent evaluations of the efficacy of office-based buprenorphine have not supported that suggestion (Fiellin et al. 2006; Weiss et al. 2011). In both of these studies, subjects were followed up closely by physician prescribers (standard medical management with brief manually guided counseling); adding other forms of more extensive counseling did not improve treatment outcome. It may well be that close physician monitoring is adequate to ensure the efficacy of this form of treatment, although more specific research is needed to establish the significance of this observation.

Methadone maintenance.   Methadone maintenance was first introduced in 1964 by Dole and Nyswander (1965). High doses of methadone alleviate craving and induce cross-tolerance to other opioids so that heroin-induced euphoria is blocked. Results with more psychologically disturbed and less-motivated patients than those treated by Dole and Nyswander, however, were less dramatic than they originally reported (Sells 1979). Nevertheless, methadone maintenance reduces heroin use, nonopioid drug use, health problems (including HIV rates), and crime (e.g., Ball and Ross 1991; Ball et al. 1988a; Gerstein and Harwood 1990; Sees et al. 2000; Senay 1985; Sullivan et al. 2005). Despite these benefits, some addicted patients have a negative attitude toward this treatment approach. They resist the controls mandated in a methadone clinic and are often misinformed about methadone itself, factors that may make them reluctant to enter into this form of treatment (Hunt et al. 1985–1986). In addition, some health professionals and members of the general public consider it a controversial treatment. Despite the extensive research documenting the efficacy of methadone maintenance, some believe its primary purpose is crime reduction; others confuse physiological dependence on methadone with addiction and see it as merely a substitution of one addiction for another. Despite these reservations, opioid maintenance treatment has been adopted independently in at least 35 countries.

Methadone is a μ opioid receptor agonist with special properties that make it particularly useful as a maintenance agent. Reliably absorbed orally, it does not reach a peak concentration until about 4 hours after administration and maintains a large extravascular reservoir (Kreek 1979). These properties minimize acute euphoric effects. The reservoir results in a plasma half-life of 1–2 days, so there are usually no rapid blood level drops that could lead to withdrawal syndromes between daily doses. Effective blood levels are in the range of 200–500 ng/mL. Trough levels of 400 ng/mL are considered optimal (Payte and Khouri 1993). There is wide variability in blood levels with identical doses (Kreek 1979), and some individuals have inadequate levels even at dosages as high as 200 mg/day (Tennant 1987; Tenore 2003).

Methadone is metabolized by enzymes in the CYP system, primarily by CYP3A4 (Shinderman et al. 2003). Hepatic enzyme-inducing drugs such as phenobarbital, phenytoin, carbamazepine, isoniazid, rifampin, nevirapine, and large doses of vitamin C may markedly reduce serum methadone concentrations (Bell et al. 1988; Kreek 1979). Drugs that raise methadone levels include ketoconazole, fluconazole, sertraline, amitriptyline, paroxetine, fluvoxamine, fluoxetine, diazepam, alprazolam, and zidovudine, which implies that CYP2D6, CYP2C9, and CYP2C19, enzymes that metabolize these drugs, as well as CYP3A4, may contribute to methadone metabolism. Even with adequate methadone plasma levels, some patients continue to abuse drugs, such as sedatives, possibly because they are seeking a form of intoxication rather than relief of opioid craving (Bell et al. 1990). Relapse to illicit drug use is also common during periods of high stress, even in patients with adequate plasma levels. Successful treatment requires that patients learn new psychological coping skills to manage these periods of stress.

Although tolerance develops to methadone, as with all opioids, some pharmacological effects of methadone may persist (Kreek 1983; also see earlier discussion in the section "Clinical Pharmacology"). Euphoria and drowsiness are generally more pronounced in the first weeks of treatment. Slight but measurable mood elevation occurs concurrently with peak plasma levels in patients stabilized on methadone and may be one reason that some patients stay in treatment (McCaul et al. 1982). Full tolerance may not develop to constipation, increased perspiration, decreased libido, and sexual dysfunction. (Opioid-induced endocrine effects usually resolve after a few months, but chronic use of opioids may lower testosterone and follicle-stimulating hormone levels. However, no strong correlation exists between these levels and sexual dysfunction.) During the early months of treatment, patients may have altered electroencephalographic sleep patterns and insomnia. Although electroencephalographic results appear to normalize, sleep disturbance may persist. There is no evidence for long-term organ damage with methadone. At higher doses (generally >100 mg), methadone may induce clinically significant prolongation of the QTc interval and lead to torsades de pointes (Kornick et al. 2003; Krantz et al. 2002, 2003). Patients at risk may require dose reductions and careful electrocardiographic monitoring.

Federal, state, and sometimes local regulations govern methadone maintenance programs. Federal standards exist for admission, frequency of urine testing, methadone dosage, quantity of take-home medication, and treatment of addiction in pregnant women. Regulations stipulate that clients must be at least 18 years old (with some exceptions), have been addicted for most of the prior year, and have at least 1 year of "physiological dependence." These regulatory requirements have not changed with the introduction of DSM-5 (American Psychiatric Association 2013), although the comparable terminology for opioid dependence is now Severe Opioid Use Disorder. Physiological dependence is not a requirement for persons recently released from prison or a chronic care institution, provided that they would have been eligible for methadone maintenance before incarceration or institutionalization, or for selected patients who have previously received methadone maintenance.

The maximum first-day dose is 30 mg, with an additional 10 mg permitted if withdrawal symptoms persist after the initial dose. Patients initially return daily for each dose of methadone. Because patients addicted to opioids often underreport their drug use (Magura et al. 1987), random urine testing is required. After 90 days of methadone treatment, patients who have been drug free for the prior 30 days are eligible for weekend take-home doses. Eventually, patients who have been drug free for the previous 9 months can qualify for up to six take-home doses per week. After 2 years of treatment, patients who remain drug free may earn up to a 30-day supply of take-home doses.

Reasons for discharge from maintenance include persistent opioid or other substance use, sporadic attendance, and aggressive behavior at the clinic. Although patients who behave in these ways undermine the treatment milieu, some clinicians are reluctant to discharge them because of concerns that they would do worse without treatment.

Although standard regulations and a common underlying philosophy result in many similarities among methadone maintenance programs, there are also several differences. Programs based on the original model of Dole and Nyswander (1965) tend to use a high methadone dosage (80–120 mg/day) or more flexible dosing to ensure cross-tolerance and suppression of craving. Because, in this model, illicit opioid use is seen as a response to a metabolic deficiency, indefinite continuation of methadone is thought to be the only way to preclude relapse. One group had good results with outpatient "medical maintenance" (Novick et al. 1988). Selected, highly successful methadone maintenance patients were seen in a physician's office every 28 days and given a take-home supply of methadone tablets at a dosage of up to 100 mg/day. The percentage of patients who relapsed, got into legal difficulty, or dropped out of treatment was very low. Another study randomly assigned 73 highly stable methadone maintenance patients to receive routine methadone maintenance, medical maintenance in a methadone clinic setting, or medical maintenance in a physician's office (King et al. 2002). Although the patients did well in all three settings, the two groups of medical maintenance patients were more satisfied and initiated more new employment or family/social activities. Despite these positive findings, medical maintenance has some important limitations. Clinicians have reported concern about the potential for diversion and serious overdose in medical maintenance programs (Wesson 1988). Furthermore, this type of medical maintenance has not proved successful for unselected addicted populations waiting for admission to standard methadone maintenance programs.

Other programs use a methadone dosage in the range of 20–60 mg/day and less flexible dosing. Clients are viewed not as having a biological illness but rather as being responsible persons who will do best if gradually shifted from maintenance to detoxification. These programs are thus less tolerant of continued drug use and are more likely to discharge clients for problem behavior. The dosages of methadone used in these programs are often not high enough to prevent heroin-induced euphoria. These programs generally had lower rates of retention in treatment (Brown et al. 1982–1983). In a study of six methadone clinics believed to be operating effectively, the percentage of patients who had used illicit injection drugs during the month before the interview ranged from 9% to 57% (Ball and Ross 1991; Ball et al. 1988a, 1988b). Even after adjustment for differences among patients, the factors associated with less injection drug use (in addition to a higher methadone dosage) were the quality of program leadership and services provided. Another important factor is variability within programs; some counselors are demonstrably more effective than others.

There are also demographic and psychological correlates of retention. Retention is better for clients who are employed, married, black, and older. Persons with criminal histories and higher levels of psychopathology tend to leave treatment sooner. However, patients who receive case management and psychiatric services show significant improvement and retention in treatment comparable to that of patients without significant psychiatric comorbidity (Cacciola et al. 2001; Grella et al. 1997). Severity and duration of opioid use per se do not appear to correlate with retention.

Treatment outcome is, of course, determined by multiple factors. Duration and severity of opioid use do not correlate with outcome. Many of the factors contributing to retention rates also affect treatment outcome. For example, patients with serious psychopathology or criminal backgrounds do less well. This is not to say, however, that such patients never improve. In one 2.5-year follow-up study, clients with criminal backgrounds showed significant improvement in substance abuse and in family, legal, and psychological problems (Kosten et al. 1987b). For patients with severe psychopathology, maintenance programs appear to be more helpful than therapeutic communities (see McLellan 1986). Opioid users with more criminality and less psychopathology appear to prefer short-term detoxification to maintenance (Kosten et al. 1986).

Buprenorphine.   In 1978, Jasinski et al. originally suggested the potential value of buprenorphine for the treatment of opioid dependence. His vision came to fruition more than two decades later when, in 2002, the FDA approved sublingual buprenorphine (Subutex) and a combination sublingual tablet of buprenorphine/naloxone (Suboxone) for the office-based treatment of opioid dependence. A comparable film strip formulation of 2/0.5 mg and 8/2 mg buprenorphine/naloxone was approved in 2010. Buprenorphine is a partial μ opioid receptor agonist, with most of the properties of morphine. It is also a strong antagonist at the κ opioid receptor. Administered at dosages of 4–24 mg/day sublingually, it attenuates or blocks opioid-induced euphoria. It is not clear whether this effect is a result of cross-tolerance or some other action at the receptor. Buprenorphine has a very high affinity for the μ receptor and can precipitate withdrawal by displacing other opioids from the receptor. However, it also dissociates very slowly from the receptor, which probably accounts for both its long duration of action (24–48 hours) and less severe withdrawal symptoms.

The efficacy of buprenorphine for the maintenance treatment of opioid dependence was established in a large multicenter, randomized clinical trial (Ling et al. 1998). In another randomized maintenance trial, buprenorphine

(16–24 mg sublingually three times a week), high-dose methadone (60–100 mg/day), and L-α-acetylmethadol (LAAM; 75–115 mg three times a week) were all effective in treating opioid dependence and superior to low-dose methadone (20 mg/day) in clinic retention and suppression of opioid use (Johnson et al. 2000). An additional benefit of buprenorphine is that risk of overdose may be low. As a partial agonist, buprenorphine has a ceiling effect on respiratory depression as the dose is increased (Ciraulo et al. 2006; Walsh et al. 1994).

To avoid precipitating severe withdrawal, patients should show clear evidence of opioid withdrawal (as determined by a withdrawal scale such as the COWS; Wesson and Ling 2003) before being given the first dose of buprenorphine. The initial dose of buprenorphine should be given at least 12–24 hours after the last dose of heroin and 36 hours after the last dose of methadone (Gunderson et al. 2010; McNicholas and Howell 2000). The methadone dosage of maintenance patients should be reduced to 30 mg/day, and the patient should be stabilized at that dosage for at least 1–2 weeks before the transfer to buprenorphine is attempted. For the first day, a sublingual buprenorphine/naloxone dose of 2/0.5–4/1 mg can be given every 2–4 hours, up to a maximum total daily dose of 8/2 mg. On the following days, the dose can be increased by 2/0.5–4/1 mg daily until the initial target maintenance dosage of 12/3–16/4 mg/day is reached (see Table 3–2). Most patients will be stabilized at a dosage of 16/4 mg/day or less. The combination buprenorphine/naloxone tablet or film strip should be used for both initiation and maintenance treatment; the buprenorphine-only tablet should be reserved for the treatment of addiction in pregnant women.

The use of buprenorphine for the office-based treatment of opioid dependence represents a major departure from the highly regulated methadone clinic system. Physicians with addiction specialist credentials or those who have completed 8 hours of approved training are eligible to receive a Drug Enforcement Administration waiver to treat up to 30 patients in their private offices. Physicians may request an increase to treat up to 100 patients after 1 year of experience in prescribing buprenorphine. Stable patients may be given prescriptions for up to a month of medication. The combination buprenorphine/naloxone tablet was developed to reduce the risk for diversion in these circumstances. When taken sublingually, as prescribed, naloxone has minimal biological activity and does not interfere with the buprenorphine dose. However, if an attempt is made to inject the drug, the physically dependent individual will experience the full antagonist effect of the naloxone. Nonetheless, injection use and diversion are still a real possibility with the combination tablets.

Buprenorphine has proved to be an acceptable treatment for a wide range of addicted individuals—especially younger individuals and those with shorter histories of dependence, thus permitting earlier intervention in the course of the addiction. Buprenorphine also offers significant advantages for patients taking antiretroviral therapy. Both methadone and buprenorphine are metabolized by CYP isoenzymes. Although most antiretrovirals can either decrease or increase methadone levels, they do not appear to affect the pharmacodynamic properties of buprenorphine, even if they alter buprenorphine levels. The only exception is atazanavir and ritonavir, both of which elevate buprenorphine levels and alter its pharmacodynamics. Nonetheless, it can be safely prescribed with appropriate observation (Gruber and McCance-Katz 2010). Clinical experience suggests that buprenorphine may be less effective for individuals with larger opioid habits or for individuals requiring opioids for chronic pain. Nonetheless, some individuals with both opioid addiction and moderate levels of chronic pain have been managed successfully with buprenorphine. Methadone remains the preferred medication for those patients.

Detoxification From Maintenance Treatment

The factors that correlate with treatment success do not clearly apply to success after detoxification from maintenance treatment. Correlates of successful detoxification include 1) less criminal behavior; 2) a more stable family; 3) more stable employment; 4) a shorter drug history; 5) a long period of maintenance with a lower dosage; and 6) discharge status, with patient and staff consensus being more favorable than unilateral discharge from treatment (Dole and Joseph 1978). In one study, addicted individuals were followed up for an average of 2 years after detoxification (Stimmel et al. 1977). Although only 28% of the total sample remained abstinent, 83% of those who had completed treatment remained abstinent. Another study of 105 patients detoxified after methadone maintenance treatment documented an 82% relapse rate within 12 months (Ball and Ross 1991). These studies suggest that clinicians should exercise caution when recommending detoxification, even for more successful maintenance patients. More recent research has failed to identify patient characteristics or clinical approaches associated with long-term abstinence following the termination of maintenance treatment (Calsyn et al. 2006). No comparable studies are available for buprenorphine-maintained patients.

When patients elect to be detoxified following maintenance, a very gradual reduction of dosage over 3–6 months is preferred, with careful monitoring of drug craving and withdrawal symptoms. Clients who need to reenter treatment at a later date often do much better than they did during their original treatment, showing less dependence, criminality, and physical disability (Kosten et al. 1986). Such findings suggest that intermittent treatment appears to be beneficial. Therefore, reentry does not necessarily indicate failure and may instead be a step toward eventual recovery. On the other hand, there is a high probability that those who discontinue opioid substitution therapy will resume injection drug use, with attendant risks for hepatitis and HIV infection (Ball et al. 1988a, 1988b).

Opioid Antagonists

Originally, behavioral principles were the basis for the use of opioid antagonists to treat addiction. In theory, drug use that was once operantly reinforced by euphoria would no longer be reinforced if the patients were given a high enough maintenance dosage of an opioid antagonist. In addition, with no regular opioid use, the association between withdrawal symptoms and the addicted person's environment would be extinct (Wikler 1980). Studies of cyclazocine, naloxone, and naltrexone showed them all to be successful in blocking opioid effects, but addicted patients generally stayed in treatment for an average of only 6–8 weeks (Capone et al. 1986; Fram et al. 1989; Resnick et al. 1980).

Oral naltrexone (Revia and generics) and depot naltrexone (Vivitrol) are the only opioid antagonists currently approved for the treatment of addiction. Naloxone is used to treat opioid overdose and to test for opioid dependence but has a short half-life and is relatively ineffective orally. When administered to treat an opioid overdose, naloxone rapidly induces a severe withdrawal syndrome, which peaks within 30 minutes and then declines rapidly. Until the antagonist is eliminated, only partial suppression of the withdrawal syndrome is possible, and then only by using very high opioid doses, which may cause respiratory depression when naloxone is metabolized.

Patients who are likely to continue to use naltrexone and to benefit from treatment are those with established careers (e.g., health professionals) and family support who are well motivated and closely monitored. Up to 70% of such clients are abstinent at 1-year follow up (Washton et al. 1984). Programs that use additional rehabilitative services have better results than those that provide minimal services. A multiclinic, double-blind study of naltrexone involving primarily heroin-addicted patients had such a high attrition rate that conclusions could not be drawn (National Research Council 1978). A more recent study compared the effect of naltrexone alone with that of naltrexone combined with either contingency management or family counseling (Carroll et al. 2001). Both study conditions improved retention and medication compliance, with the most significant effect seen in the subgroup that attended family counseling.

Oral naltrexone is a long-acting medication that may be given at a dosage of 50 mg/day or three times a week, at a dosage of 100 mg/day on weekdays and 150 mg/day on a weekend day. Some authors recommend that naltrexone be started slowly and only after a waiting period (e.g., a maximum starting dosage of 50 mg/day only after the patient is heroin free for 7 days or methadone free for 10 days, confirmed by a negative naloxone challenge) (Ginzburg 1984). Unfortunately, patients are at significant risk for relapse during such a waiting period. There has been some success with the rapid induction of naltrexone during clonidine detoxification from opioids (see subsection "Opioid Detoxification" earlier in this chapter). Patients who start naltrexone immediately after detoxification often complain of insomnia, gastrointestinal distress, hyperalgesia, anergia, anxiety, and dysphoria (the "naltrexone flu"). Adjunctive treatment with selective serotonin reuptake inhibitors may improve retention. These symptoms usually clear in 2–4 weeks, but the dropout rate is high during this period. Oral naltrexone can be expected to lead to retention of 20%–30% of patients at 6 months.

In 2010, an injectable depot formulation of naltrexone (380 mg given intramuscularly monthly) was approved for the treatment of opioid dependence. Efficacy was confirmed in a large Russian study (Krupitsky et al. 2011), although questions have been raised regarding the applicability of these finding to the U.S. addicted population. Behavioral therapy strategies can improve retention with both oral and depot naltrexone (Rothenberg et al. 2002; Sullivan 2011); 6-month retention rates near 30% have been described for the depot formulation, approaching those of buprenorphine maintenance (Sullivan 2011).

At the dosages of naltrexone used, the effects of as much as 25 mg of injected heroin are blocked. Although toxicity of naltrexone in heroin-addicted individuals is low, there have been some reported subtle adverse effects, such as decreased energy (Hollister et al. 1981). Nonaddicted obese subjects have been known to develop markedly elevated transaminase levels at a dosage of 300 mg/day (Mitchell et al. 1987). The inference has been drawn that high doses of the drug are potentially hepatotoxic (Pfohl et al. 1986), so naltrexone is contraindicated in patients with liver failure or acute hepatitis.

Conclusion

Opioid dependence has been recognized as a problem in the United States since the end of the nineteenth century. The introduction of methadone maintenance treatment in 1964 showed that patients whose addiction was treated could be returned to productive lives and ushered in a new era of scientific and medical interest in opioid addiction. There has been major progress in our understanding of the actions of the opioids and of the risk factors associated with dependence. The last 50 years have seen the development of a range of treatment options. They include detoxification, usually followed by drug-free outpatient counseling; opioid substitution therapy with methadone or buprenorphine; antagonist therapy, both oral and a long-acting formulation; therapeutic communities; and 12-step programs. Success in methadone substitution therapy is associated with adequate dosage (80–120 mg/day), extended time in treatment, and provision of professional counseling services.

The approval of buprenorphine for use in the private office setting represents a significant shift in public policy for the management of opioid dependence. This option has significantly increased the number of patients in treatment and has attracted many individuals in the early stages of illness who have traditionally avoided methadone treatment. Furthermore, the recent approval of depot naltrexone mitigates the compliance problem with oral naltrexone and adds another potentially useful treatment option. These new treatment options, coupled with recognition of the need to treat co-occurring psychiatric conditions in opioid-addicted patients, hold great promise for the development of a more effective treatment system for this major public health problem.

References

Aghajanian GK, Kogan JH, Moghaddam B: Opiate withdrawal increases glutamate and aspartate efflux in the locus coeruleus: an in vivo microdialysis study. Brain Res 636:126–130, 1994

American Psychiatric Association: American Psychiatric Association Practice Guidelines for the Treatment of Psychiatric Disorders: Compendium 2006. Washington, DC, American Psychiatric Association, 2006

American Psychiatric Association: Diagnostic and Statistical Manual of Mental Disorders, 5th Edition. Arlington, VA, American Psychiatric Association, 2013

Ball JC, Ross A: The Effectiveness of Methadone Maintenance Treatment. New York, Springer-Verlag, 1991

Ball J, Corty E, Bond H, et al: The reduction of intravenous heroin use, non-opiate use and crime during methadone maintenance treatment: further findings. NIDA Res Monogr 81:224–230, 1988a

Ball JC, Lange WR, Myers CP, et al: Reducing the risk of AIDS through methadone maintenance treatment. J Health Soc Behav 29:214–226, 1988b

Bekkering GE, Soares-Weiser K, Reid K, et al: Can morphine still be considered to be the standard for treating chronic pain? A systematic review including pair-wise and network meta-analysis. Curr Med Res Opin 27:1477–1499, 2011

Bell J, Seres V, Bowron P, et al: The use of serum methadone levels in patients receiving methadone maintenance. Clin Pharmacol Ther 43:623–629, 1988

Bell J, Bowron P, Lewis J, et al: Serum levels of methadone in maintenance clients who persist in illicit drug use. Br J Addict 85:1599–1602, 1990

Bickel WK, Johnson RE, Stitzer ML, et al: A clinical trial of buprenorphine, I: comparison with methadone in the detoxification of heroin addicts, II: examination of its opioid blocking properties. NIDA Res Monogr 76:182–188, 1987

Bohn LM, Gainetdinov RR, Lin FT, et al: Mu-opioid receptor desensitization by beta-arrestin-2 determines morphine tolerance but not dependence. Nature 408:720–723, 2000

Brewer C, Maksoud NA: Opiate detoxification under anesthesia. JAMA 278:1318–1319, 1997

Brewer C, Williams J, Rendueles EC, et al: Unethical promotion of rapid opiate detoxification under anaesthesia (RODA) (letter). Lancet 351:218, 1998

Brown BS, Watters JK, Iglehart AS: Methadone maintenance dosage levels and program retention. Am J Drug Alcohol Abuse 9:129–139, 1982–1983

Cacciola JS, Alterman AI, Rutherford MJ, et al: The relationship of psychiatric comorbidity to treatment outcomes in methadone maintained patients. Drug Alcohol Depend 61:271–280, 2001

Callaly T, Trauer T, Munro L, et al: Prevalence of psychiatric disorder in a methadone maintenance population. Aust NZJ Psychiatry 35:601–605, 2001

Calsyn DA, Malcy JA, Saxon AJ: Slow tapering from methadone maintenance in a program encouraging indefinite maintenance. J Subst Abuse Treat 30:159–163, 2006

Cami J, Farre M: Drug addiction. N Engl J Med 349:975–986, 2003

Cao JL, Vialou VF, Lobo MK, et al: Essential role of the cAMP-cAMP response-element binding protein pathway in opiate-induced homeostatic adaptations of locus coeruleus neurons. Proc Natl Acad Sci USA 107:17011–17016, 2010

Capone T, Brahen L, Condren R, et al: Retention and outcome in a narcotic antagonist treatment program. J Clin Psychol 42:825–833, 1986

Carroll KM, Ball SA, Nich C, et al: Targeting behavioral therapies to enhance naltrexone treatment of opioid dependence. Arch Gen Psychiatry 58:755–761, 2001

Charney DS, Steinberg DE, Kleber HD, et al: The clinical use of clonidine in abrupt withdrawal from methadone. Arch Gen Psychiatry 38:1273–1277, 1981

Charney DS, Heninger OR, Kleber HD: The combined use of clonidine and naltrexone as a rapid, safe, and effective treatment of abrupt withdrawal from methadone. Am J Psychiatry 143:831–837, 1986

Cheatle MD, O'Brien CP: Opioid therapy in patients with chronic noncancer pain: diagnostic and clinical challenges. Adv Psychosom Med 30:61–91, 2011

Cheskin LJ, Fudala PJ, Johnson RE: A controlled comparison of buprenorphine and clonidine for acute detoxification from opioids. Drug Alcohol Depend 36:115–121, 1994

Childress AR, McLellan AT, Ehrman R, et al: Classically conditioned responses in opioid and cocaine dependence: a role in relapse? NIDA Res Monogr 84:25–43, 1988

Christie MJ: Cellular neuroadaptations to chronic opioids: tolerance, withdrawal and addiction. Br J Pharmacol 154:384–396, 2008

Ciraulo DA, Ciraulo AN: Substance abuse, in Handbook of Clinical Psychopharmacology. Edited by Tupin JP, Shader RI, Harnett DS. Northvale, NJ, Jason Aronson, 1988, p 143

Ciraulo DA, Hitzemann RJ, Somoza E, et al: Pharmacokinetics and pharmacolodynamics of multiple sublingual buprenorphine tablets in dose-escalation trials. J Clin Pharmacol 46:179–192, 2006

Clayton RR, Voss HL: Young men and drugs in Manhattan: a causal analysis. NIDA Res Monogr 39:1–187, 1981

Cushman P, Dole VP: Detoxification of rehabilitated methadone-maintained patients. JAMA 226:747–752, 1973

Dang VC, Christie MJ: Mechanisms of rapid opioid receptor desensitization, resensitization and tolerance in brain neurons. Br J Pharmacol 165:1704–1716, 2012

Delfs JM, Zhu Y, Druhan JP, et al: Noradrenaline in the ventral forebrain is critical for opiate withdrawal-induced aversion. Nature 403:430–434, 2000

Dietis N, Rowbotham DJ, Lambert DG: Opioid receptor subtypes: fact or artifact? Br J Anaesth 107:8–18, 2011

Dole VP: Implications of methadone maintenance for theories of narcotic addiction. JAMA 260:3025–3029, 1988

Dole VP, Joseph H: Long-term outcome of patients treated with methadone. Ann NY Acad Sci 311:181–189, 1978

Dole VP, Nyswander MN: A medical treatment for diacetylmorphine (heroin) addiction. JAMA 193:646–650, 1965

Dole VP, Nyswander MN: Heroin addiction: a metabolic disease. Arch Intern Med 120:19–24, 1967

Dupont RL, McLellan AT, Carr G, et al: How are addicted physicians treated? A national survey of physician health programs, J Subst Abuse Treat 37:1–7, 2009

Farrell AD, White KS: Peer influences and drug use among urban adolescents: family structure and parent-adolescent relationship as protective factors. J Consult Clin Psychol 66:248–258, 1998

Fiellin DA, Pantalon MV, Chawarski MC, et al: Counseling plus buprenorphine-naloxone maintenance therapy for opioid dependence. N Engl J Med 355:365–374, 2006

Fram DH, Marmo J, Holden R: Naltrexone treatment: the problem of patient acceptance. J Subst Abuse Treat 6:119–122, 1989

Fudala PJ, Jaffe JH, Dax EM, et al: Use of buprenorphine in the treatment of opioid addiction, II: physiologic and behavioral effects of daily and alternate-day administration and abrupt withdrawal. Clin Pharmacol Ther 47:525–534, 1990

Gerstein DR, Harwood HJ (eds): Treating Drug Problems, Vol 1: A Study of the Evolution, Effectiveness, and Financing of Public and Private Drug Treatment Systems. Washington, DC, National Academy Press, 1990

Ginzburg HM: Naltrexone: its clinical utility (NIDA Treatment Research Report ADM-84-1358). Washington, DC, U.S. Government Printing Office, 1984

Gold MS, Redmond DE, Kleber HD: Clonidine in opiate withdrawal. Lancet 1:929–930, 1978

Gordon DB, Stevenson KK, Griffie J, et al: Opioid equianalgesic calculations. J Palliat Med 2:209–218, 1999

Gossop M, Bradley B, Phillips GT: An investigation of withdrawal symptoms shown by opiate addicts during and subsequent to a 21-day in-patient methadone detoxification procedure. Addict Behav 12:1–6, 1987

Green L, Gossop M: Effects of information on the opiate withdrawal syndrome. Br J Addict 83:305–309, 1988

Grella CE, Wugalter SE, Anglin MD: Predictors of treatment retention in enhanced and standard methadone maintenance treatment for HIV risk reduction. J Drug Issues 27:203–224, 1997

Groer CE, Schmid CL, Jaeger AM, et al: Agonist-directed interactions with specific beta-arrestins determine mu-opioid receptor trafficking, ubiquitination, and dephosphorylation. J Biol Chem 286:31731–31741, 2011

Gruber VA, McCance-Katz EF: Methadone, buprenorphine, and street drug interactions with antiretroviral medications. Curr HIV/AIDS Rep 7:152–160, 2010

Gunderson EW, Levin FR, Rombone MM, et al: Improving temporal efficiency of outpatient buprenorphine induction. Am J Addict 20:397–404, 2010

Gutstein HB, Akil H: Opioid analgesics, in Goodman and Gilman's The Pharmacological Basis of Therapeutics, 10th Edition. Edited by Hardman JG, Limbird LE, Gilman AG. New York, McGraw-Hill, 2001, pp 569–619

Heishman SJ, Stitzer ML, Bigelow GE, et al: Acute opioid physical dependence in postaddict humans: naloxone dose effects after brief morphine exposure. J Pharmacol Exp Ther 248:127–134, 1989

Hien DA, Nunes E, Levin FR, et al: Posttraumatic stress disorder and short-term outcome in early methadone treatment. J Subst Abuse Treat 19:31–37, 2000

Himmelsbach CK: The morphine abstinence syndrome, its nature and treatment. Ann Intern Med 15:829–839, 1941

Hollister LE, Johnson K, Bowkhabza, et al: Aversive effects of naltrexone in subjects not dependent on opiates. Drug Alcohol Depend 8:37–41, 1981

Horspool MJ, Seivewright N, Armitage CJ, et al: Post-treatment outcomes of buprenorphine detoxification in community settings: a systematic review. Eur Addict Res 14:179–185, 2008

Hser YI, Hoffman V, Grella CE, et al: A 33-year follow-up of narcotic addicts. Arch Gen Psychiatry 58:503–508, 2001

Hubbard RL, Marsden ME, Rachal JV, et al: Drug Abuse Treatment: A National Study of Effectiveness. Chapel Hill, University of North Carolina Press, 1989

Hunt DE, Lipton DS, Goldsmith DS, et al: "It takes your heart": the image of methadone maintenance in the addict world and its effect on recruitment into treatment. Int J Addict 20:1751–1771, 1985–1986

Institute of Medicine: Relieving Pain in America: A Blueprint for Transforming Prevention, Care, Education, and Research. June 29, 2011. Available at: http://www.iom.edu/Reports/2011/Relieving-Pain-in-America-A-Blueprint-for-transforming-Prevention-Care-Education-Research.aspx. Accessed November 19, 2012.

Jaffe J, Knapp CM, Ciraulo DA: Opiates: clinical aspects, in Substance Abuse: A Comprehensive Textbook. Edited by Lowinson JH, Ruiz P, Millman RB, et al. New York, Lippincott Williams & Wilkins, 2004, pp 158–165

Jasinski DR, Pevnick JS, Griffith JD: Human pharmacology and abuse potential of the analgesic buprenorphine: a potential agent for treating narcotic addiction. Arch Gen Psychiatry 35:501–516, 1978

Jasinski DR, Johnson RE, Kocher TR: Clonidine in morphine withdrawal: differential effects on signs and symptoms. Arch Gen Psychiatry 42:1063–1066, 1985

Johnson RE, Chutuape MA, Strain EC, et al: A comparison of levomethadyl acetate, buprenorphine, and methadone for opioid dependence. N Engl J Med 343:1290–1297, 2000

Jones RT: Dependence in non-addict humans after a single dose of morphine, in Endogenous and Exogenous Opiate Agonists and Antagonists. Edited by Way EL. New York, Pergamon, 1979, pp 557–560

Kakko J, Svanborg KD, Kreek MJ, et al: 1-Year retention and social functioning after buprenorphine-assisted relapse prevention treatment for heroin dependence in Sweden: a randomized, placebo-controlled trial. Lancet 361:662–668, 2003

Kandel D, Yamaguchi K: From beer to crack: developmental patterns of drug involvement. Am J Public Health 83:851–855, 1993

King VL, Stoller KB, Hayes M, et al: A multicenter randomized evaluation of methadone medical maintenance. Drug Alcohol Depend 65:137–148, 2002

Kleber HD: Detoxification from narcotics, in Substance Abuse: Clinical Problems and Perspectives. Edited by Lowinson J, Ruiz P. Baltimore, MD, Williams & Wilkins, 1981, pp 317–338

Kleber HD: Ultrarapid opiate detoxification. Addiction 93:1629–1633, 1998

Kleber HD: Pharmacologic treatments for opioid dependence: detoxification and maintenance options. Dialogues Clin Neurosci December 9:455–470, 2007

Kleber HD, Riordan CE, Rounsaville BJ, et al: Clonidine in outpatient detoxification from methadone maintenance. Arch Gen Psychiatry 42:391–394, 1985

Kleber HD, Topazian M, Gaspari J, et al: Clonidine and naltrexone in the outpatient treatment of heroin withdrawal. Am J Drug Alcohol Abuse 13:1–17, 1987

Kornetsky C: Brain stimulation reward, morphine-induced stereotypy, and sensitization: implications for abuse. Neurosci Biobehav Rev 27:777–786, 2004

Kornick CA, Kilborn MJ, Santiago-Palma J, et al: QTc interval prolongation associated with intravenous methadone. Pain 105:499–506, 2003

Kosten TR, Kleber HD: Buprenorphine detoxification from opioid dependence: a pilot study. Life Sci 42:635–641, 1988

Kosten TR, Rounsaville BJ, Kleber HD: A 2.5 year follow-up of treatment retention and reentry among opioid addicts. J Subst Abuse Treat 3:181–189, 1986

Kosten TR, Rounsaville BJ, Kleber HD: Multidimensionality and prediction of treatment outcome in opioid addicts: 2.5-year follow-up. Compr Psychiatry 28:3–13, 1987a

Kosten TR, Rounsaville BJ, Kleber HD: Predictors of 2.5-year outcome in opioid addicts: pretreatment source of income. Am J Drug Alcohol Abuse 13:19–32, 1987b

Krantz MJ, Lewkowiez L, Hays H, et al: Torsade de pointes associated with very-high-dose methadone. Ann Intern Med 137:501–504, 2002

Krantz MJ, Kutinsky IB, Robertson AD, et al: Dose-related effects of methadone on QT prolongation in a series of patients with torsade de pointes. Pharmacotherapy 23:802–805, 2003

Krausz M, Degkwitz P, Kuhne A, et al: Comorbidity of opiate dependence and mental disorders. Addict Behav 23:767–783, 1998

Krausz M, Verthein U, Degkwitz P: Psychiatric comorbidity in opiate addicts. Eur Addict Res 5:55–62, 1999

Kreek MJ: Methadone in treatment: physiological and pharmacological issues, in Handbook on Drug Abuse. Edited by Dupont RL, Goldstein A, O'Donnell J. Washington, DC, U.S. Government Printing Office, 1979, pp 57–86

Kreek MJ: Health consequences associated with the use of methadone, in Research on the Treatment of Narcotic Addiction: State of the Art (NIDA Research Monograph ADM-83-1281). Edited by Cooper JR, Altman R, Brown BS, et al. Washington, DC, U.S. Government Printing Office, 1983, pp 456–482

Kroslak T, Laforge KS, Gianotti RJ, et al: The single nucleotide polymorphism A118G alters functional properties of the human mu opioid receptor. J Neurochem 103:77–87, 2007

Krupitsky E, Nunes E, Ling W, et al: Injectable extended-release naltrexone for opioid dependence: a double-blind, placebo-controlled, multicentre randomised trial. Lancet 377:1506–1513, 2011

La Vincente SF, White JM, Somogyi AA, et al: Enhanced buprenorphine analgesia with the addition of ultra-low-dose naloxone in healthy subjects. Clin Pharmacol Ther 83:144–152, 2008

Ling W, Charuvastra C, Collins JF, et al: Buprenorphine maintenance treatment of opiate dependence: a multi-center, randomized clinical trial. Addiction 93:475–486, 1998

Ling W, Hillhouse M, Domier C, et al: Buprenorphine tapering schedule and illicit opioid use. Addiction 104:256–265, 2009

Magura S, Goldsmith D, Casriel C, et al: The validity of methadone clients' self-reported drug use. Int J Addict 22:727–749, 1987

Maldonado R, Blendy JA, Tzavara E, et al: Reduction of morphine abstinence in mice with a mutation in the gene encoding CREB. Science 273:657–659, 1996

Malinoff HL, Barkini RL, Wilson G: Sublingual buprenorphine is effective in the treatment of chronic pain syndrome. Am J Ther 12:379–384, 2005

Marsden J, Gossop M, Stewart D, et al: Psychiatric symptoms among clients seeking treatment for drug dependence: intake data from the National Treatment Outcome Research Study. Br J Psychiatry 176:285–289, 2000

Martin WR, Jasinski DR, Haertzen CA, et al: Methadone: a reevaluation. Arch Gen Psychiatry 28:286–295, 1973

Mayer P, Höllt V: Allelic and somatic variations in the endogenous opioid system of humans. Pharmacol Ther 91:167–177, 2001

McCaul ME, Bigelow GE, Stitzer ML, et al: Short-term effects of oral methadone in methadone maintenance subjects. Clin Pharmacol Ther 31:753–761, 1982

McLellan AT: "Psychiatric severity" as a predictor of outcome from substance abuse treatments, in Psychopathology and Addictive Disorders. Edited by Meyer RE. New York, Guilford, 1986, pp 97–139

McLellan AT, Childress AR, Ehrman R, et al: Extinguishing conditioned responses during opiate dependence treatment: turning laboratory findings into clinical procedures. J Subst Abuse Treat 3:33–40, 1986

McLellan AT, Skipper GS, Campbell M, et al: Five year outcomes in a cohort study of physicians treated for substance use disorders in the United States. BMJ 337:a2038, 2008

McNicholas L, Howell EF: Buprenorphine Clinical Practice Guidelines, Field Review Draft November 17, 2000. Rockville, MD, U.S. Department of Health and Human Services, Substance Abuse and Mental Health Services Administration, Center for Substance Abuse Treatment, Office of Pharmacologic and Alternative Therapies, 2000

Mello NK, Mendelson JH: Buprenorphine suppresses heroin use by heroin addicts. Science 207:657–659, 1980

Meyer RE, Mirin SM: The Heroin Stimulus: Implication for a Theory of Addiction. New York, Plenum, 1979

Milby JB, Sims, MK, Khuder S, et al: Psychiatric comorbidity: prevalence in methadone maintenance treatment. Am J Drug Alcohol Abuse 22:95–107, 1996

Mitchell JE, Morley JE, Levine AS, et al: High dose naltrexone therapy and dietary counseling for obesity. Biol Psychiatry 22:35–42, 1987

Morgan MM, Christie MJ: Analysis of opioid efficacy, tolerance, addiction and dependence from cell culture to human. Br J Pharmacol 164:1322–1334, 2011

National Research Council: Clinical evaluation of naltrexone treatment of opiate-dependent individuals: report of the National Research Council Committee on Clinical Evaluation of Narcotic Antagonists. Arch Gen Psychiatry 35:335–340, 1978

Nestler EJ, Hyman SE, Malenka RC: Molecular Neuropharmacology: A Foundation for Clinical Neuroscience. New York, McGraw-Hill, 2001

Novick DM, Pascarelli EF, Joseph H, et al: Methadone maintenance patients in general medical practice: a preliminary report. JAMA 259:3299–3302, 1988

O'Brien CP, Woody GE, McLellan AT: Enhancing the effectiveness of methadone using psychotherapeutic interventions. NIDA Res Monogr 150:5–8, 1995

O'Connor PG, Carroll KM, Shi JM, et al: Three methods of opioid detoxification in a primary care setting: a randomized trial. Ann Intern Med 127:526–530, 1997

O'Connor PG, Kosten TR: Rapid and ultrarapid opioid detoxification techniques. JAMA 279:229–234, 1998

Payte J, Khouri E: Principles of methadone dose determination, in State Methadone Treatment Guidelines. Treatment Improvement Protocol (TIP) Series 1 (DHHS Publ No SMA-93-1991). Edited by Parrino MW. Rockville, MD, U.S. Department of Health and Human Services, Center for Substance Abuse Treatment, 1993

Pergolizzi J, Aloisi AM, Dahan A, et al: Current knowledge of buprenorphine and its unique pharmacological profile. Pain Pract 10:428–450, 2010

Pfohl DN, Allen JI, Atkinson RL, et al: Naltrexone hydrochloride (Trexan): a review of serum transaminase elevations at high dosage. NIDA Res Monogr 67:66–72, 1986

Portenoy PM, Foley KM: Chronic use of opioid analgesics in non-malignant pain: report of 38 cases. Pain 25:171–186, 1986

Rabinowitz J, Cohen H, Kotler M: Outcomes of ultrarapid opiate detoxification combined with naltrexone maintenance and counseling. Psychiatr Serv 49:831–833, 1998

Regier DA, Farmer ME, Rae DS, et al: Comorbidity of mental disorders with alcohol and other drug abuse. JAMA 264:2511–2518, 1990

Resnick RB, Schuyten-Resnick E, Washton AM: Assessment of narcotic antagonists in the treatment of opioid dependence. Annu Rev Pharmacol Toxicol 20:463–474, 1980

Ripamonti C, Groff L, Brunelli C, et al: Switching from morphine to oral methadone in treating cancer pain: what is the equianalgesic dose ratio? J Clin Oncol 16:3216–3221, 1998

Roehrich H, Gold MS: Propranolol as adjunct to clonidine in opiate detoxification. Am J Psychiatry 144:1099–1100, 1987

Roozen HG, Kerhof AJ, van den Brink W: Experiences with an outpatient relapse program (community reinforcement approach) combined with naltrexone in the treatment of opioid-dependence: effect on addictive behaviors and the predictive value of psychiatric comorbidity. Eur Addict Res 9:53–58, 2003

Rothenberg JL, Sullivan MA, Church SH, et al: Behavioral naltrexone therapy: an integrated treatment for opiate dependence. J Subst Abuse Treat 23:351–360, 2002

Rounsaville BJ, Kleber HD: Untreated opiate addicts. Arch Gen Psychiatry 42:1072–1077, 1985

Rounsaville BJ, Kosten TR, Kleber HD: The antecedents and benefits of achieving abstinence in opioid addicts: a 2.5-year follow-up study. Am J Drug Alcohol Abuse 13:213–229, 1987

San L, Arranz B: Pros and cons of ultrarapid opiate detoxification. Addiction 94:1240–1241, 1999

Schulz S, Mayer D, Pfeiffer M, et al: Morphine induces terminal mu-opioid receptor desensitization by sustained phosphorylation of serine-375. The EMBO Journal 23:3282–3289, 2004

Seecof R, Tennant FS: Subjective perceptions to the intravenous "rush" of heroin and cocaine in opioid addicts. Am J Drug Alcohol Abuse 12:79–87, 1987

Sees KL, Delucci KL, Masson C, et al: Methadone maintenance vs. 180-day psychosocially enriched detoxification for treatment of opioid dependence: a randomized controlled trial. JAMA 283:1303–1310, 2000

Selley DE, Liu Q, Childers SR: Signal transduction correlates of mu opioid agonist intrinsic efficacy: receptor-stimulated [35S]GTP gamma S binding in mMOR-CHO cells and rat thalamus. J Pharmacol Exp Ther 285:496–505, 1998

Selley DE, Herbert JT, Morgan D, et al: Effect of strain and sex on mu opioid receptor-mediated G-protein activation in rat brain. Brain Res Bull 60:201–208, 2003

Sells SB: Treatment effectiveness, in Handbook on Drug Abuse. Edited by Dupont RE, Goldstein A, O'Donnell J. Washington, DC, U.S. Government Printing Office, 1979, pp 105–118

Senay EC: Methadone maintenance treatment. Int J Addict 20:803–821, 1985

Senay EC, Dorus W, Goldberg F, et al: Withdrawal from methadone maintenance: rate of withdrawal and expectation. Arch Gen Psychiatry 34:361–367, 1977

Shaw-Lutchman TZ, Barrot M, Wallace T, et al: Regional and cellular mapping of cAMP response element-mediated transcription during naltrexone-precipitated morphine withdrawal. J Neurosci 22:3663–3672, 2002

Shinderman M, Maxwell S, Brawand-Arney M, et al: Cytochrome P4503A4 metabolic activity, methadone blood concentrations, and methadone doses. Drug Alcohol Depend 69:205–211, 2003

Shreeram SS, McDonald T, Dennison S: Psychosis after ultrarapid opiate detoxification (letter). Am J Psychiatry 158:970, 2001

Simpson DD, Marsh KL: Relapse and recovery among opioid addicts 12 years after treatment. NIDA Res Monogr 72:86–103, 1986

Simpson DD, Joe GW, Bracy SA: Six-year follow-up of opioid addicts after admission to treatment. Arch Gen Psychiatry 39:1318–1323, 1982

Smith B, Hoffman V, Fan J, et al: Years of potential life lost among heroin addicts 33 years after treatment. Prev Med 44:369–374, 2007

Stephenson J: Experts debate merits of 1-day opiate detoxification under anesthesia. JAMA 277:363–364, 1997

Stimmel B, Goldberg J, Rotkopf E, et al: Ability to remain abstinent after methadone detoxification: a six year study. JAMA 237:1216–1220, 1977

Strang J, Bearn J, Gossop M: Lofexidine for opiate detoxification: review of recent randomized and open controlled trials. Am J Addict 8:337–348, 1999

Substance Abuse and Mental Health Services Administration: Overview of Findings From the 2002 National Survey on Drug Use and Health: National Findings (Office of Applied Sciences, NHSDA Series H-22, DHHS Publ No SMA-03-3863). Rockville, MD, Substance Abuse and Mental Health Services Administration, 2003

Substance Abuse and Mental Health Services Administration: Results from the 2010 National Survey on Drug Use and Health: Summary of National Findings (NSDUH Series H-41, HHS Publ No SMA-11-4658. Rockville, MD, Substance Abuse and Mental Health Services Administration, 2011a. Available at: http://www.samhsa.gov/data/NSDUH/2k10NSDUH/2k10Results.htm#Fig5.2. Accessed November 19, 2012.

Substance Abuse and Mental Health Services Administration: Results from the 2010 National Survey on Drug Use and Health: Summary of National Findings (NSDUH Series H-41, HHS Publ No SMA-11-4658). (Table 1.1A) Rockville, MD, Substance Abuse and Mental Health Services Administration, 2011b. Available at: http://oas.samhsa.gov/NSDUH/2k10NSDUH/2k10/tabs/Sect1peTabs1to46.htm. Accessed November 19, 2012.

Substance Abuse and Mental Health Services Administration: Results from the 2010 National Survey on Drug Use and Health: Summary of National Findings (NSDUH Series H-41, HHS Publ No SMA-11-4658). Rockville, MD, Substance Abuse and Mental Health Services Administration, 2011c. Available at: http://www.samhsa.gov/data/NSDUH/2k10NSDUH/2k10Results.htm#Fig2-4. Accessed November 19, 2012.

Substance Abuse and Mental Health Services Administration, Results from the 2011 National Survey on Drug Use and Health: Summary of National Findings, NSDUH Series H-44, HHS Publ No SMA 12-4713. (Figure 5.2) Rockville, MD, Substance Abuse and Mental Health Services Administration, 2012. Available at: http://www.samhsa.gov.data/NSDUH/2k11Results/NSDUHresults2011.htm#fig5-2. Accessed June 27, 2013.

Sullivan LE, Metzger DS, Fudala PJ, et al: Decreasing international HIV transmission: the role of expanding access to opioid agonist therapies for injection drug users. Addiction 100:150–158, 2005

Sullivan MA: Antagonist maintenance for opioid dependence: the naltrexone story. Presented at the 22nd Annual Meeting of the American Academy of Addiction Psychiatry, Scottsdale, AZ, December 10, 2011

Tennant FS: Inadequate plasma concentrations in some high-dose methadone maintenance patients. Am J Psychiatry 144:1349–1350, 1987

Tenore PL: Guidance on optimal methadone dosing. Addiction Treatment Forum 12:3, 2003

Vining E, Kosten TR, Kleber H: Clinical utility of rapid clonidine-naltrexone detoxification for opioid abusers. Br J Addict 83:567–575, 1988

Walsh SL, Preston KL, Stitzer ML, et al: Clinical pharmacology of buprenorphine: ceiling effects at high doses. Clin Pharmacol Ther 55:569–580, 1994

Washton AM, Pottash AC, Gold MS: Naltrexone in addicted business executives and physicians. J Clin Psychiatry 45:39–41, 1984

Weiss RD, Potter JS, Fiellin DA, et al: Adjunctive counseling during brief and extended buprenorphine-naloxone treatment of prescription opioid dependence: a 2-phase randomized controlled trial. Arch Gen Psychiatry 68:1238–1246, 2011

Wesson DR: Revival of medical maintenance in the treatment of heroin dependence (editorial). JAMA 259:3314–3315, 1988

Wesson DR, Ling W: The Clinical Opiate Withdrawal Scale (COWS). J Psychoactive Drugs 35:253–259, 2003

Wikler A: Opioid Dependence: Mechanisms and Treatment. New York, Plenum, 1980

Williams JT, Christie MJ, Manzoni O: Cellular and synaptic adaptations mediating opioid dependence. Physiol Rev 81:299–343, 2001

Woody GE, McLellan AT, Liborsky L, et al: Psychotherapy in community methadone programs: a validation study. Am J Psychiatry 152:1302–1308, 1995

Zhang J, Ferguson SS, Barak LS, et al: Role for G protein-coupled receptor kinase in agonist-specific regulation of mu-opioid receptor responsiveness. Proc Natl Acad Sci USA 95:7157–7162, 1998

4

Cannabis

John J. Mariani, M.D.
Frances R. Levin, M.D.

History

Cannabis is one of the oldest psychotropic drugs known to humans, with the earliest evidence of its use dating to 4000 B.C. Cannabis plants have been used as food, fuel, fiber, and intoxicant. Controversy persists as to whether cannabis exists as one or multiple species (Russo 2007), and cultivation and breeding for particular traits continue to shape the characteristics of cannabis plants. Marijuana (dried leaves and flowers of the plant) and hashish (viscous resin) are the two main psychotropic preparations derived from cannabis. Selective breeding has apparently doubled the potency of cannabis plants in the United States over a 10-year period (McLaren et al. 2008).

Epidemiology

Marijuana is the most widely used illicit drug in the United States, with approximately 17.4 million individuals reporting past-month use, according to the 2010 National Survey on Drug Use and Health (NSDUH) (Substance Abuse and Mental Health Services Administration [SAMHSA] 2011). The 2001–2002 National Epidemiologic Survey on Alcohol and Related Conditions estimated past-year and lifetime prevalence of cannabis abuse to be 1.1% and 7.2%, respectively, and past-year and lifetime prevalence of cannabis dependence to be 0.3% and 1.3%, respectively (Stinson et al. 2005, 2006).

Cannabis use disorders generally begin in late adolescence and early adulthood. Every day, approximately 6,600 individuals try cannabis for the first time (SAMHSA 2011), and 58.3% of new marijuana users are younger than 18. Within 24 months, an estimated 3.9% of recent-onset users of marijuana develop a cannabis dependence syndrome (Chen et al. 2005), with excess risk concentrated among those whose first use of cannabis occurred before late adolescence, those with low family income, and those who had used three or more drugs (e.g., tobacco, alcohol, and other drugs) before using cannabis.

The prevalence of cannabis use peaks in early adulthood. Cannabis use is widespread in colleges: in a 1-year period, approximately 30% of college students use cannabis, and the prevalence of cannabis use disorders is 9.4% in first-year students and 24.6% in past-year cannabis users (Caldeira et al. 2008). Cannabis abuse develops from a combination of genetic and environmental risk factors, with cannabis availability being among the most important risk factors (Gillespie et al. 2009).

Pharmacology

The endocannabinoid neurotransmitter system consists of two known cannabinoid receptor types (CB_1 and CB_2) and endogenous ligands (endocannabinoids), the best known of which are 2-arachidonoylglycerol and anandamide. In mammals, CB_1 receptors are most highly concentrated in the hippocampus, neocortex, basal ganglia, cerebellum, and anterior olfactory nucleus (Glass et al. 1997; Herkenham et al. 1991; Matsuda et al. 1993). This distribution is consistent with the function of the endocannabinoid system in mediating pain, mood, motivation, and cognition (Piomelli 2003; Viveros et al. 2005). CB_2 receptors are present in immune cells and possibly the brain stem (Gong et al. 2006; Van Sickle et al. 2005), although the precise function of this receptor subtype is not fully known (Ishiguro et al. 2007; Onaivi et al. 2006).

Cannabinoids—chemicals that interact with cannabinoid receptors—can be classified into three groups: the phytocannabinoids, which are produced in the cannabis plant; the endocannabinoids, which are endogenous ligands that interact with cannabinoid receptors; and the synthetic cannabinoids, which do not occur in nature but interact with cannabinoid receptors (Sun and Bennett 2007). Cannabis plants produce at least several dozen different phytocannabinoids, which have not been detected in any other plant; new phytocannabinoids continue to be isolated (Radwan et al. 2009). The most important known cannabinoids include 1) cannabidiol, a CB_1 and CB_2 antagonist; 2) delta-9-tetrahydrocannabivarin, which acts as a partial agonist in vitro and an antagonist in vivo; and 3) delta-9-tetrahydrocannabinol (THC), which is a CB_1 and CB_2 receptor partial agonist (Pertwee 2008). The psychotropic effects of cannabis are produced mainly by THC, although other cannabinoids may modify its effects (Elsohly and Slade 2005). One such modifier is cannabidiol, which potentiates the pharmacological effects of THC via a CB_1 receptor-dependent mechanism (Hayakawa et al. 2008). THC potency varies widely among different samples of cannabis (McLaren et al. 2008), and the ratios of the major cannabinoids vary as well (Hillig and Mahlberg 2004). Potency is commonly measured by THC content, but the psychoactive effect also may depend on levels of other cannabinoids, which may interact with one another.

Synthetic cannabinoid receptor agonists are a large family of chemically unrelated molecules that act on cannabinoid receptors, often with greater potency than that of THC (Vardakou et al. 2010). Synthetic cannabinoids can be found in over-the-counter products marketed as "incense not intended for human consumption" and sold under labels such as "Spice" and "K2." Synthetic cannabinoids that have been reported in "Spice" and other similar products include JWH-018, JWH-073, JWH-398, JWH-250, HU-210, and CP 47,497 (Vardakou et al. 2010). In contrast to THC, which is a partial agonist, many of the synthetic cannabinoids act as full agonists at cannabinoid receptors. Because the full-agonist actions of synthetic cannabinoids may yield a higher potential for adverse behavioral effects, governments around the world are acting to ban or control synthetic cannabinoids. At present, standard toxicology testing does not detect the most commonly available synthetic cannabinoids.

Two cannabinoids are available by prescription in the United States. Dronabinol is synthetically produced but chemically identical to THC found in cannabis plants, and it is licensed for the treatment of anorexia associated with weight loss caused by AIDS and nausea and vomiting resulting from cancer chemotherapy not responsive to standard treatments. Dronabinol is a Schedule III controlled drug in the United States. Nabilone, a synthetic cannabinoid, acts as a partial agonist at cannabinoid receptors and, like dronabinol, is licensed for the treatment of nausea and vomiting resulting from chemotherapy not responsive to standard treatments. Nabilone is a Schedule II controlled drug in the United States, although reports of abuse of nabilone are extremely rare (Ware and St. Arnaud-Trempe 2010). A third agent, rimonabant (Acomplia), is a synthetic CB_1 antagonist. Rimonabant was not approved by the U.S. Food and Drug Administration (FDA) as an antiobesity medication because of an adverse psychiatric symptom profile (Butler and Korbonits 2009). Although approved in Europe for this indication, it was subsequently withdrawn from the market.

Neurobiology

Cannabis shares characteristics with other addictive substances—that is, reinforcement is mediated via the nucleus accumbens (Bossong et al. 2009), and cessation is associated with a withdrawal syndrome (Budney et al. 1999; Haney et al. 1999). THC—the psychoactive component of marijuana—interacts with cannabinoid receptors (CB_1 and CB_2). In both animal and human self-administration studies, THC has been shown to have reinforcing properties (Hart et al. 2005; Justinova et al. 2003). Controlled studies have reported an increase in withdrawal discomfort throughout periods of abstinence, with a return to baseline with either marijuana smoking (Budney et al. 2001) or dronabinol administration (Haney et al. 1999). Chronic THC administration in rats is associated with CB_1 receptor downregulation and desensitization (Breivogel et al. 2003), suggesting a potential mechanism for the development of the withdrawal syndrome in humans (i.e., following chronic exposure and downregulation of the endocannabinoid system, abstinence leads to an abrupt decrease in activity of the endocannabinoid system). Positron emission tomography data in humans indicate that THC facilitates dopamine release in the striatum (Bossong et al. 2009), thereby sharing a key feature of all drugs with a confirmed abuse liability.

In rats, long-term exposure to THC blocks synaptic plasticity in the nucleus accumbens and reduces the sensitivity of γ-aminobutyric acid (GABA)ergic and glutamatergic synapses to both cannabinoids and opioids (Hoffman et al. 2003), demonstrating how chronic THC exposure induces functional synaptic changes in neurotransmitter systems other than the endocannabinoid system. CB_1 is coexpressed with serotonin and dopamine receptors and interacts with the serotonin and dopamine neurotransmitter systems (Best and Regehr 2008; Melis et al. 2004).

Accumulating evidence suggests that chronic cannabis use induces changes in brain functioning, but these changes appear to be reversible with cessation of use. Functional neuroimaging studies of chronic or acute cannabis use suggest that the drug modulates global and prefrontal metabolism, but minimal evidence of effects on brain structure has been found (Martin-Santos et al. 2010). Cognitive deficits associated with heavy cannabis use appear to be reversible and related to recent cannabis exposure rather than irreversible and related to cumulative lifetime use (Pope et al. 2001). Chronic users of cannabis develop tolerance to the psychotomimetic and amnestic effects of THC (D'Souza et al. 2008).

When a regular user of cannabis reduces or ceases use, a withdrawal syndrome may develop. Cannabis withdrawal symptoms are common and clinically significant among regular users of cannabis (Cornelius et al. 2008; Hasin et al. 2008).

Psychotherapeutic Approaches

Although this chapter is focused on pharmacological strategies to treat cannabis dependence, psychotherapeutic approaches have been more extensively studied. Moreover, the most effective treatment approach may be the combination of psychotherapy and pharmacotherapy. Although aversive approaches (e.g., emetic agents and electric shock [Morakinyo 1983; Smith et al. 1988]) have been used to treat cannabis dependence, as with dependence on alcohol and other drugs of abuse, these approaches are now largely discredited. The most commonly used therapies are motivational interviewing (Lang et al. 2000; Walker et al. 2011), 12-step facilitation counseling, cognitive-behavioral therapy (CBT) (Copeland et al. 2001; Marijuana Treatment Project Research Group 2004; Stephens et al. 2000), and contingency management strategies (Budney et al. 2000, 2006, 2007; Carroll and Rounsaville 2007; Kadden et al. 2007). Other approaches that are currently being evaluated include aerobic exercise interventions (Buchowski et al. 2011) and computerized delivery of commonly used therapies (Budney et al. 2010).

Psychotherapeutic approaches that do not include contingency management strategies are not as effective in promoting abstinence as those that use such strategies alone or in combination with motivational enhancement therapy (MET) or CBT. However, the reduction or cessation of marijuana use elicited by contingency management is often not maintained after active treatment is ended. At least in adults, this can be mitigated by the addition of MET/CBT and abstinence-based voucher incentives. One criticism of voucher incentives is that they cannot be easily implemented in community treatment settings. However, prized-based contingency methods may be more cost-effective than vouchers and have been used with good effect (Olmstead and Petry 2009; Petry et al. 2007). These, along with other practical strategies, might allow the translation and implementation of these incentivized approaches into community treatment settings.

Pharmacological Interventions

The psychotherapeutic approaches described in the previous section often require a significant allocation of time and clinical expertise. Furthermore, most marijuana abusers will continue to use the drug, despite intensive interventions. Therefore, effective medications have an important potential role. Psychotherapeutic approaches, used in conjunction with medications, could promote medication adherence and help to establish patient-centered goals. In substance abuse treatment settings, psychotherapeutic interventions, such as MET and CBT, and community reinforcement approaches are likely to be enhanced by effective medications. At present, no FDA-approved pharmacotherapies are available for cannabis dependence. Substantially less research effort has been dedicated to evaluating pharmacological agents to treat cannabis dependence than for other substances of abuse (e.g., alcohol, cocaine, opioids). This is partially because of the lack of awareness that a clear-cut withdrawal syndrome is associated with chronic, heavy cannabis use and that dependence on the drug is more common than either cocaine or heroin dependence.

Animal Studies

Although several animal studies have evaluated withdrawal symptoms (Aceto et al. 1995; Tsou et al. 1995) and precipitation of withdrawal with cannabinoid antagonists (Huang et al. 2010; Lichtman et al. 1998; Tzavara et al. 2000), preclinical investigation of pharmacological agents to mitigate cannabis withdrawal symptoms is limited. In one study, lithium inhibited cannabis withdrawal symptoms in animals pretreated with a cannabinoid agonist (Cui et al. 2001). Evaluating the effect of pharmacological agents in animal models of addiction has been limited by the difficulty in training animals to self-administer THC (Gardner et al. 2002). Despite this, some investigators have successfully trained animals to self-administer intravenous THC or other cannabinoids (Braida et al. 2001; Fattore et al. 2001; Justinova et al. 2005; Martellotta et al. 1998; Tanda et al. 2000). Martellotta et al. (1998) used the CB_1 antagonist S141716A to train mice to self-administer a synthetic cannabinoid (WIN 55,212-2). Justinova et al. (2005) found that pretreating squirrel monkeys with the narcotic antagonist naltrexone reduced self-administration of intravenous THC, suggesting that this approach might be used to test the therapeutic utility of various proposed agents. However, most of the research assessing the effect of pharmacological agents on cannabinoid self-administration has been conducted in humans.

Human Laboratory Studies

In general, clinical pharmacological studies have focused on non-treatment-seeking heavy marijuana users in controlled laboratory settings or marijuana abusers seeking treatment in outpatient settings. Human laboratory studies might be considered a bridge between preclinical and clinical studies in which one can 1) test the subjective effects of smoked marijuana and cannabinoids, 2) assess withdrawal symptoms associated with the cessation of smoked marijuana or oral THC, and 3) assess the effect of pharmacological agents on subjective effects of smoked or oral THC, withdrawal symptoms, or the self-administration of smoked or oral THC. These studies most frequently use within-subject, inpatient, placebo-controlled designs and are conducted with a small number of non-treatment-seeking drug users. Laboratory studies permit controlled conditions in which participants can be monitored closely to ensure that no other concomitant alcohol or drug use is present. Generally, research participants remain on an inpatient unit for 2–3 weeks. Research participants are told that the marijuana or capsule strength that they are given may change while they are enrolled in the trial. However, they are not told that the characterization of subjective effects, withdrawal symptoms, or self-administration and the effects of maintenance medications on these parameters are objectives of the study.

Table 4–1 shows the laboratory studies of various pharmacological agents for cannabis dependence that have been conducted to date. These agents include inhibitors of noradrenergic or noradrenergic/dopamine reuptake (atomoxetine, bupropion), serotonin type 1A (5-HT$_{1A}$) receptor partial agonists (buspirone), α_2-adrenergic agonists (clonidine, lofexidine), cannabinoid CB$_1$ receptor partial agonists (dronabinol), selective serotonin reuptake inhibitors (fluoxetine), 5-HT$_2$ receptor antagonists (nefazodone), GABA$_B$ receptor agonists (baclofen) and mixed GABA agonist/N-methyl-D-aspartate antagonists (valproic acid), CB$_1$ receptor antagonists (rimonabant), medications with unclear mechanisms of action (lithium), dual mechanism agents (venlafaxine), and agents that modulate glutamate transmission (N-acetylcysteine [NAC]).

Several antidepressants have been studied to assess their effect on withdrawal and relapse. Nefazodone was shown to decrease a subset of withdrawal symptoms (anxiety and muscle pain) but not other symptoms (Haney et al. 2003b). Bupropion reduced ratings of "high" from smoked marijuana but worsened mood withdrawal and aggravated other withdrawal symptoms such as irritability, restlessness, and trouble sleeping (Haney et al. 2004). More recently, Haney et al. (2010) evaluated mirtazapine and found that it improved sleep during abstinence and increased food intake but had no effect on other withdrawal symptoms and did not decrease self-administration after a period of marijuana abstinence. In the same article, the potential utility of baclofen was also evaluated. Baclofen reduced craving, but mood symptoms were not affected, and it did not reduce cannabis self-administration. Baclofen's effect on withdrawal symptoms could not be assessed because these were minimal for the sample enrolled.

Another agent, modafinil, reduced the euphoria associated with oral THC (Sugarman et al. 2011), and further investigation of the drug is warranted. Although divalproex decreased ratings of marijuana craving during withdrawal, it increased ratings of anxiety, irritability, and tiredness (Haney et al. 2004).

Table 4–1. Laboratory studies: pharmacological treatment of cannabis dependence

Study	Medication	N	Dosage	Mechanism of action	Design	Result
Haney et al. 2010	Baclofen	10	60, 90 mg/day	GABA$_B$ receptor agonist and antispasmodic	Randomized, double-blind, placebo-controlled, crossover	Dose-dependently decreased craving for tobacco and marijuana but did not decrease relapse; worsened cognitive performance
	Mirtazapine	11	30 mg/day	Antagonist at multiple 5-HT receptor antagonists and α_2 receptors; enhances noradrenergic and serotonergic transmission		Improved sleep during abstinence and increased food intake but no effect on withdrawal symptoms and marijuana relapse
Haney et al. 2001	Bupropion SR	10	300 mg/day	Noradrenergic and dopamine reuptake inhibitor	Randomized, double-blind, placebo-controlled, crossover	Worsened measures of irritability, restlessness, and depression; difficulty sleeping

Table 4–1. Laboratory studies: pharmacological treatment of cannabis dependence *(continued)*

Study	Medication	N	Dosage	Mechanism of action	Design	Result
Cone et al. 1988	Clonidine	3	0.1–0.4 mg pretreatment dose over 4 days	α_2 Agonist	Single-blind, placebo-controlled	No changes in subjective effects from smoked marijuana
Haney et al. 2004	Divalproex sodium	7	1,500 mg/day	Enhances neurotransmission of GABA, histone deacetylase inhibitor	Randomized, double-blind, placebo-controlled, crossover	Decreased ratings of marijuana craving but increased ratings of anxiety, irritability, and tiredness
Bowen et al. 2005	Lithium	9	600 mg on day 4, 900 mg on days 5–8, and 600 mg on day 9	Unknown	Open-label	Variable self-reported improvement in withdrawal
Winstock et al. 2009	Lithium	20	500 mg/day for 7 inpatient days	Unknown	Open-label	High percentage of days abstinent after inpatient detoxification

Table 4–1. Laboratory studies: pharmacological treatment of cannabis dependence *(continued)*

Study	Medication	N	Dosage	Mechanism of action	Design	Result
Haney et al. 2008	Lofexidine and oral THC	8	2.4 mg/day 60 mg/day	Lofexidine: α_2 agonist Oral THC: partial CB_1 receptor agonist	Randomized, double-blind, placebo-controlled, crossover	Reduced withdrawal and relapse alone and in combination with dronabinol, although combination superior to other groups on some measures; marijuana craving and relapse most reduced with combination
Sugarman et al. 2011	Modafinil and oral THC	12	400 mg/day 15 mg/day	Modafinil: enhancement of glutamate release and inhibition of GABA release as well as dopamine and noradrenergic transporter inhibition Oral THC: partial CB_1 agonist	Double-blind, placebo-controlled, crossover	No marijuana administered; modafinil increased vigor and tension; oral THC increased feeling of high and sedation; combination had significantly less euphoria than other conditions

Table 4–1. Laboratory studies: pharmacological treatment of cannabis dependence *(continued)*

Study	Medication	N	Dosage	Mechanism of action	Design	Result
Haney et al. 2003b	Nefazodone	7	450 mg/day	Serotonin and noradrenergic reuptake inhibitor, 5-HT$_2$ receptor antagonist	Randomized, double-blind, placebo-controlled, crossover	Reduced anxiety but not other withdrawal symptoms and did not change subjective effects of smoked marijuana
Greenwald and Stitzer 2000	Naltrexone	5	50 mg/day or 200 mg/day	μ Opioid receptor antagonist	Randomized, double-blind, placebo-controlled, crossover	Marijuana alone produced dose-dependent antinociception; opioid antagonist had no effect on smoked marijuana–induced antinociception
Wachtel and de Wit 2000	Naltrexone and oral THC	14	0 mg/day and 50 mg/day	μ Opioid receptor antagonist	Randomized, double-blind, placebo-controlled, crossover	Naltrexone did not alter the subjective, physiological, or behavioral effects of oral THC
Haney et al. 2003a	Naltrexone	9	50 mg/day	μ Opioid receptor antagonist	Randomized, double-blind, placebo-controlled	Naltrexone increased high-dose oral THC pleasurable effects

Table 4–1. Laboratory studies: pharmacological treatment of cannabis dependence (*continued*)

Study	Medication	N	Dosage	Mechanism of action	Design	Result
Haney 2007	Naltrexone	Study 1: marijuana smokers: 22; Study 2: marijuana non-smokers: 21	12 mg/day	μ Opioid receptor antagonist	Randomized, double-blind, placebo-controlled, crossover	Low-dose naltrexone decreased subjective effects of low-dose oral THC (20 mg) and increased anxiety at higher THC dose (40 mg) in heavy marijuana smokers; in nonmarijuana smokers, low-dose naltrexone increased subjective effects of low-dose oral THC (2.5 mg) and decreased anxiety at higher THC dose (10 mg)
Cooper and Haney 2010	Naltrexone	29	12, 25, 50, or 100 mg/day	μ Opioid antagonist	Randomized, double-blind, placebo-controlled	Naltrexone decreased performance on cognitive tasks, and all doses increased positive subjective and physiological effects of smoked marijuana

Table 4–1. Laboratory studies: pharmacological treatment of cannabis dependence (*continued*)

Study	Medication	N	Dosage	Mechanism of action	Design	Result
Haney et al. 2003b	Nefazodone	7	450 mg/day	Noradrenaline and serotonin reuptake inhibitor, 5-HT$_2$ receptor antagonist	Randomized, double-blind, placebo-controlled, crossover	Nefazodone decreased ratings of anxiety and muscle pain but not total withdrawal severity or subjective effects of smoked marijuana
Hart et al. 2002	Oral THC	12	10, 40, 80 mg/day	Partial CB$_1$ agonist	Single-blind, placebo-controlled	Good drug effect and high of smoked marijuana reduced by oral THC; neither dose of oral THC affected self-administration of marijuana
Haney et al. 2004	Oral THC	7	10 mg 5 times/day	Partial CB$_1$ agonist	Randomized, double-blind, placebo-controlled, crossover	Oral THC decreased ratings of marijuana withdrawal and craving and reversed decreases in food intake

Table 4–1. Laboratory studies: pharmacological treatment of cannabis dependence *(continued)*

Study	Medication	N	Mechanism of action	Dosage	Design	Result
Budney et al. 2007	Oral THC	8	Partial CB$_1$ agonist	0, 10, 30 mg 3 times/day	Randomized, double-blind, placebo-controlled, crossover	Lower dose reduced some withdrawal symptoms; higher dose produced additional suppression of withdrawal symptoms
Huestis et al. 2007	Rimonabant	42	CB$_1$ antagonist	40 mg/day for 15 days; placebo for 14 days, then rimonabant 90 mg for 1 day; placebo for 15 days	Randomized, double-blind, placebo-controlled	Lower-dose rimonabant partially blocked acute effects of smoked marijuana at 8 days of administration, but neither repeated lower dose nor single higher dose significantly blocked acute smoked marijuana effects at 15 days
Huestis et al. 2001	Rimonabant	63	CB$_1$ receptor antagonist	1–90 mg/day	Randomized, double-blind, placebo-controlled	Partially blocked acute effects of smoked marijuana

Note. CB=cannabinoid receptor; GABA=γ-aminobutyric acid; 5-HT=serotonin; SR=sustained release; THC=delta-9-tetrahydrocannabinol.

At present, naltrexone and oral THC (dronabinol) have been the most extensively studied in the human laboratory. Naltrexone was initially investigated because a series of animal studies found that it decreased THC's discriminative effects (Solinas and Goldberg 2005) and reduced cannabinoid self-administration (Justinova et al. 2004). In one human laboratory study, naltrexone did not alter the subjective, physiological, or behavioral effects of oral THC (Wachtel and de Wit 2000). Haney (2007) and colleagues (Haney et al. 2003a, 2003b) extensively studied naltrexone at low and higher doses and found that it did not reduce the subjective effects of oral THC; moreover, at a range of doses, naltrexone enhanced the pleasurable effects of smoked marijuana (Cooper and Haney 2010). It is notable that these studies used naltrexone for pretreatment but did not continue naltrexone prior to marijuana administration, which could have affected the results. In a different line of investigation, Greenwald and Stitzer (2000) found that the opioid antagonist did not affect smoked marijuana–induced antinociception. Although these studies suggest that naltrexone has little promise as a therapeutic agent for the treatment of cannabis dependence, a trial of an extended period of dosing may be indicated before concluding that naltrexone has no therapeutic value for the disorder.

Given that agonist approaches have been effective in treating opioid and nicotine dependence (Amato et al. 2005; Berrettini and Lerman 2005), it is not surprising that they have been extensively studied in heavy marijuana users. Hart et al. (2002) found that oral THC reduced the positive subjective effects of smoked marijuana. Haney et al. (2004) found that oral THC also decreased ratings of marijuana withdrawal and craving. In a subsequent study with higher, less frequent dosing, oral THC again significantly reduced withdrawal symptoms but also was associated with greater drug liking, latency to sleep, and irritability than was placebo (Haney et al. 2008). Notably, in an outpatient study of non-treatment-seeking heavy marijuana users, Budney et al. (2007) found that a high dose of oral THC (30 mg three times daily) alleviated withdrawal symptoms so effectively that individuals who ceased using smoked marijuana had no more withdrawal symptoms than did those in the smoking-as-usual condition. Of note, the high dose was easily distinguished from placebo, whereas the low dose (10 mg three times daily) was not. Despite these promising results, oral THC has not been found to reduce self-administration (Hart et al. 2002), even after a period of abstinence (Haney et al. 2010).

Limitations of these studies were that the alternative reinforcer (a $2 voucher) or the maintenance period on oral THC (3 days) may not have been adequate to alter behavior. Subsequently, in a study in which it was more costly for subjects to take an initial puff of marijuana after a period of abstinence and the maintenance period was extended, oral THC still did not maintain abstinence better than placebo (Haney et al. 2008).

Another therapeutic strategy is to block rather than simply reduce the subjective effects of marijuana, similar to the use of naltrexone to treat opioid dependence. Huestis and colleagues (2001) conducted two important proof-of-concept studies evaluating the subjective effects of smoked marijuana in individuals administered rimonabant. The first study found that pretreatment with rimonabant significantly reduced (but did not eliminate) the subjective and physiological effects of smoked marijuana (Huestis et al. 2001). In the second study, repeated administration of a lower dose of rimonabant (40 mg) partially blocked the acute effects of smoked marijuana after 8 days of administration, but repeated dosing did not significantly block the effects of smoked marijuana after 2 weeks. Furthermore, single administration of a high dose of rimonabant (90 mg) reduced smoked marijuana–induced tachycardia but did not substantially reduce subjective effects. Although the use of an antagonist may provide a useful treatment strategy, other antagonists should be considered because rimonabant has been associated with a risk of precipitating depression and suicidal ideation (Huestis et al. 2007). Individuals often are not compliant with antagonists because they neither induce positive subjective effects nor alleviate withdrawal, and withdrawal symptoms may be precipitated by antagonist treatment; therefore, this approach may be of value only in patients with a high level of motivation to stop their marijuana use.

Similar to other areas of medicine, there has been interest in developing combined pharmacotherapies. Given that oral THC might have some therapeutic utility, and lofexidine, an α_2-adrenergic receptor agonist available in the United Kingdom, has been found useful to treat opioid withdrawal, each medication alone and in combination was compared with placebo in reducing withdrawal symptoms and self-administration of marijuana after a period of marijuana abstinence. The combination of oral THC and lofexidine was superior to the other conditions in treating withdrawal. Both the combination treatment and lofexidine alone were superior to placebo in reducing self-administration of marijuana.

In summary, some medications have shown promise in the laboratory and have been safely administered in conjunction with smoked marijuana (e.g., modafinil, oral THC, the combination of oral THC and lofexidine, nabilone, cannabinoid antagonists). However, these agents should be evaluated in clinical trials to assess their efficacy.

Pharmacological Clinical Trials Evaluating Marijuana Abusers Seeking Treatment

Although marijuana is the most commonly abused illicit drug, it is striking that there have been so few controlled pharmacological clinical trials. There have been fewer than 11 published case reports, open trials, and double-blind, placebo-controlled studies (Table 4–2). Four of these trials targeted cannabis-dependent individuals with psychiatric comorbidity. The trials conducted have examined the efficacy of attention-deficit/hyperactivity disorder (ADHD) medications (atomoxetine), antidepressants (bupropion, nefazodone, venlafaxine, fluoxetine), anxiolytic agents (buspirone), mood stabilizers (divalproex sodium), antipsychotics (quetiapine), partial cannabinoid agonists (oral THC, dronabinol), and glutaminergic enhancers (NAC).

Because this treatment literature is nascent, few of these pharmacological agents have been studied in more than one trial. Atomoxetine, a medication approved for the treatment of adult ADHD, was evaluated because individuals with cannabis dependence have difficulties with concentration, memory, and executive functioning (Grant et al. 2012; Solowij et al. 2002; Thoma et al. 2011) and therefore might benefit from a medication that enhances attention and concentration (Tirado et al. 2008). Although atomoxetine produced a modest reduction in drug use, it was poorly tolerated, with substantial gastrointestinal distress.

Buspirone was studied with the hope that it might reduce withdrawal-induced anxiety and facilitate abstinence. An open trial conducted with the drug showed that treatment reduced craving and irritability. However, only 2 of the 10 patients enrolled completed the study, making it difficult to draw any conclusions (McRae et al. 2006). The same research group conducted a double-blind treatment trial, analyzing the data from 50 participants with a modified intent-to-treat analysis. They found a trend toward a greater percentage of negative urine test results in the active treatment arm, but there were no differences in self-reported days of use (McRae-Clark et al. 2009).

Table 4–2. Clinical studies: pharmacological treatment of adults with cannabis use disorders

Study	Medication	N	Dosage	Mechanism of action	Design	Result
Tirado et al. 2008	Atomoxetine	13 (8 included in the analysis)	25–80 mg/day	Selective noradrenergic reuptake inhibitor	Open-label	Trend for reduction in use and increase in percentage of days abstinent; no effect on urine drug screens, with 94% positive during study; troublesome adverse effects (gastrointestinal)
McRae et al. 2006	Buspirone	11 (10 included in the analysis)	Up to 60 mg/day	5-HT$_{1A}$ receptor partial agonist	Open-label	Reduced cannabis use, craving, and irritability, but only 2 of 10 participants completed 12-week trial

Table 4–2. Clinical studies: pharmacological treatment of adults with cannabis use disorders *(continued)*

Study	Medication	N	Dosage	Mechanism of action	Design	Result
McRae-Clark et al. 2009	Buspirone	59 (50 included in the analysis)	Up to 60 mg/day	5-HT$_{1A}$ receptor partial agonist	Randomized, double-blind, placebo-controlled	Modified intent-to-treat sample (patients who gave at least one urine sample postrandomization); trend for negative urine drug screen results to be higher in treatment group; no difference in self-reported days of use; completers analysis (less than half of randomized sample) found higher negative urine drug screen results in treatment group
Levin et al. 2004	Divalproex sodium	25	1,500–2,000 mg/day	Mechanism unknown	Randomized, double-blind, placebo-controlled, crossover	No difference between drug and placebo in any measure of marijuana use

Table 4–2. Clinical studies: pharmacological treatment of adults with cannabis use disorders (*continued*)

Study	Medication	N	Dosage	Mechanism of action	Design	Result
Levin and Kleber 2008	Oral THC	2	20–40 mg/day, other medications provided clinically	Partial CB_1 receptor agonist	Case reports	Helped attain long-term marijuana abstinence
Levin et al. 2011	Oral THC	156	20 mg twice a day	Partial CB_1 receptor agonist	Randomized, double-blind, placebo-controlled	Reduced marijuana withdrawal symptoms and improved retention but failed to improve abstinence
Carpenter et al. 2009	Nefazodone	106	Up to 300 mg twice a day	Noradrenergic and serotonergic reuptake inhibitor and $5\text{-}HT_{2A}$ receptor antagonist	Randomized, double-blind, placebo-controlled	Overall reductions in marijuana use and marijuana dependence severity, but no differences were found between either drug or placebo in terms of abstinence or withdrawal symptoms
	Bupropion		Up to 150 mg twice a day	Noradrenergic reuptake inhibitor and dopaminergic reuptake inhibitor		

Note. CB=cannabinoid receptor; 5-HT=serotonin; THC=delta-9-tetrahydrocannabinol.

Concurrent with the work conducted in a laboratory setting (Haney et al. 2004), Levin et al. (2004) conducted a small double-blind trial comparing divalproex sodium with placebo for relapse prevention. Although both groups reduced their marijuana use, there was no difference between groups, and adherence was poor. Another treatment study, conducted in conjunction with and then subsequent to the laboratory work (Haney et al. 2001, 2003b), compared nefazodone and bupropion with placebo in a randomized controlled trial. Although patients in all three treatment arms improved, none of the treatments was proved to be superior (Carpenter et al. 2009).

A medication that has been recently investigated for the treatment of cannabis dependence is the mucolytic agent NAC. NAC reduced reinstatement of drug-seeking behavior in animals, perhaps through modification of glutaminergic transmission via the cystine-glutamate exchanger (Kalivas 2009; Kau et al. 2008). NAC is hypothesized to reduce the use of various drugs of abuse, including marijuana. An open trial in adolescents showed that the agent was well tolerated, with a reduction in self-reported use, although urine test results did not change.

As mentioned previously, agonist approaches in the laboratory have been shown to reduce withdrawal symptoms but not self-administration. Two case reports suggested that oral THC might have some clinical utility in reducing marijuana use and facilitating abstinence (Levin and Kleber 2008). In the largest randomized controlled pharmacological trial to date in cannabis-dependent adults, oral THC was compared with placebo (Levin et al. 2011) in 156 outpatients. The investigators found that treatment with oral THC was associated with greater treatment retention and a reduction in withdrawal symptoms. However, no group differences in abstinence rates were seen. Nonetheless, treatment with oral THC shows promise and warrants further investigation, either in combination with more intensive psychotherapies or in combination with other medications (such as lofexidine). An alternative approach would be to use potent partial agonists (such as nabilone).

Psychiatric Comorbidity

Although most clinical treatment trials have excluded cannabis-dependent individuals with psychiatric comorbidity, a substantial number of cannabis-dependent individuals have mood and/or anxiety disorders (Chen et al. 2002; Degenhardt et al. 2003), ADHD (Dennis et al. 2004), and, less commonly, schizophrenia (Arseneault et al. 2002; Moore et al. 2007). Patients with un-recognized or untreated psychiatric symptoms have been repeatedly shown to do less well in substance abuse treatment (Kranzler et al. 1996; Levin et al. 2004; Rooke et al. 2011). It has been hypothesized that when the underlying psychiatric illness is effectively treated, patients with dual diagnoses may be more likely to respond to substance abuse treatment. Although numerous tri-als have evaluated various pharmacotherapies for dual disorders, many of these studies included mixed samples of patients who identified alcohol, mar-ijuana, or other drugs as their primary drug of abuse (Baker et al. 2010; Riggs et al. 2010) (Table 4–3).

In a small open-label trial, cannabis-dependent individuals with bipolar ill-ness or schizophrenia reduced their marijuana use when taking quetiapine (Potvin et al. 2004). Two studies have evaluated treatment with fluoxetine in depressed individuals. One study was a secondary analysis of adult marijuana users entering a randomized, double-blind, placebo-controlled trial for de-pressed alcoholic patients (Cornelius et al. 1999). Those receiving fluoxetine were more likely to reduce the amount and frequency of their marijuana use compared with the placebo group. A subsequent study in depressed adolescents seeking treatment for their problematic marijuana use found that fluoxetine was not superior to placebo in reducing depressive symptoms or marijuana use (Cornelius et al. 2010). The placebo response rate in this trial was high, per-haps lessening the likelihood of detecting a group difference.

McRae-Clark and colleagues (2010) used a modified intent-to-treat analy-sis to assess atomoxetine in a randomized, double-blind, placebo-controlled de-sign in 50 adults with ADHD. No significant differences in ADHD symptom improvement occurred between the two treatment arms, and no reduction in marijuana use was found, again suggesting that noradrenergic agents may not be beneficial in cannabis-dependent populations (McRae-Clark et al. 2010).

Conclusion

There has been limited study of medications to treat cannabis dependence. To date, few double-blind, placebo-controlled treatment trials have been con-ducted, with most of the controlled research occurring primarily in laboratory settings with those who are not seeking treatment. Although the capacity to generalize results from the laboratory to clinical settings is limited, they can

Table 4–3.   Pharmacological treatment of adults with cannabis use disorder and comorbid psychiatric disorders

Study	Medication	N	Dosage	Mechanism of action	Design	Result
McRae-Clark et al. 2010	Atomoxetine	78 with adult ADHD (38 in the analysis, those who were randomized and returned for at least one postrandomization visit)	100 mg/day	Selective noradrenergic reuptake inhibitor	Double-blind, placebo-controlled	Decreased ADHD symptoms but not superior to placebo on most outcome measures; did not reduce marijuana use
Cornelius et al. 1999	Fluoxetine	22 with depression (primary alcoholic patients who are heavy marijuana users)	20–40 mg/day	Selective serotonin reuptake inhibitor	Randomized, double-blind, placebo-controlled	The placebo group used 20 times more marijuana cigarettes and had 5 times more days of use during the trial
Cornelius et al. 2010	Fluoxetine	70 with depression (participants ages 14–25)	20 mg/day	Selective serotonin reuptake inhibitor	Double-blind, placebo-controlled	Decreased depressive symptoms but not superior to placebo; no reduction in marijuana use

Table 4–3. Pharmacological treatment of adults with cannabis use disorder and comorbid psychiatric disorders *(continued)*

Study	Medication	N	Dosage	Mechanism of action	Design	Result
Potvin et al. 2004	Quetiapine	8 (4 with schizophrenia and 4 with bipolar disorder)	100–1,200 mg/day	Antagonist at multiple 5-HT receptor subtypes, α_2 receptor antagonist	Open trial	Reduction in weekly amount of marijuana use

Note. ADHD=attention-deficit/hyperactivity disorder; 5-HT=serotonin.

provide data on how well tolerated various pharmacological agents are in combination with the controlled administration of oral THC and smoked marijuana and how effective these agents might be in reducing withdrawal symptoms, the subjective effects of marijuana, and self-administration. Ultimately, the clinical utility of these agents needs to be tested in treatment trials with diverse patient samples and varying types and intensity of behavioral interventions. To date, partial agonists have been studied most extensively and show promise as a therapeutic approach for cannabis dependence. Other agents worthy of future investigation include those that modulate glutaminergic transmission, increase dopamine synaptic concentration, or act as 5-HT_{1A} receptor partial agonists or serotonin receptor antagonists.

References

Aceto MD, Scates SM, Lowe JA, et al: Cannabinoid precipitated withdrawal by the selective cannabinoid receptor antagonist, SR 141716A. Eur J Pharmacol 282:R1–R2, 1995

Amato L, Davoli M, Perucci CA, et al: An overview of systematic reviews of the effectiveness of opiate maintenance therapies: available evidence to inform clinical practice and research. J Subst Abuse Treat 28:321–329, 2005

Arseneault L, Moffit TE, Caspi A, et al: The targets of violence committed by young offenders with alcohol dependence, marijuana dependence and schizophrenia-spectrum disorders: findings from a birth cohort. Crim Behav Ment Health 12:155–168, 2002

Baker AL, Hides L, Lubman DI: Treatment of cannabis use among people with psychotic or depressive disorders: a systematic review. J Clin Psychiatry 71:247–254, 2010

Berrettini WH, Lerman CE: Pharmacotherapy and pharmacogenetics of nicotine dependence. Am J Psychiatry 162:1441–1451, 2005

Best AR, Regehr WG: Serotonin evokes endocannabinoid release and retrogradely suppresses excitatory synapses. J Neurosci 28:6508–6515, 2008

Bossong MG, van Berckel BN, Boellaard R, et al: Delta9-tetrahydrocannabinol induces dopamine release in the human striatum. Neuropsychopharmacology 34:759–766, 2009

Bowen R, McIlwrick J, Baetz M, Zhang X: Lithium and marijuana withdrawal. Can J Psychiatry 50:240–241, 2005

Braida D, Pozzi M, Parolaro D, et al: Intracerebral self-administration of the cannabinoid receptor agonist CP 55,940 in the rat: interaction with the opioid system. Eur J Pharmacol 413:227–234, 2001

Breivogel CS, Scates SM, Beletskaya IO, et al: The effects of delta9-tetrahydrocannabinol physical dependence on brain cannabinoid receptors. Eur J Pharmacol 459:139–150, 2003

Buchowski MS, Meade NN, Charboneau E, et al: Aerobic exercise training reduces cannabis craving and use in non-treatment seeking cannabis-dependent adults. PLoS One 6:E17465, 2011

Budney AJ, Novy PL, Hughes JR: Marijuana withdrawal among adults seeking treatment for marijuana dependence. Addiction 94:1311–1322, 1999

Budney AJ, Higgins ST, Radonovich KJ, et al: Adding voucher-based incentives to coping skills and motivational enhancement improves outcomes during treatment for marijuana dependence. J Consult Clin Psychol 68:1051–1061, 2000

Budney AJ, Hughes JR, Moore BA, et al: Marijuana abstinence effects in marijuana smokers maintained in their home environment. Arch Gen Psychiatry 58:917–924, 2001

Budney AJ, Moore BA, Rocha HL, et al: Clinical trial of abstinence-based vouchers and cognitive-behavioral therapy for cannabis dependence. J Consult Clin Psychol 74:307–316, 2006

Budney AJ, Vandrey RG, Hughes JR, et al: Oral delta-9-tetrahydrocannabinol suppresses cannabis withdrawal symptoms. Drug Alcohol Depend 86:22–29, 2007

Budney AJ, Fearer S, Walker DD, et al: An initial trial of a computerized behavioral intervention for cannabis use disorder. Drug Alcohol Depend 115:74–79, 2010

Butler H, Korbonits M: Cannabinoids for clinicians: the rise and fall of the cannabinoid antagonists. Eur J Endocrinol 161:655–662, 2009

Caldeira KM, Arria AM, O'Grady KE, et al: The occurrence of cannabis use disorders and other cannabis-related problems among first-year college students. Addict Behav 33:397–411, 2008

Carpenter KM, McDowell D, Brooks DJ, et al: A preliminary trial: double-blind comparison of nefazodone, bupropion-SR, and placebo in the treatment of cannabis dependence. Am J Addict 18:53–64, 2009

Carroll KM, Rounsaville BJ: A perfect platform: combining contingency management with medications for drug abuse. Am J Drug Alcohol Abuse 33:343–365, 2007

Chen CY, Wagner FA, Anthony JC: Marijuana use and the risk of major depressive episode: epidemiological evidence from the United States National Comorbidity Survey. Soc Psychiatry Psychiatr Epidemiol 37:199–206, 2002

Chen CY, O'Brien MS, Anthony JC: Who becomes cannabis dependent soon after onset of use? Epidemiological evidence from the United States: 2000–2001. Drug Alcohol Depend 79:11–22, 2005

Compton WM, Grant BF, Colliver JD, et al: Prevalence of marijuana use disorders in the United States: 1991–1992 and 2001–2002. JAMA 291:2114–2121, 2004

Cone EJ, Welch P, Lange WR: Clonidine partially blocks the physiologic effects but not the subjective effects produced by smoking marijuana in male human subjects. Pharmacol Biochem Behav 29:649–652, 1988

Cooper ZD, Haney M: Opioid antagonism enhances marijuana's effects in heavy marijuana smokers. Psychopharmacology (Berl) 211:141–148, 2010

Copeland J, Swift W, Roffman R, et al: A randomized controlled trial of brief cognitive-behavioral interventions for cannabis use disorder. J Subst Abuse Treat 21:55–64; discussion 65–56, 2001

Cornelius JR, Salloum IM, Haskett RF, et al: Fluoxetine versus placebo for the marijuana use of depressed alcoholics. Addict Behav 24:111–114, 1999

Cornelius JR, Chung T, Martin C, et al: Cannabis withdrawal is common among treatment-seeking adolescents with cannabis dependence and major depression, and is associated with rapid relapse to dependence. Addict Behav 33:1500–1505, 2008

Cornelius JR, Bukstein OG, Douaihy AB, et al: Double-blind fluoxetine trial in comorbid MDD-CUD youth and young adults. Drug Alcohol Depend 112:39–45, 2010

Cui SS, Bowen RC, Gu GB, et al: Prevention of cannabinoid withdrawal syndrome by lithium: involvement of oxytocinergic neuronal activation. J Neuroscience 21:9867–9876, 2001

Degenhardt L, Hall W, Lynskey M: Exploring the association between cannabis use and depression. Addiction 98:1493–1504, 2003

Dennis M, Godley SH, Diamond G, et al: The Cannabis Youth Treatment (CYT) Study: main findings from two randomized trials. J Subst Abuse Treat 27:197–213, 2004

D'Souza DC, Ranganathan M, Braley G, et al: Blunted psychotomimetic and amnestic effects of delta-9-tetrahydrocannabinol in frequent users of cannabis. Neuropsychopharmacology 33:2505–2516, 2008

Elsohly MA, Slade D: Chemical constituents of marijuana: the complex mixture of natural cannabinoids. Life Sci 78:539–548, 2005

Fattore L, Cossu G, Martellotta CM, et al: Intravenous self-administration of the cannabinoid CB1 receptor agonist WIN 55,212–2 in rats. Psychopharmacology (Berl) 156:410–416, 2001

Gardner B, Zu LX, Sharma S, et al: Autocrine and paracrine regulation of lymphocyte CB2 receptor expression by TGF-beta. Biochem Biophys Res Commun 290:91–96, 2002

Gillespie NA, Neale MC, Kendler KS: Pathways to cannabis abuse: a multi-stage model from cannabis availability, cannabis initiation and progression to abuse. Addiction 104:430–438, 2009

Glass M, Dragunow M, Faull RL: Cannabinoid receptors in the human brain: a detailed anatomical and quantitative autoradiographic study in the fetal, neonatal and adult human brain. Neuroscience 77:299–318, 1997

Gong JP, Onaivi ES, Ishiguro H, et al: Cannabinoid CB2 receptors: immunohistochemical localization in rat brain. Brain Res 1071:10–23, 2006

Grant JE, Chamberlain SR, Schreiber L, et al: Neuropsychological deficits associated with cannabis use in young adults. Drug Alcohol Depend 121:159–162, 2012

Greenwald MK, Stitzer ML: Antinociceptive, subjective and behavioral effects of smoked marijuana in humans. Drug Alcohol Depend 59:261–275, 2000

Haney M: Opioid antagonism of cannabinoid effects: differences between marijuana smokers and nonmarijuana smokers. Neuropsychopharmacology 32:1391–1403, 2007

Haney M, Ward AS, Comer SD, et al: Abstinence symptoms following oral THC administration to humans. Psychopharmacology (Berl) 141:385–394, 1999

Haney M, Ward AS, Comer SD, et al: Bupropion SR worsens mood during marijuana withdrawal in humans. Psychopharmacology (Berl) 155:171–179, 2001

Haney M, Bisaga A, Foltin RW: Interaction between naltrexone and oral THC in heavy marijuana smokers. Psychopharmacology (Berl) 166:77–85, 2003a

Haney M, Hart CL, Ward AS, et al: Nefazodone decreases anxiety during marijuana withdrawal in humans. Psychopharmacology (Berl) 165:157–165, 2003b

Haney M, Hart CL, Vosburg SK, et al: Marijuana withdrawal in humans: effects of oral THC or divalproex. Neuropsychopharmacology 29:158–170, 2004

Haney M, Hart CL, Vosburg SK, et al: Effects of THC and lofexidine in a human laboratory model of marijuana withdrawal and relapse. Psychopharmacology (Berl) 197:157–168, 2008

Haney M, Hart CL, Vosburg SK, et al: Effects of baclofen and mirtazapine on a laboratory model of marijuana withdrawal and relapse. Psychopharmacology (Berl) 211:233–244, 2010

Hart CL, Haney M, Ward AS, et al: Effects of oral THC maintenance on smoked marijuana self-administration. Drug Alcohol Depend 67:301–309, 2002

Hart CL, Haney M, Vosburg SK, et al: Reinforcing effects of oral Delta9-THC in male marijuana smokers in a laboratory choice procedure. Psychopharmacology (Berl) 181:237–243, 2005

Hasin DS, Keyes KM, Alderson D, et al: Cannabis withdrawal in the United States: results from NESARC. J Clin Psychiatry 69:1354–1363, 2008

Hayakawa K, Mishima K, Hazekawa M, et al: Cannabidiol potentiates pharmacological effects of Delta(9)-tetrahydrocannabinol via CB(1) receptor-dependent mechanism. Brain research 1188:157–164, 2008

Herkenham M, Lynn AB, Johnson MR, et al: Characterization and localization of cannabinoid receptors in rat brain: a quantitative in vitro autoradiographic study. J Neurosci 11:563–583, 1991

Hillig KW, Mahlberg PG: A chemotaxonomic analysis of cannabinoid variation in cannabis (Cannabaceae). Am J Bot 91:966–975, 2004

Hoffman AF, Oz M, Caulder T, et al: Functional tolerance and blockade of long-term depression at synapses in the nucleus accumbens after chronic cannabinoid exposure. J Neurosci 23:4815–4820, 2003

Huang P, Liu-Chen LY, Kirby LG: Anxiety-like effects of SR141716-precipitated delta9-tetrahydrocannabinol withdrawal in mice in the elevated plus-maze. Neurosci Lett 475:165–168, 2010

Huestis MA, Gorelick DA, Heishman SJ, et al: Blockade of effects of smoked marijuana by the CB1-selective cannabinoid receptor antagonist SR141716. Arch Gen Psychiatry 58:322–328, 2001

Huestis MA, Boyd SJ, Heishman SJ, et al: Single and multiple doses of rimonabant antagonize acute effects of smoked cannabis in male cannabis users. Psychopharmacology (Berl) 194:505–515, 2007

Ishiguro H, Iwasaki S, Teasenfitz L, et al: Involvement of cannabinoid CB2 receptor in alcohol preference in mice and alcoholism in humans. Pharmacogenomics J 7:380–385, 2007

Justinova Z, Tanda G, Redhi GH, et al: Self-administration of delta9-tetrahydrocannabinol (THC) by drug naive squirrel monkeys. Psychopharmacology (Berl) 169:135–140, 2003

Justinova Z, Tanda G, Munzar P, et al: The opioid antagonist naltrexone reduces the reinforcing effects of Delta 9 tetrahydrocannabinol (THC) in squirrel monkeys. Psychopharmacology (Berl) 173:186–194, 2004

Justinova Z, Goldberg SR, Heishman SJ, et al: Self-administration of cannabinoids by experimental animals and human marijuana smokers. Pharmacol Biochem Behav 81:285–299, 2005

Kadden RM, Litt MD, Kabela-Cormier E, et al: Abstinence rates following behavioral treatments for marijuana dependence. Addict Behav 32:1220–1236, 2007

Kalivas PW: The glutamate homeostasis hypothesis of addiction. Nat Rev Neurosci 10:561–572, 2009

Kau KS, Madayag A, Mantsch JR, et al: Blunted cystine-glutamate antiporter function in the nucleus accumbens promotes cocaine-induced drug seeking. Neuroscience 155:530–537, 2008

Kranzler HR, Del Boca FK, Rounsaville BJ: Comorbid psychiatric diagnosis predicts three-year outcomes in alcoholics: a posttreatment natural history study. J Stud Alcohol 57:619–626, 1996

Lang E, Engelander M, Brooke T: Report of an integrated brief intervention with self-defined problem cannabis users. J Subst Abuse Treat 19:111–116, 2000

Levin FR, Kleber HD: Use of dronabinol for cannabis dependence: two case reports and review. Am J Addict 17:161–164, 2008

Levin FR, McDowell D, Evans SM, et al: Pharmacotherapy for marijuana dependence: a double-blind, placebo-controlled pilot study of divalproex sodium. Am J Addict 13:21–32, 2004

Levin FR, Mariani J, Brooks DJ, et al: Dronabinol for the treatment of cannabis dependence: a randomized, double-blind, placebo-controlled trial. Drug Alcohol Depend 116:142–150, 2011

Lichtman AH, Wiley JL, LaVecchia KL, et al: Effects of SR 141716A after acute or chronic cannabinoid administration in dogs. Eur J Pharmacol 357:139–148, 1998

Marijuana Treatment Project Research Group: Brief treatments for cannabis dependence: findings from a randomized multisite trial. J Consult Clin Psychol 72:455–466, 2004

Martellotta MC, Cossu G, Fattore L, et al: Self-administration of the cannabinoid receptor agonist WIN 55,212–2 in drug-naive mice. Neuroscience 85:327–330, 1998

Martin-Santos R, Fagundo AB, Crippa JA, et al: Neuroimaging in cannabis use: a systematic review of the literature. Psychol Med 40:383–398, 2010

Matsuda LA, Bonner TI, Lolait SJ: Localization of cannabinoid receptor mRNA in rat brain. J Comp Neurol 327:535–550, 1993

McLaren J, Swift W, Dillon P, et al: Cannabis potency and contamination: a review of the literature. Addiction 103:1100–1109, 2008

McRae AL, Brady KT, Carter RE: Buspirone for treatment of marijuana dependence: a pilot study. Am J Addict 15:404, 2006

McRae-Clark AL, Carter RE, Killeen TK, et al: A placebo-controlled trial of buspirone for the treatment of marijuana dependence. Drug Alcohol Depend 105:132–138, 2009

McRae-Clark AL, Carter RE, Killeen TK, et al: A placebo-controlled trial of atomoxetine in marijuana-dependent individuals with attention deficit hyperactivity disorder. Am J Addict 19:481–489, 2010

Melis M, Pistis M, Perra S, et al: Endocannabinoids mediate presynaptic inhibition of glutamatergic transmission in rat ventral tegmental area dopamine neurons through activation of CB1 receptors. J Neurosci 24:53–62, 2004

Moore TH, Zammit S, Lingford-Hughes A, et al: Cannabis use and risk of psychotic or affective mental health outcomes: a systematic review. Lancet 370:319–328, 2007

Morakinyo O: Aversion therapy of cannabis dependence in Nigeria. Drug Alcohol Depend 12:287–293, 1983

Olmstead TA, Petry NM: The cost-effectiveness of prize-based and voucher-based contingency management in a population of cocaine- or opioid-dependent outpatients. Drug Alcohol Depend 102:108–115, 2009

Onaivi ES, Ishiguro H, Gong JP, et al: Discovery of the presence and functional expression of cannabinoid CB2 receptors in brain. Ann N Y Acad Sci 1074:514–536, 2006

Pertwee RG: The diverse CB1 and CB2 receptor pharmacology of three plant cannabinoids: delta9-tetrahydrocannabinol, cannabidiol and delta9-tetrahydrocannabivarin. Br J Pharmacol 153:199–215, 2008

Petry NM, Alessi SM, Hanson T, et al: Randomized trial of contingent prizes versus vouchers in cocaine-using methadone patients. J Consult Clin Psychol 75:983–991, 2007

Piomelli D: The molecular logic of endocannabinoid signalling. Nat Rev Neurosci 4:873–884, 2003

Pope HG Jr, Gruber AJ, Hudson JI, et al: Neuropsychological performance in long-term cannabis users. Arch Gen Psychiatry 58:909–915, 2001

Potvin S, Stip E, Roy JY: The effect of quetiapine on cannabis use in 8 psychosis patients with drug dependency. Can J Psychiatry 49:711, 2004

Radwan MM, Elsohly MA, Slade D, et al: Biologically active cannabinoids from high-potency Cannabis sativa. J Nat Prod 72:906–911, 2009

Riggs PD, Winhusen T, Davies RD, et al: Randomized controlled trial of osmotic-release methylphenidate with cognitive-behavioral therapy in adolescents with attention-deficit/hyperactivity disorder and substance use disorders. J Am Acad Child Adolesc Psychiatry 50:903–914, 2010

Rooke SE, Norberg MM, Copeland J: Successful and unsuccessful cannabis quitters: comparing group characteristics and quitting strategies. Subst Abuse Treat Prev Policy 6:30, 2011

Russo EB: History of cannabis and its preparations in saga, science, and sobriquet. Chem Biodivers 4:1614–1648, 2007

Smith JW, Schmeling G, Knowles PL: A marijuana smoking cessation clinical trial utilizing THC-free marijuana, aversion therapy, and self-management counseling. J Subst Abuse Treat 5:89–98, 1988

Solinas M, Goldberg SR: Involvement of mu-, delta- and kappa-opioid receptor subtypes in the discriminative-stimulus effects of delta-9-tetrahydrocannabinol (THC) in rats. Psychopharmacology (Berl) 179:804–812, 2005

Solowij N, Stephens RS, Roffman RA, et al: Cognitive functioning of long-term heavy cannabis users seeking treatment. JAMA 287:1123–1131, 2002

Stephens RS, Roffman RA, Curtin L: Comparison of extended versus brief treatments for marijuana use. J Consult Clin Psychol 68:898–908, 2000

Stinson FS, Grant BF, Dawson DA, et al: Comorbidity between DSM-IV alcohol and specific drug use disorders in the United States: results from the National Epidemiologic Survey on Alcohol and Related Conditions. Drug Alcohol Depend 80:105–116, 2005

Stinson FS, Ruan WJ, Pickering R, et al: Cannabis use disorders in the USA: prevalence, correlates and co-morbidity. Psychol Med 36:1447–1460, 2006

Substance Abuse and Mental Health Services Administration: Results from the 2010 National Survey on Drug Use and Health: Summary of National Findings (NSDUH Series H-41, HHS Publ No SMA 11-4658). Rockville, MD, Substance Abuse and Mental Health Services Administration, 2011. Available at: http://www.samhsa.gov/data/NSDUH/2k10NSDUH/2k10Results.htm#Fig5.2. Accessed November 19, 2012.

Sugarman DE, Poling J, Sofuoglu M: The safety of modafinil in combination with oral 9-tetrahydrocannabinol in humans. Pharmacol Biochem Behav 98:94–100, 2011

Sun Y, Bennett A: Cannabinoids: a new group of agonists of PPARs. PPAR Res 2007:23513, 2007

Tanda G, Munzar P, Goldberg SR: Self-administration behavior is maintained by the psychoactive ingredient of marijuana in squirrel monkeys. Nat Neurosci 3:1073–1074, 2000

Thoma RJ, Monnig MA, Lysne PA, et al: Adolescent substance abuse: the effects of alcohol and marijuana on neuropsychological performance. Alcohol Clin Exp Res 35:39–46, 2011

Tirado CF, Goldman M, Lynch K, et al: Atomoxetine for treatment of marijuana dependence: a report on the efficacy and high incidence of gastrointestinal adverse events in a pilot study. Drug Alcohol Depend 94:254–257, 2008

Tsou K, Patrick SL, Walker JM: Physical withdrawal in rats tolerant to delta 9-tetrahydrocannabinol precipitated by a cannabinoid receptor antagonist. Eur J Pharmacol 280:R13–15, 1995

Tzavara ET, Valjent E, Firmo C, et al: Cannabinoid withdrawal is dependent upon PKA activation in the cerebellum. Eur J Neurosci 12:1038–1046, 2000

Van Sickle MD, Duncan M, Kingsley PJ, et al: Identification and functional characterization of brainstem cannabinoid CB2 receptors. Science 310:329–332, 2005

Vardakou I, Pistos C, Spiliopoulou C: Spice drugs as a new trend: mode of action, identification and legislation. Toxicol Lett 197:157–162, 2010

Viveros MP, Marco EM, File SE: Endocannabinoid system and stress and anxiety responses. Pharmacol Biochem Behav 81:331–342, 2005

Wachtel SR, de Wit H: Naltrexone does not block the subjective effects of oral Delta(9)-tetrahydrocannabinol in humans. Drug Alcohol Depend 59:251–260, 2000

Walker DD, Stephens R, Roffman R, et al: Randomized controlled trial of motivational enhancement therapy with nontreatment-seeking adolescent cannabis users: a further test of the teen marijuana check-up. Psychol Addict Behav 25:474–484, 2011

Ware MA, St Arnaud-Trempe E: The abuse potential of the synthetic cannabinoid nabilone. Addiction 105:494–503, 2010

Winstock AR, Lea T, Copeland J: Lithium carbonate in the management of cannabis withdrawal in humans: an open-label study. J Psychopharmacol 23:84–93, 2009

5

Stimulants

Kyle M. Kampman, M.D.

Stimulant, including cocaine, dependence is a significant public health problem. Although the rates of current cocaine and amphetamine use have declined since 2005, there are still 1.5 million regular cocaine users and about 353,000 regular methamphetamine users in the United States (Substance Abuse and Mental Health Services Administration 2011b). Cocaine and methamphetamine abuse and dependence continue to place a great deal of demand on the health care system. The Drug Abuse Warning Network Survey in 2008 reported that emergency department visits associated with drug use increased by 70% from 2004 to 2008. Cocaine was involved in nearly half (48.5%) of the 2 million emergency department visits involving illicit drugs, with methamphetamine use accounting for 9.3% of the emergency department visits (Substance Abuse and Mental Health Services Administration 2011a).

The demand for treatment of cocaine and other stimulant dependence remains high. The rate of admission to drug treatment programs for cocaine dependence ranked third among illicit drugs, behind only marijuana and heroin dependence. The rate of admission for stimulant dependence was fifth highest among the illicit drugs (see Table 5–1) (Substance Abuse and Mental Health Services Administration 2011c). So, despite some decline in the number of regular users of cocaine and amphetamine, abuse and dependence on these drugs result in a great deal of morbidity and place a significant burden on health care resources.

Although progress has been made in developing new psychosocial treatments for stimulant dependence, standard psychotherapy alone does not provide substantial benefit for many patients (Alterman et al. 1996; Carroll 2004; Kampman et al. 2001). Thus, medications have been sought to augment psychosocial treatment. Although no medications are currently approved to treat cocaine or amphetamine dependence, progress in the understanding of the neurobiology of stimulant dependence has led to the discovery of several promising medications that have already shown encouraging results in controlled clinical trials. Novel compounds, currently in early clinical studies, have shown promise and should soon be available for testing in controlled clinical trials.

Neurobiology of Cocaine and Amphetamine Dependence

Both cocaine and amphetamine increase arousal, alertness, and motor activity and are highly reinforcing in humans. Both drugs act—by different mechanisms—to increase transmission of the monoamine neurotransmitters dopamine, norepinephrine, and serotonin. Although cocaine and amphetamine affect all three neurotransmitters, their activity on dopamine neurotransmission has been most closely associated with their reinforcing effects. Thus, the dopaminergic system has been the main focus of pharmacological strategies to treat cocaine and amphetamine dependence. In addition, chronic cocaine use has been shown to modify other neurotransmitter systems such as those involving γ-aminobutyric acid (GABA) and glutamate. These neurotransmitter systems also have been targeted to treat cocaine and amphetamine dependence.

Cocaine increases monoamine transmission by blocking the reuptake of norepinephrine, serotonin, and dopamine into presynaptic neurons (White and Kalivas 1998). By increasing synaptic levels of dopamine in certain brain regions, such as the nucleus accumbens, cocaine induces a strong sense of pleasure. Activation of the nucleus accumbens by natural reinforcers, such as food and sex, ensures that these survival-associated behaviors are maintained.

Table 5–1.   Rates of admission to substance abuse treatment programs for various substances, per 100,000 persons age 12 and older

Drug	Rate of admission per 100,000
Alcohol	314
Marijuana	136
Heroin	108
Cocaine	71
Prescription pain relievers	53
Stimulants	44

Source.   Substance Abuse and Mental Health Services Administration 2011c.

Cocaine artificially elevates dopamine levels in the nucleus accumbens much higher than levels generated by natural stimuli, inducing a tremendous euphoria that far exceeds pleasure resulting from natural reinforcers (Nestler 2005). Laboratory animals given unlimited access to cocaine have been known to use it until they starve (Wise and Bozarth 1985).

Although blockade of norepinephrine reuptake and serotonin reuptake may not be crucial to the euphorigenic and reinforcing properties of cocaine or amphetamine, these neurotransmitter systems may be important in maintaining cocaine and amphetamine dependence, making them potential targets for pharmacotherapy. For example, norepinephrine may be critically important in stress-induced relapse to cocaine. α_2-Noradrenergic agonists have been shown to decrease stress-induced relapse to cocaine seeking in rats (Erb et al. 2000). Norepinephrine also appears to be critical for the development of stimulant sensitization, a process thought to be important for development of stimulant dependence. Mice lacking α_1-noradrenergic receptors do not develop this sensitization (Drouin et al. 2002). Likewise, lesioning noradrenergic neurons in the locus coeruleus or depleting central norepinephrine will also block the development of amphetamine sensitization (Archer et al. 1986; Kostowski et al. 1982). (See Sofuoglu and Sewell [2008] for a review.) Serotonin reuptake appears to play an important role in shaping cocaine's euphorigenic and reinforcing properties, although the data are complicated, and no consensus exists for a clear direction for pharmacological intervention (Nonkes et al. 2011).

Nonmonoaminergic neurotransmitter effects of cocaine use have been identified and may be used as pharmacological targets in medication development. Chronic cocaine use leads to profound changes in glutamatergic neurotransmission in the limbic system, particularly the nucleus accumbens. These changes appear to be critical in mediating behaviors characteristic of addiction, including drug craving and relapse. Acutely, cocaine administration has little or no effect on extracellular glutamate levels in the nucleus accumbens, but withdrawal from chronic cocaine use reduces basal extracellular glutamate levels (Schmidt and Pierce 2010). Normalization of basal extracellular glutamate levels has been shown to prevent reinstatement of drug-seeking behavior induced by a priming dose of cocaine (Schmidt and Pierce 2010). In rats pretreated with repeated cocaine administrations, cocaine administration increased glutamate release in the nucleus accumbens core. Blockade of the α-amino-3-hydroxy-5-methyl-4-isoxazolepropionic acid (AMPA)–type glutamate receptors blocked the reinstatement of cocaine-primed drug-seeking behavior (Park et al. 2002). Thus, chronic cocaine use appears to alter glutamate activity in the nucleus accumbens, changes that appear to be associated with the relapse process.

Amphetamine and methamphetamine also increase monoaminergic neurotransmission, but their mechanism of action is somewhat different from that of cocaine. Cocaine acts primarily by reuptake blockade, whereas amphetamines both block the reuptake of monoamines and stimulate the release of catecholamines from nerve terminals. Amphetamine and methamphetamine increase cytosolic dopamine and reverse the normal activity of the dopamine transporter, which causes the transporter to release dopamine into the synapse (Brown et al. 2001; Khoshbouei et al. 2003). Amphetamines also appear to stimulate the release of norepinephrine (Azzaro et al. 1974). Amphetamine has much greater activity at the norepinephrine transporter compared with cocaine, and this may have implications for pharmacological treatments. In humans, the subjective effects of amphetamine are closely related to its ability to stimulate the release of norepinephrine (Rothman et al. 2001). Medications that affect noradrenergic neurotransmission may hold more promise to treat amphetamine or methamphetamine dependence.

Cocaine and amphetamine/methamphetamine also differ in their duration of action. The half-life of amphetamine and methamphetamine is considerably longer than that of cocaine. This may lead to a different pattern of use for amphetamine and cocaine that could have implications for their associated toxicities and the development of effective medications.

Behavioral Effects of Cocaine and Amphetamines

Cocaine and amphetamine are central nervous system stimulants. They produce dose-dependent increases in heart rate and blood pressure along with increased arousal, alertness, and sense of well-being. Higher doses produce euphoria. Often, the brief period of euphoria is followed by a strong urge to repeat the dose. Involuntary motor activity, stereotyped behavior, and psychosis can occur after repeated doses. Repeated use of cocaine and amphetamine can lead to addiction. Characteristics of this addiction include behavioral sensitization and physical dependence with a characteristic withdrawal syndrome.

Behavioral sensitization is a long-lasting increase in behavioral response occurring on repeated presentation of a stimulus that reliably elicits a response at its initial presentation (Koob 1996). In this model of drug dependence, intermittent administration of cocaine leads to an increase in the subjective effects of cocaine and cocaine craving, leading to a loss of control over use, and finally, addiction. Some preclinical studies and human laboratory studies have shown the development of sensitization to stimulants under controlled conditions (Ahmed and Cador 2006; Schenk and Partridge 1997). However, cocaine-dependent patients rarely report an increase in the subjective effects of cocaine over time. This observation has led researchers to suggest that the *hedonic dysregulation* model better explains cocaine addiction. In this model, adaptive processes within the body lead to decreased subjective effects of the drug (tolerance) and a negative affective state when drug use is stopped (withdrawal). Tolerance and withdrawal arise from neurochemical changes in brain reward and stress pathways, inducing a negative motivation state that drives addiction (Koob 1996, 2006). Other investigators have tried to find a middle ground, proposing that drug craving (the desire to use a drug) and drug liking (the euphoric effects of the drug) are differentially regulated in a model called *incentive sensitization.* They suggest that brain systems that mediate incentive salience (craving) become sensitized to drugs and associated stimuli while the reward system that regulates euphoric effects becomes tolerant to drugs. The

uncoupling of these feelings results in intense craving and drug-seeking behavior without enjoyment of the drugs being sought (Robinson and Berridge
1993, 2001; Small et al. 2009).

Cocaine withdrawal symptoms include dysphoric mood, fatigue, sleep
disturbance, appetite changes, and irritability (Kampman et al. 1998). Patients entering treatment with severe cocaine withdrawal symptoms often
drop out of treatment prematurely and are less likely to attain abstinence from
cocaine in outpatient treatment programs (Kampman et al. 1998, 2001,
2002; Mulvaney et al. 1999). Because cocaine-dependent patients who have
withdrawal symptoms (cocaine withdrawal syndrome) experience cocaine differently, poor treatment outcomes may result. Several investigators have noted
that cocaine-dependent patients who experience cocaine withdrawal symptoms report a greater high from experimentally administered cocaine (Newton et al. 2003; Sofuoglu et al. 2003; Uslaner et al. 1999). The increased
euphoria that patients with cocaine withdrawal syndrome experience may
make the drug more rewarding and therefore more difficult to give up.

Amphetamine and methamphetamine dependence, like cocaine dependence, has been linked to a withdrawal syndrome. Amphetamine withdrawal
symptoms are similar to cocaine withdrawal symptoms and include increased
appetite, increased sleep, and dysphoria. McGregor and colleagues (2005)
characterized the nature and time course of amphetamine withdrawal. They
reported a two-phase syndrome, with an acute phase lasting 7–10 days during
which patients experienced an increased appetite, increased sleep, depression,
fatigue, anhedonia, and dysphoria. These symptoms peaked during the first
24 hours after the last use of amphetamine and declined linearly over time.
The second, or subacute, phase lasted 2–3 weeks and consisted of similar but
more attenuated symptoms. Older patients, patients with more severe dependence, and patients with a longer history of amphetamine use had more severe
withdrawal symptoms.

Use of both cocaine and amphetamine has been associated with the development of psychotic symptoms, including both delusions and hallucinations (Brady et al. 1991; McKetin et al. 2006; Satel et al. 1991). Among
cocaine users, psychotic symptoms have been reported in more than half of
the patients admitted to inpatient treatment programs (Brady et al. 1991; Satel et al. 1991). Delusions and hallucinations occur with equal frequency, and
no clear association is found between amount and duration of cocaine use and

the presence of psychotic symptoms. Among methamphetamine users, the rate of psychotic symptoms has been shown to be 11 times greater than the rate of psychotic symptoms in the general public (McKetin et al. 2006). In a trial that compared the psychotic symptoms reported by both amphetamine and cocaine users, Mahoney and colleagues (2008) found that methamphetamine users were more likely to report psychotic symptoms compared with cocaine users. This may be a result of the different mechanism of action of amphetamine (monoamine release as opposed to reuptake blockade for cocaine) or the longer half-life of amphetamine (11 hours vs. 90 minutes for cocaine).

Pharmacological Treatments

Although no medications are currently approved to treat cocaine dependence or amphetamine dependence, several medications have shown potential efficacy in controlled clinical trials for cocaine dependence, and a few have shown efficacy for the treatment of amphetamine dependence. Others appear promising based on more preliminary trials. Medications to treat cocaine dependence and amphetamine dependence are discussed separately. First, I describe medications that have potential efficacy reported in controlled clinical trials, which are grouped according to the neurotransmitter system they are thought to target. Vaccines are discussed next, followed by promising medications. Finally, I discuss medications found to be efficacious only when used in conjunction with a novel psychosocial treatment called contingency management.

Medications to Treat Cocaine Dependence

Dopamine Agonists

Agonist treatments have been used successfully to treat both opioid and nicotine dependence. Ideally, in agonist treatment, the medication used should be one that binds to the same receptor as the abused drug, exerts similar effects, and has pharmacological properties that render it less susceptible to abuse than the drug for which it is being substituted. Effective agonist treatments for opioid dependence include methadone, because of its slow onset, and buprenorphine, because of its partial agonist activity at the opioid receptors. Likewise, the transdermal nicotine patch's slow absorption contributes to its effectiveness in the treatment of nicotine dependence. Cocaine has diverse effects in the brain and, unlike nicotine and opiates, does not have a single molecular target. Therefore, finding an effective agonist treatment for cocaine dependence has been more challenging.

Agonist treatments for cocaine dependence have thus far focused on the dopaminergic properties of cocaine. Methylphenidate, an amphetamine analog, was ineffective for the treatment of cocaine dependence in one trial (Grabowski et al. 1997). However, Levin and colleagues (2007) found that among cocaine-dependent patients with comorbid attention-deficit/hyperactivity disorder (ADHD), methylphenidate therapy was associated with decreased cocaine use. Limited success has been achieved with amphetamine and methamphetamine to treat cocaine dependence. In 2001, Grabowski and colleagues published results of the first pilot trial evaluating dextroamphetamine to treat cocaine dependence. In this 12-week trial, 128 cocaine-dependent patients were randomly assigned to placebo, low-dose dextroamphetamine (30 mg/day), or high-dose dextroamphetamine (60 mg/day). Treatment retention was significantly better in the low-dose amphetamine group. Cocaine use was nonsignificantly lower in the high-dose amphetamine group. Dropout rates for all groups were high. In a subsequent trial by the same group involving 120 cocaine- and opioid-dependent patients stabilized on methadone, significant reductions in cocaine use were seen in patients taking 60 mg of dextroamphetamine compared with placebo or 30 mg. Again, treatment retention in this trial was poor, with fewer than 50% of the subjects completing the trial (Grabowski et al. 2004). Most recently, a trial of immediate- and sustained-release methamphetamine was conducted. In this trial, the sustained-release methamphetamine group submitted significantly fewer cocaine-positive urine drug screen results during the trial (29% sustained-release vs. 66% immediate-release vs. 60% placebo). However, the dropout rate in this trial was high, with only 32% of the patients completing the trial (Mooney et al. 2009). Although results, in general, favor amphetamine and methamphetamine, high dropout rates in all the trials make the results difficult to interpret.

Modafinil, a medication approved to treat narcolepsy and shift work sleep disorder, is under investigation to treat cocaine dependence. Proposed uses include the reduction of cocaine withdrawal symptoms, reduction in cocaine craving, and reduction in cocaine-induced euphoria. As a mild stimulant, modafinil may be able to reduce cocaine withdrawal symptoms (Dackis and O'Brien 2003). Modafinil has been shown to increase dopaminergic neurotransmission by blocking the dopamine transporter, and this may account for its ability to reduce cocaine withdrawal symptoms (Volkow et al. 2009). Modafinil also enhances glutamate neurotransmission (Touret et al. 1994). It may therefore be efficacious for cocaine dependence by ameliorating glutamate depletion seen in chronic cocaine users (Dackis and O'Brien 2003). Improved baseline glutamatergic tone in the nucleus accumbens prevents reinstatement of cocaine self-administration in an animal model of relapse (Baker et al. 2003).

Modafinil was found to block the euphoric effects of cocaine in three independent human laboratory studies (Dackis et al. 2003; Hart et al. 2007; Malcolm et al. 2002). First, Dackis and colleagues conducted a double-blind, placebo-controlled cocaine-modafinil interaction trial. In this trial, cocaine-dependent patients were given modafinil 200 mg, 400 mg, or placebo and then challenged with 30 mg of intravenous cocaine. Pretreatment with modafinil significantly blunted cocaine-induced euphoria in one of the subjective measures (Dackis et al. 2003). In a separate, but very similar, human laboratory trial, Malcolm and colleagues found that modafinil at both 400 and 800 mg significantly reduced the response to cocaine, as measured by visual analog scale ratings of "High," "Any drug effect," and "Worth in dollars," compared with cocaine alone (Malcolm et al. 2002). Most recently, Hart and colleagues evaluated the effect of modafinil on the self-administration of cocaine in a human laboratory trial. In this trial, the effects of modafinil maintenance (0, 200, and 400 mg/day) on response to smoked cocaine (0, 12, 25, and 50 mg) were examined in non-treatment-seeking cocaine-dependent individuals ($n=8$). Cocaine significantly increased self-administration, subjective-effect ratings, and cardiovascular measures (i.e., systolic and diastolic blood pressure, heart rate); modafinil at both doses (200 and 400 mg/day) markedly attenuated these effects (Hart et al. 2007).

A double-blind, placebo-controlled pilot trial of modafinil involving 62 cocaine-dependent patients was completed in 2004. In this trial, modafinil-treated patients submitted significantly more cocaine metabolite–free urine samples compared with placebo-treated patients (42% vs. 22%). Modafinil-treated patients were also rated as more improved compared with placebo-treated patients (Dackis et al. 2005).

The results of the pilot trial were partly replicated in a larger multicenter trial involving 210 cocaine-dependent patients. In this 16-week trial, cocaine-dependent patients received modafinil at a dosage of either 200 mg/day or

400 mg/day, or placebo. In contrast to the pilot trial, in which none of the patients were both cocaine and alcohol dependent, in this trial 41% of the patients were both alcohol and cocaine dependent. In the group as a whole, modafinil was not superior to placebo in promoting abstinence from cocaine. However, among patients who were not also alcohol dependent, both doses of modafinil were superior to placebo for promoting abstinence from cocaine (Anderson et al. 2009). Modafinil may be efficacious in only cocaine-dependent patients without alcohol dependence.

Enthusiasm for modafinil was somewhat dampened by the results of a clinical trial recently completed by Dackis and colleagues (2012). In this trial, 210 cocaine-dependent patients who were actively using cocaine at baseline were randomly assigned to 8 weeks of modafinil (0 mg/day, 200 mg/day, or 400 mg/day) combined with once-weekly cognitive-behavioral therapy. The investigators found no effect of modafinil at either dose on cocaine use or cocaine craving. Currently, two other clinical trials of modafinil are yet to be completed. The utility of modafinil to treat cocaine dependence has not been established.

Disulfiram, an approved treatment for alcohol dependence, is also a promising medication for the treatment of cocaine dependence. Its mechanism of action in the treatment of alcohol dependence is based on its blockade of the enzyme aldehyde dehydrogenase and the subsequent buildup of the toxic metabolite acetaldehyde when alcohol is ingested, which produces a characteristic unpleasant reaction. Disulfiram also blocks the degradation of cocaine and dopamine by the enzyme dopamine β-hydroxylase, which leads to extremely high cocaine and dopamine levels when cocaine is ingested (Karamanakos et al. 2001; McCance-Katz et al. 1998). This may affect cocaine use by decreasing the reinforcing properties of cocaine or by making cocaine use aversive (Hameedi et al. 1995; McCance-Katz et al. 1998).

In three of four placebo-controlled clinical trials, disulfiram reduced cocaine use in cocaine-dependent patients (Carroll et al. 1998, 2004; George et al. 2000; Petrakis et al. 2000). Petrakis and colleagues compared disulfiram with placebo in 67 cocaine- and opioid-dependent patients maintained on methadone. They found that disulfiram-treated patients self-reported significantly less cocaine use in a 12-week trial (Petrakis et al. 2000). In a smaller trial done with cocaine- and opioid-dependent patients maintained on buprenorphine, disulfiram was significantly better than placebo in reducing cocaine use measured by urine drug screens (George et al. 2000). In a trial of 130 cocaine-dependent patients not dependent on opioids, disulfiram was associated with less cocaine use measured by urine drug screens. In this trial, patients without a history of alcohol use responded better to disulfiram, confirming disulfiram's specific effect on cocaine use (Carroll et al. 2004). More recently, disulfiram at a dosage of 250 mg/day was not found to be superior to placebo in reducing cocaine use in a trial involving 161 cocaine- and opioid-dependent patients maintained on methadone. Moreover, lower dosages of disulfiram (62.5 or 125 mg/day) were associated with significantly more cocaine use than was placebo (Oliveto et al. 2011). Although Carroll found disulfiram alone to be ineffective in patients with comorbid cocaine and alcohol dependence, Pettinati and colleagues (2008) found the combination of disulfiram and naltrexone to be better than placebo in promoting sustained abstinence from both cocaine and alcohol in patients with dual cocaine and alcohol dependence.

GABAergic and Glutamatergic Medications

Mesocortical dopaminergic neurons receive modulatory inputs from both GABAergic and glutamatergic neurons. GABA is primarily an inhibitory neurotransmitter in the central nervous system, and activation of GABAergic neurons tends to decrease activation in the dopaminergic reward system. Preclinical trials of medications that foster GABAergic neurotransmission have suggested that these compounds reduce the dopamine response to both cocaine administration and conditioned reminders of prior cocaine use (Dewey et al. 1992, 1997; Gerasimov et al. 1999). GABAergic medications also reduce the self-administration of cocaine in animal models (Kushner et al. 1999; Roberts et al. 1996). Therefore, GABAergic medications could prevent relapse either by blocking cocaine-induced euphoria or by reducing craving caused by exposure to conditioned reminders of prior cocaine use. Some promising GABAergic medications include vigabatrin, tiagabine, and topiramate.

Vigabatrin is an antiepileptic widely available worldwide for several years. It irreversibly inhibits GABA transaminase, elevating brain GABA concentrations. An association between the use of vigabatrin and visual field defects has limited its usefulness as an anticonvulsant. However, data suggest that visual field defects associated with vigabatrin occur after relatively long-term exposure and are less commonly associated with brief treatments (Manuchehri et al. 2000; Schmitz et al. 2002).

Preclinical trials of vigabatrin have been promising. Vigabatrin has been shown to block cocaine and cocaine cue–induced increases of dopamine in the nucleus accumbens (Dewey et al. 1997; Morgan and Dewey 1998). Vigabatrin has been shown to block cocaine self-administration in rodents (Kushner et al. 1999).

There have been three clinical trials of vigabatrin to treat stimulant dependence. The first two were small open-label trials involving 20 cocaine-dependent and 30 amphetamine-dependent patients (Brodie et al. 2003, 2005). In these trials, treatment completers showed significant reductions in drug use. In the first trial, 8 of 20 patients completed treatment and reported drug-free periods ranging from 46 to 58 days. In the second trial, 18 of 30 subjects completed treatment. Of these 18 subjects, 16 had negative drug test results for amphetamine and cocaine for the last 6 weeks of the trial.

The third trial was a double-blind, placebo-controlled study of vigabatrin in 106 cocaine-dependent subjects. After 1–3 weeks of a baseline/screening period, subjects were randomly assigned to receive either 3 g/day of vigabatrin or matching placebo during a 9-week medication phase. Significantly more vigabatrin-treated subjects achieved abstinence during the last 3 weeks of the trial compared with placebo-treated subjects (28% vs. 7%). In addition, for subjects who reported recent alcohol use at baseline, those taking vigabatrin were seven times more likely than those taking placebo to report full end-of-trial alcohol abstinence (43.5% vs. 6.3%; $P \leq 0.03$). Vigabatrin was safe and well tolerated (Brodie et al. 2009).

Tiagabine, another GABAergic medication, may be promising for the treatment of cocaine dependence. Tiagabine is a selective blocker of the presynaptic GABA reuptake transporter type 1; it is currently approved to treat seizures (Schachter 1999). Tiagabine was well tolerated and moderately effective for improving abstinence in a pilot study that included 45 cocaine- and opiate-dependent patients participating in a methadone maintenance program. In this 10-week trial, the number of cocaine metabolite–free urine samples increased by 33% in the group taking tiagabine 24 mg/day and decreased by 14% in the placebo-treated group (Gonzalez et al. 2003). In a more recent trial, Gonzalez et al. (2007) compared tiagabine with gabapentin and placebo in 76 cocaine- and opiate-dependent patients maintained on methadone. In this trial, tiagabine at 24 mg/day was superior to both placebo and gabapentin in promoting cocaine abstinence (Gonzalez et al. 2007). However, Winhusen and colleagues (2007) did not find tiagabine (20 mg/day) to be superior to placebo in 79 cocaine-dependent patients in a 12-week double-blind, placebo-controlled trial.

Topiramate, based on its effects on both GABA neurotransmission and glutamate neurotransmission, is under investigation for the relapse prevention treatment of cocaine dependence. Topiramate increases cerebral levels of GABA and facilitates GABA neurotransmission (Kuzniecky et al. 1998; Petroff et al. 1999). Topiramate also inhibits glutamate neurotransmission through a blockade of AMPA/kainate receptors (Gibbs et al. 2000). In animal models of cocaine relapse, blockade of AMPA receptors in the nucleus accumbens prevented reinstatement of cocaine self-administration (Cornish and Kalivas 2000).

In a 13-week double-blind, placebo-controlled pilot trial of topiramate for cocaine dependence involving 40 cocaine-dependent patients, topiramate-treated patients were significantly more likely to be abstinent during the last 5 weeks of the trial compared with placebo-treated patients. In addition, among patients who returned for at least one visit after receiving medications, topiramate-treated patients were significantly more likely to achieve at least 3 weeks of continuous abstinence from cocaine compared with placebo-treated patients (59% vs. 26%), and topiramate-treated patients were significantly more likely than placebo-treated patients to be rated very much improved at their last visit (71% vs. 32%) (Kampman et al. 2004).

Vaccines for Cocaine Dependence

The vaccine TA-CD works by stimulating the production of cocaine-specific antibodies that bind to cocaine molecules and prevent them from crossing the blood-brain barrier. Because cocaine is inhibited from entering the brain, its euphoric and reinforcing effects are reduced. Animal trials of TA-CD have shown that the vaccine produces cocaine-specific antibodies and decreases self-administration of cocaine in rodents (Kantak et al. 2000).

Human trials of TA-CD have been promising. Outcome data from two early human trials showed that the vaccine was well tolerated, stimulated high antibody titers, and reduced the euphoric effects of cocaine (Kosten et al. 2002; Martell et al. 2005). In a double-blind, placebo-controlled trial conducted in 115 cocaine- and opiate-dependent patients maintained on methadone, patients who received the vaccine and also achieved high immunoglobulin G antibody levels were significantly more likely to achieve abstinence from cocaine than were patients who received a placebo injection (Martell et al. 2009). A multicenter Phase III trial of TA-CD is ongoing.

Newer Medications for Cocaine Dependence

Several new compounds—including neurokinin-1 receptor (NK1R) antagonists, dopamine D_3 receptor antagonists, and N-acetylcysteine (NAC)—have been identified in preclinical trials as potentially useful treatments for cocaine dependence. These medications, which have not yet been studied in controlled clinical trials, are potential relapse prevention medications that may reduce cocaine-induced euphoria, craving for cocaine, or relapse to cocaine caused by stress.

Substance P is a neuropeptide that has been implicated in the response to stress, as well as reward-related behaviors. Substance P and its preferred receptor, NK1R, are highly expressed in brain areas involved in stress response and drug reward such as the hypothalamus, amygdala, and nucleus accumbens (Mantyh et al. 1984). NK1R antagonists such as aprepitant may be useful to treat cocaine dependence. Blockade of central NK1R results in antidepressant-related and anxiolytic-like activity in several animal models (Holmes et al. 2003). NK1R antagonists have been shown to reduce symptoms of social anxiety (Furmark et al. 2005), and the NK1R antagonist MK-869 was shown to be superior to placebo in the treatment of major depression (Kramer et al. 1998). That NK1R is involved in drug reward was first suggested by the fact that genetically altered mice without NK1R showed reduced alcohol consumption compared with wild-type control mice (George et al. 2008). NK1R antagonists also reduce striatal dopamine release provoked by cocaine administration (Loonam et al. 2003). Finally, activation of central NK1R induces reinstatement of cocaine-seeking behavior (Placenza et al. 2005).

Evidence supporting a direct effect of NK1R antagonists on cocaine reward is mixed. In one trial, the NK1R antagonist WIN51708 blocked the acquisition of sensitization to repeated doses of cocaine (Davidson et al. 2004). However, in a series of other trials, NK1R antagonists did not block cocaine-induced increases in locomotor activity, cocaine self-administration, or cocaine-induced reinstatement of drug-seeking behavior (Placenza et al. 2005, 2006). In addition, in mice with a genetic deletion of NK1R, neither the locomotor-activating effects of cocaine nor sensitization was altered (Ripley et al. 2002).

Although NK1R antagonists may not have a significant effect on cocaine reward, their effects on stress reduction may make them useful in preventing relapse, primarily through reductions in stress-induced craving. Stress has been shown to be a powerful inducer of cocaine craving and relapse. In human laboratory trials, stress has been shown to provoke cocaine craving, and patients with more stress-induced craving had greater corticotropin and cortisol response to stress. In this trial, stress-induced craving was associated with a shorter time to relapse during a 90-day period after discharge from inpatient treatment (Sinha et al. 2006). In clinical trials, patients with more cocaine withdrawal symptoms have worse outcomes in outpatient treatment compared with cocaine-dependent patients without cocaine withdrawal symptoms (Kampman et al. 2002; Mulvaney et al. 1999). Thus, NK1R antagonists may be useful in reducing stress-induced craving and relapse in cocaine-dependent patients.

Dopamine is central to the reinforcing effects of all drugs of abuse, including alcohol and cocaine. Among the first medications considered for the treatment of cocaine dependence were dopamine antagonists. The two main groups of dopamine receptors are the D_1–D_5 family and the D_2–D_3 family. Several representatives of antagonists to both groups of dopamine receptors have been evaluated for cocaine dependence treatment and have not been found to be efficacious. D_1 receptor antagonists such as ecopipam were simply ineffective (McCance-Katz et al. 2001). D_2 antagonists, although sometimes effective at reducing either cocaine or cue-induced craving in human laboratory studies, either had intolerable side effects or proved ineffective in clinical trials (Amato et al. 2007; Grabowski et al. 2000; Kampman et al. 2003; Loebl et al. 2008; Sayers et al. 2005).

D_3 receptor antagonists may be more effective than D_2 receptor antagonists. The high concentration of D_3 receptors in limbic structures suggests that these receptors may be most important in drug reward and addiction (Heidbreder et al. 2005). D_3 receptors have the highest affinity of all dopamine receptors for exogenous dopamine, again suggesting a predominant role for these receptors in reward and addiction (Levant 1997; Sokoloff et al. 2006). The net effect of D_3 receptor antagonism is a slight increase in dopaminergic tone, which may be useful in chronic cocaine users who generally have decreased dopaminergic tone (Heidbreder et al. 2005). Thus, D_3 receptor antagonism may be a better strategy than D_1 or D_2 receptor blockade to treat cocaine dependence.

The preclinical trials with D_3 receptor antagonists predict clinical usefulness. In almost every animal model of addiction, D_3 receptor antagonists appear to be useful to treat cocaine dependence. The D_3 receptor antagonist SB-277011 blocked both the acquisition and the expression of cocaine-induced conditioned place preference (Vorel et al. 2002). D_3 receptor antagonists also reduced cocaine-induced reinstatement of self-administration as well as conditioned cue-induced reinstatement of cocaine self-administration (Di Ciano et al. 2003; Vorel et al. 2002) and lowered the breakpoint in progressive ratio self-administration models (Xi et al. 2006). They also reduced stress-induced reinstatement of cocaine self-administration (Xi et al. 2004). Clinical trials with D_3 receptor antagonists are currently being planned.

The last of the promising medications ready for controlled clinical trials is NAC. NAC is an amino acid and a cysteine prodrug. In preclinical and some early pilot clinical trials, NAC has shown potential utility in the treatment of addictive disorders. Preclinical studies have suggested that levels of glutamate in the nucleus accumbens mediate reward-seeking behavior (Kalivas and Volkow 2005; McFarland et al. 2003). Low levels of extracellular glutamate in the nucleus accumbens are associated with chronic cocaine exposure. Through stimulation of the cysteine-glutamate antiporters, NAC may increase extracellular glutamate. This modulates the release of glutamate in response to drug taking via stimulation of metabotropic glutamate autoreceptors. This reduction in glutamate release may block drug-seeking behaviors and drug craving. In rats, NAC pretreatment blocked the reinstatement of drug-seeking behavior induced by cocaine or conditioned cues of cocaine (Baker et al. 2003). In a human laboratory trial, NAC reduced cocaine craving in non-treatment-seeking cocaine-dependent men and women (LaRowe et al. 2007). In an open-label trial, NAC was safe and well tolerated in cocaine-dependent patients (LaRowe et al. 2006).

Medications to Treat Amphetamine Dependence

The effort to find medications to treat amphetamine and methamphetamine dependence started much more recently than the search for a medication to treat cocaine dependence. Consequently, fewer medications have been tested. Similarities between the mechanisms of action of amphetamine and methamphetamine and cocaine have suggested that medications effective for cocaine dependence also may be effective for amphetamine and methamphetamine dependence, and several medications tested for treatment of cocaine dependence are currently undergoing or are about to undergo testing for treatment of methamphetamine dependence. So far, only bupropion has shown evidence of potential efficacy in controlled clinical trials.

Bupropion, an antidepressant medication, acts primarily as a reuptake inhibitor of dopamine and norepinephrine. It has also been shown to be effective in treating nicotine dependence. Bupropion's mechanism of action in the treatment of nicotine and methamphetamine dependence may be related to its effects on dopamine reuptake. It is thought to potentially alleviate stimulant withdrawal symptoms by facilitating dopamine neurotransmission. Bupropion was tested for treatment of cocaine dependence in the past and found to be ineffective (Margolin et al. 1995). For methamphetamine dependence, bupropion has been shown to be more promising.

Bupropion was tested for the treatment of methamphetamine dependence in 151 methamphetamine-dependent patients. In the group as a whole, methamphetamine treatment resulted in a nonsignificant trend toward more weeks of abstinence compared with placebo. In a subgroup of patients with less methamphetamine use at baseline, bupropion treatment was associated with significantly more weeks of abstinence for methamphetamine compared with placebo treatment (Elkashef et al. 2008). This finding was replicated in a subsequent trial involving 73 methamphetamine-dependent outpatients. Among light methamphetamine users (defined as 0–2 of 6 amphetamine-positive urine samples during a 2-week baseline), bupropion-treated patients had significantly more methamphetamine-free weeks measured by negative urine drug screen results than did placebo-treated patients (Shoptaw et al. 2008). This suggests that bupropion may be efficacious for less severe amphetamine users.

Combining Contingency Management With Medications

Voucher-based reinforcement therapy (VBRT) is a behavioral treatment intervention for substance use disorders in which patients receive vouchers redeemable for goods and services in the community contingent on achieving a predetermined therapeutic goal. VBRT has been shown to be highly effective in promoting initial abstinence from cocaine among cocaine-dependent patients (Higgins et al. 1994). Recently, researchers have begun to combine

VBRT with medications to augment medication response in cocaine-dependent patients. In several trials, patients receiving the combination of VBRT and medications have responded better than patients receiving either medications alone or VBRT alone. For example, Kosten and colleagues (2003) tested the efficacy of desipramine and VBRT in cocaine- and opiate-dependent patients maintained on buprenorphine. Previously, desipramine had not been found to be consistently efficacious for the treatment of cocaine dependence when combined with standard psychosocial treatment. In this trial, patients received desipramine or placebo with VBRT or a noncontingent voucher control. Cocaine-free and combined cocaine- and opiate-free urine samples increased more rapidly over time in those subjects receiving desipramine or VBRT. Those receiving both VBRT and desipramine had significantly more drug-free urine samples than did the other three groups (Kosten et al. 2003). In a double-blind, placebo-controlled trial of bupropion and VBRT, the combination of bupropion and VBRT was superior to bupropion alone, placebo, and VBRT alone in promoting abstinence from cocaine in cocaine-dependent patients (Poling et al. 2006). Similar results were found for the combination of the serotonin reuptake inhibitor (SRI) citalopram and VBRT (Moeller et al. 2007). Several SRIs have been tested to treat cocaine dependence, but, like desipramine, SRIs have not been found to be consistently efficacious for the treatment of cocaine dependence when used in association with standard psychosocial treatment. The use of VBRT as a psychosocial treatment platform appears to be highly effective in increasing the efficacy of certain medications to treat cocaine dependence.

Conclusion

The goal of finding an effective medication to treat cocaine or amphetamine dependence remains to be achieved. Nevertheless, several medications to treat cocaine dependence have shown promise in controlled trials and continue to be studied. Dopamine agonists and vigabatrin appear to be most promising at this point. Preliminary results also have shown a consistent response to bupropion among amphetamine-dependent patients with less severe disease. Many more trials are needed to identify medications to treat amphetamine dependence, because the process of medication development for this disorder is not as far along as that for cocaine dependence.

References

Ahmed SH, Cador M: Dissociation of psychomotor sensitization from compulsive cocaine consumption. Neuropsychopharmacology 31:563–571, 2006

Alterman AI, McKay JR, Mulvaney FD, et al: Prediction of attrition from day hospital treatment in lower socioeconomic cocaine-dependent men. Drug Alcohol Depend 40:227–233, 1996

Amato L, Minozzi S, Pani PP, et al: Antipsychotic medications for cocaine dependence. Cochrane Database of Systematic Reviews 2007, Issue 3. Art. No.: CD006306. DOI: 10.1002/14651858.CD006306.pub2.

Anderson AL, Reid MS, Li SH, et al: Modafinil for the treatment of cocaine dependence. Drug Alcohol Depend 104:133–139, 2009

Archer T, Fredriksson A, Jonsson G, et al: Central noradrenaline depletion antagonizes aspects of d-amphetamine-induced hyperactivity in the rat. Psychopharmacology (Berl) 88:141–146, 1986

Azzaro AJ, Ziance RJ, Rutledge CO: The importance of neuronal uptake of amines for amphetamine-induced release of 3H-norepinephrine from isolated brain tissue. J Pharmacol Exp Ther 189:110–118, 1974

Baker DK, McFarland K, Lake RW, et al: N-acetyl cysteine-induced blockade of cocaine-induced reinstatement. Ann NY Acad Sci 1003:349–351, 2003

Brady KT, Lydiard RB, Malcolm, R, et al: Cocaine-induced psychosis. J Clin Psychiatry 52:509–512, 1991

Brodie JD, Figueroa E, Dewey SL: Treating cocaine addiction: from preclinical to clinical trial experience with gamma-vinyl GABA. Synapse 50:261–265, 2003

Brodie JD, Figueroa E, Laska EM, et al: Safety and efficacy of gamma-vinyl GABA (GVG) for the treatment of methamphetamine and/or cocaine addiction. Synapse 55:122–125, 2005

Brodie JD, Case BG, Figueroa E, et al: Randomized, double-blind, placebo-controlled trial of vigabatrin for the treatment of cocaine dependence in Mexican parolees. Am J Psychiatry 166:1269–1277, 2009

Brown JM, Hanson GR, Fleckenstein AE: Regulation of the vesicular monoamine transporter-2: a novel mechanism for cocaine and other psychostimulants. J Pharmacol Exp Ther 296:762–767, 2001

Caroll K: Behavioral therapies for co-occurring substance use and mood disorders. Biol Psychiatry 56:778–784, 2004

Carroll K, Nich C, Ball, SA, et al: Treatment of cocaine and alcohol dependence with psychotherapy and disulfiram. Addiction 93:713–727, 1998

Carroll K, Fenton L, Ball SA, et al: Efficacy of disulfiram and cognitive behavioral therapy in cocaine dependent outpatients: a randomized placebo-controlled trial. Arch Gen Psychiatry 61:264–272, 2004

Cornish JL, Kalivas PW: Glutamate transmission in the nucleus accumbens mediates relapse in cocaine addiction. J Neurosci 20:RC89, 2000

Dackis C, O'Brien CP: Glutamatergic agents for cocaine dependence. Ann NY Acad Sci 1003:328–345, 2003

Dackis CA, Lynch KG, Yu E, et al: Modafinil and cocaine: a double-blind, placebo-controlled drug interaction study. Drug Alcohol Depend 70:29–37, 2003

Dackis C, Kampman KM, Lynch KG, et al: A double-blind, placebo-controlled trial of modafinil for cocaine dependence. Neuropsychopharmacology 30:205–211, 2005

Dackis CA, Kampman KM, Lych KG, et al: A double-blind, placebo-controlled trial of modafinil for cocaine dependence. J Subst Abuse Treat 43:303–312, 2012

Davidson C, Lee TH, Ellinwood EH: The NK(1) receptor antagonist WIN51708 reduces sensitization after chronic cocaine. Eur J Pharmacol 499:355–356, 2004

Dewey S, Smith G, Logan J, et al: GABAergic inhibition of endogenous dopamine release measured in vivo with 11c-raclopride and positron emission tomography. J Neurosci 12:3773–3780, 1992

Dewey SL, Chaurasia CS, Chen C, et al: GABAergic attenuation of cocaine-induced dopamine release and locomoter activity. Synapse 25:393–398, 1997

Di Ciano P, Underwood RJ, Hagan J, et al: Attenuation of cue-controlled cocaine-seeking by a selective D3 dopamine receptor antagonist SB-277011-A. Neuropsychopharmacology 28:329–338, 2003

Drouin C, Darracq L, Trovero F, et al: Alpha1b-adrenergic receptors control locomotor and rewarding effects of psychostimulants and opiates. J Neurosci 22:2873–2884, 2002

Elkashef AM, Rawson RA, Anderson AL, et al: Bupropion for the treatment of methamphetamine dependence. Neuropsychopharmacology 33:1162–1170, 2008

Erb S, Hitchcott PK, Rajabi H, et al: Alpha-2 adrenergic receptor agonists block stress-induced reinstatement of cocaine seeking. Neuropsychopharmacology 23:138–150, 2000

Furmark T, Appel L, Michelgard A, et al: Cerebral blood flow changes after treatment of social phobia with the neurokinin-1 antagonist GR205171, citalopram, or placebo. Biol Psychiatry 58:132–142, 2005

George DT, Gilman J, Hersh J, et al: Neurokinin 1 receptor antagonism as a possible therapy for alcoholism. Science 319:1536–1539, 2008

George TP, Chawarski MC, Pakes J, et al: Disulfiram versus placebo for cocaine dependence in buprenorphine-maintained subjects: a preliminary trial. Biol Psychiatry 47:1080–1086, 2000

Gerasimov MR, Ashby CR, Gardner EL, et al: Gamma-vinyl-GABA inhibits methamphetamine, heroin, or ethanol-induced increases in nucleus accumbens dopamine. Synapse 34:11–19, 1999

Gibbs J, Sombati S, DeLorenzo RJ, et al: Cellular actions of topiramate: blockade of kainate-evoked inward currents in cultured hippocampal neurons. Epilepsia 41 (suppl 1):S10–S16, 2000

Gonzalez G, Sevarino K, Sofuoglu M, et al: Tiagabine increases cocaine-free urines in cocaine-dependent methadone treated patients: results of a randomized pilot study. Addiction 98:1625–1632, 2003

Gonzalez G, Desai R, Sofuoglu, M, et al: Clinical efficacy of gabapentin versus tiagabine for reducing cocaine use among cocaine dependent methadone-treated patients. Drug Alcohol Depend 87:1–9, 2007

Grabowski J, Roache JD, Schmitz JM, et al: Replacement medication for cocaine dependence: methylphenidate. J Clin Psychopharmacol 17:485–488, 1997

Grabowski J, Rhoades H, Silverman P, et al: Risperidone for the treatment of cocaine dependence: randomized, double-blind trial. J Clin Psychopharmacol 20:305–310, 2000

Grabowski J, Rhoades H, Schmitz J, et al: Dextroamphetamine for cocaine-dependence treatment: a double-blind randomized clinical trial. J Clin Psychopharmacol 21:522–526, 2001

Grabowski J, Rhoades H, Stotts A, et al: Agonist-like or antagonist-like treatment for cocaine dependence with methadone for heroin dependence: two double-blind randomized clinical trials. Neuropsychopharmacology 29:969–981, 2004

Hameedi F, Rosen M, McCance-Katz EF, et al: Behavioral, physiological, and pharmacological interaction of cocaine and disulfiram in humans. Biol Psychiatry 37:560–563, 1995

Hart CL, Haney M, Vosberg SK, et al: Smoked cocaine self-administration is decreased by modafinil. Neuropsychopharmacology 33:761–768, 2007

Heidbreder CA, Gardner EL, Xi ZX, et al: The role of central dopamine D3 receptors in drug addiction: a review of pharmacological evidence. Brain Res Brain Res Rev 49:77–105, 2005

Higgins ST, Budney AJ, Bickel WK, et al: Incentives improve outcome in outpatient behavioral treatment of cocaine dependence. Arch Gen Psychiatry 51:568–576, 1994

Holmes A, Heilig M, Rupniak N, et al: Neuropeptide systems as novel therapeutic targets for depression and anxiety disorders. Trends Pharmacol Sci 24:580–588, 2003

Kalivas PW, Volkow ND: The neural basis of addiction: a pathology of motivation and choice. Am J Psychiatry 162:1403–1413, 2005

Kampman KM, Volpicelli JR, McGinnis DE, et al: Reliability and validity of the Cocaine Selective Severity Assessment. Addict Behav 23:449–461, 1998

Kampman KM, Alterman AI, Volpicelli JR, et al: Cocaine withdrawal symptoms and initial urine toxicology results predict treatment attrition in outpatient cocaine dependence treatment. Psychol Addict Behav 15:52–59, 2001

Kampman KM, Volpicelli JR, Mulvany FD, et al: Cocaine withdrawal severity and urine toxicology results from treatment entry predict outcome in medication trials for cocaine dependence. Addict Behav 27:251–260, 2002

Kampman KM, Pettinati H, Lynch KG, et al: A pilot trial of olanzapine for the treatment of cocaine dependence. Drug Alcohol Depend 70:265–273, 2003

Kampman KM, Pettinati H, Lynch KG, et al: A pilot trial of topiramate for the treatment of cocaine dependence. Drug Alcohol Depend 75:233–240, 2004

Kantak K, Collins S, Lipman EG, et al: Evaluation of anti-cocaine antibodies and a cocaine vaccine in a rat self-administration model. Psychopharmacology (Berl) 148:251–262, 2000

Karamanakos P, Pappas P, Stephanou P, et al: Differentiation of disulfiram effects on central catecholamines and hepatic ethanol metabolism. Pharmacol Toxicol 88:106–110, 2001

Khoshbouei, H, Wang H, Lechleiter JD, et al: Amphetamine-induced dopamine efflux: a voltage-sensitive and intracellular Na+-dependent mechanism. J Biol Chem 278:12070–12077, 2003

Koob GF: Drug addiction: the yin and yang of hedonic homeostasis. Neuron 16:893–896, 1996

Koob GF: The neurobiology of addiction: a neuroadaptational view relevant for diagnosis. Addiction 101 (suppl 1):23–30, 2006

Kosten T, Rosen M, Bond J, et al: Human therapeutic cocaine vaccine: safety and immunogenicity. Vaccine 20:1196–1204, 2002

Kosten T, Oliveto A, Feingold A, et al: Desipramine and contingency management for cocaine and opiate dependence in buprenorphine maintained patients. Drug Alcohol Depend 70:315–325, 2003

Kostowski W, Płaźnik A, Puciłowski O, et al: Effect of lesions of the brain noradrenergic systems on amphetamine-induced hyperthermia and locomotor stimulation. Acta Physiol Pol 33:383–387, 1982

Kramer MS, Cutler N, Feighner J, et al: Distinct mechanism for antidepressant activity by blockade of central substance P receptors. Science 281:1640–1645, 1998

Kushner SA, Dewey SL, Kornetsky C: The irreversible γ-aminobutyric acid (GABA) transaminase inhibitor γ-vinyl-GABA blocks cocaine self-administration in rats. J Pharmacol Exp Ther 290:797–802, 1999

Kuzniecky R, Hetherington H, Ho S, et al: Topiramate increases cerebral GABA in healthy humans. Neurology 51:627–629, 1998

LaRowe SD, Mardikian P, Malcolm R, et al: Safety and tolerability of N-acetylcysteine in cocaine-dependent individuals. Am J Addict 15:105–110, 2006

LaRowe SD, Myrick H, Hedden S, et al: Is cocaine desire reduced by N-acetylcysteine? Am J Psychiatry 164:1115–1117, 2007

Levant B: The D3 dopamine receptor: neurobiology and potential clinical relevance. Pharmacol Rev 49:231–252, 1997

Levin FR, Evans SM, Brooks DJ, et al: Treatment of cocaine dependent treatment seekers with adult ADHD: double-blind comparison of methylphenidate and placebo. Drug Alcohol Depend 87:20–29, 2007

Loebl T, Angarita GA, Pachas GN, et al: A randomized, double-blind, placebo-controlled trial of long-acting risperidone in cocaine-dependent men. J Clin Psychiatry 69:480–486, 2008

Loonam TM, Noailles PA, Yu J, et al: Substance P and cholecystokinin regulate neurochemical responses to cocaine and methamphetamine in the striatum. Life Sci 73:727–739, 2003

Mahoney JJ, Kalechstein AD, De La Garza R, et al: Presence and persistence of psychotic symptoms in cocaine- versus methamphetamine-dependent participants. Am J Addict 17:83–98, 2008

Malcolm RJ, Donovan CL, Devane A, et al: Influence of modafinil, 400 or 800 mg/day on subjective effects of intravenous cocaine in non-treatment seeking volunteers. Drug Alcohol Depend 66 (suppl 1):S110, 2002

Mantyh PW, Hunt SP, Maggio JE: Substance P receptors: localization by light microscopic autoradiography in rat brain using [3H]SP as the radioligand. Brain Res 307:147–165, 1984

Manuchehri K, Goodman S, Siviter L, et al: A controlled study of vigabatrin and visual abnormalities. Br J Ophthalmol 84:499–505, 2000

Margolin A, Kosten TR, Avants SK, et al: A multicenter trial of bupropion for cocaine dependence in methadone-maintained patients. Drug Alcohol Depend 40:125–131, 1995

Martell B, Mitchell E, Poling J, et al: Vaccine pharmacotherapy for the treatment of cocaine dependence. Biol Psychiatry 58:158–164, 2005

Martell BA, Orson FM, Poling J, et al: Cocaine vaccine for the treatment of cocaine dependence in methadone-maintained patients: a randomized, double-blind, placebo-controlled efficacy trial. Arch Gen Psychiatry 66:1116–1123, 2009

McCance-Katz E, Kosten T, Jatlow P: Disulfiram effects on acute cocaine administration. Drug Alcohol Depend 52:27–39, 1998

McCance-Katz EF, Kosten TA, Kosten TR: Going from the bedside back to the bench with ecopipam: a new strategy for cocaine pharmacotherapy development. Psychopharmacology 155:327–329, 2001

McFarland K, Lapish CC, Kalivas PW: Prefrontal glutamate release into the core of the nucleus accumbens mediates cocaine-induced reinstatement of drug-seeking behavior. J Neurosci 23:3531–3537, 2003

McGregor C, Srisurapanont M, Jittiwutikarn J, et al: The nature, time course and severity of methamphetamine withdrawal. Addiction 100:1320–1329, 2005

McKetin R, McLaren J, Lubman DI, et al: The prevalence of psychotic symptoms among methamphetamine users. Addiction 101:1473–1478, 2006

Moeller FG, Schmitz JM, Steinberg JL, et al: Citalopram combined with behavioral treatment reduces cocaine use: a double-blind, placebo-controlled trial. Am J Drug Alcohol Abuse 33:367–378, 2007

Mooney ME, Herin DV, Schmitz JM, et al: Effects of oral methamphetamine on cocaine use: a randomized, double-blind, placebo-controlled trial. Drug Alcohol Depend 101:34–41, 2009

Morgan AE, Dewey SL: Effects of pharmacologic increases in brain GABA levels on cocaine-induced changes in extracellular dopamine. Synapse 28:60–65, 1998

Mulvaney FD, Alterman AI, Boardman C, et al: Cocaine abstinence symptomatology and treatment attrition. J Subst Abuse Treat 16:129–135, 1999

Nestler EJ: The neurobiology of cocaine addiction. Sci Pract Perspect 3:4–10, 2005

Newton TA, Kalechstein AD, Tervo KE, et al: Irritability following abstinence from cocaine predicts euphoric effects of cocaine administration. Addict Behav 28:817–821, 2003

Nonkes L, van Bussell I, Verheil, MM, et al: The interplay between brain 5-hydroxytryptamine levels and cocaine addiction. Behav Pharmacol 22:723–738, 2011

Oliveto A, Poling J, Mancino MJ, et al: Randomized, double blind, placebo-controlled trial of disulfiram for the treatment of cocaine dependence in methadone-stabilized patients. Drug Alcohol Depend 113:184–191, 2011

Park WK, Bari AA, Jey AR, et al: Cocaine administered into the medial prefrontal cortex reinstates cocaine-seeking behavior by increasing AMPA receptor-mediated glutamate transmission in the nucleus accumbens. J Neurosci 22:2916–2925, 2002

Petrakis I, Carroll K, Nich C, et al: Disulfiram treatment for cocaine dependence in methadone-maintained opioid addicts. Addiction 95:219–228, 2000

Petroff OA, Hyder F, Mattson RH, et al: Topiramate increases brain GABA, homocarnasine, and pyrrolidinone in patients with epilepsy. Neurology 52:473–478, 1999

Pettinati HM, Kampman KM, Lynch KG, et al: A double blind, placebo-controlled trial that combines disulfiram and naltrexone for treating co-occurring cocaine and alcohol dependence. Addict Behav 33:651–667, 2008

Placenza FM, Vaccarino FJ, Fletcher PJ, et al: Activation of central neurokinin-1 receptors induces reinstatement of cocaine-seeking behavior. Neurosci Lett 390:42–47, 2005

Placenza FM, Fletcher PJ, Vaccarino F, et al: Effects of central neurokinin-1 receptor antagonism on cocaine- and opiate-induced locomotor activity and self-administration behaviour in rats. Pharmacol Biochem Behav 84:94–101, 2006

Poling J, Oliveto A, Petry N, et al: Six-month trial of bupropion with contingency management for cocaine dependence in a methadone-maintained population. Arch Gen Psychiatry 63:219–228, 2006

Ripley TL, Gadd CA, De Felipe C, et al: Lack of self-administration and behavioural sensitisation to morphine, but not cocaine, in mice lacking NK1 receptors. Neuropharmacology 43:1258–1268, 2002

Roberts DC, Andrews, MM, Vickers GJ: Baclofen attenuates the reinforcing effects of cocaine in rats. Neuropsychopharmacology 15:417–423, 1996

Robinson TE, Berridge KC: The neural basis of drug craving: an incentive-sensitization theory of addiction. Brain Res Brain Res Rev 18:247–291, 1993

Robinson TE, Berridge KC: Incentive-sensitization and addiction. Addiction 96:103–114, 2001

Rothman RB, Baumann MH, Dersch CM, et al: Amphetamine-type central nervous system stimulants release norepinephrine more potently than they release dopamine and serotonin. Synapse 39:32–41, 2001

Satel SL, Southwick SM, Gawin FH: Clinical features of cocaine-induced paranoia. Am J Psychiatry 148:495–498, 1991

Sayers SL, Campbell EC, Kondrich J, et al: Cocaine abuse in schizophrenic patients treated with olanzapine versus haloperidol. J Nerv Ment Dis 193:379–386, 2005

Schachter S: Tiagabine. Epilepsia 40:S17–S22, 1999

Schenk S, Partridge B: Sensitization and tolerance in psychostimulant self-administration. Pharmacol Biochem Behav 57:543–550, 1997

Schmidt HD, Pierce RC: Cocaine-induced neuroadaptations in glutamate transmission: potential therapeutic targets for craving and addiction. Ann N Y Acad Sci 1187: 35–75, 2010

Schmitz B, Schmidt T, Jokiel, B, et al: Visual field constriction in epilepsy patients treated with vigabatrin and other antiepileptic drugs: a prospective study. J Neurol 249:469–475, 2002

Shoptaw S, Heinzerling KG, Rotheram-Fuller E, et al: Randomized, placebo-controlled trial of bupropion for the treatment of methamphetamine dependence. Drug Alcohol Depend 96:222–232, 2008

Sinha R, Garcia M, Paliwal P, et al: Stress-induced cocaine craving and hypothalamic-pituitary-adrenal responses are predictive of cocaine relapse outcomes. Arch Gen Psychiatry 63:324–331, 2006

Small AC, Kampman KM, Plebani J, et al: Tolerance and sensitization to the effects of cocaine use in humans: a retrospective study of long-term cocaine users in Philadelphia. Subst Use Misuse 44:1888–1898, 2009

Sofuoglu M, Sewell RA: Norepinephrine and stimulant addiction. Addict Biol 14:119–129, 2008

Sofuoglu MS, Dudish-Poulsen S, Brown SB, et al: Association of cocaine withdrawal symptoms with more severe dependence and enhanced subjective response to cocaine. Drug Alcohol Depend 69:273–282, 2003

Sokoloff P, Diaz J, Le Foll B, et al: The dopamine D3 receptor: a therapeutic target for the treatment of neuropsychiatric disorders. CNS Neurol Disord Drug Targets 5:25–43, 2006

Substance Abuse and Mental Health Services Administration: Drug Abuse Warning Network, 2009: National Estimates of Drug-Related Emergency Department Visits (HHS Publ No SMA-11-4659). Rockville, MD, Substance Abuse and Mental Health Services Administration, 2011a. Available at: http://www.samhsa.gov/data/2k11/dawn/2k9dawned/html/dawn2k9ed.htm. Accessed November 26, 2012.

Substance Abuse and Mental Health Services Administration: Results From the 2010 National Survey on Drug Use and Health: Summary of National Findings (NSDUH Series H-41, HHS Publ No SMA-11-4658). Rockville, MD, Substance Abuse and Mental Health Services Administration, 2011b. Available at: http://www.samhsa.gov/data/nsduh/2k10nsduh/2k10results.htm. Accessed November 26, 2012.

Substance Abuse and Mental Health Services Administration: Treatment Episode Dataset (TEDS):1999–2009. State Admissions to Substance Abuse Treatment Services. DASIS Series S-58 (HHS Publ No SMA-11-4663). Rockville, MD, Substance Abuse and Mental Health Services Administration, 2011c. Available at: http://www.samhsa.gov/data/DASIS/teds09st/teds2009stweb.pdf. Accessed November 26, 2012.

Touret M, Sallanon-Moulin M, Fages C, et al: Effects of modafinil-induced wakefulness on glutamine synthetase regulation in the rat brain. Brain Res Mol Brain Res 26:123–128, 1994

Uslaner J, Kalechstein A, Richter T, et al: Association of depressive symptoms during abstinence with the subjective high produced by cocaine. Am J Psychiatry 156:1444–1446, 1999

Volkow ND, Fowler JS, Logan J, et al: Effects of modafinil on dopamine and dopamine transporters in the male human brain: clinical implications. JAMA 301:1148–1154, 2009

Vorel SR, Ashby CR, Paul M, et al: Dopamine D3 receptor antagonism inhibits cocaine-seeking and cocaine-enhanced brain reward in rats. J Neuroscience 22:9595–9603, 2002

White FJ, Kalivas PW: Neuroadaptations involved in amphetamine and cocaine addiction. Drug Alcohol Depend 51:141–153, 1998

Winhusen T, Somoza E, Ciraulo DA, et al: A double-blind, placebo-controlled trial of tiagabine for the treatment of cocaine dependence. Drug Alcohol Depend 91:141–148, 2007

Wise RA, Bozarth MA: Brain mechanisms of drug reward and euphoria. Psychiatr Med 3:445–460, 1985

Xi Z-X, Gilbert J, Campos A, et al: Blockade of mesolimbic dopamine D3 receptors inhibits stress-induced reinstatement of cocaine-seeking in rats. Psychopharmacology (Berl) 176:57–65, 2004

Xi Z-X, Newman AH, Gilbert J, et al: The novel dopamine D3 receptor antagonist NGB 2904 inhibits cocaine's rewarding effects and cocaine-induced reinstatement of drug-seeking behavior in rats. Neuropsychopharmacology 31:1393–1405, 2006

6

Sedatives, Hypnotics, and Anxiolytics

Domenic A. Ciraulo, M.D.

Drugs that are classified as sedatives, hypnotics, or anxiolytics represent a pharmacologically diverse group of compounds. Those that have abuse potential produce antianxiety effects that are on a continuum with their hypnotic actions. The liability for abuse is certainly correlated with these actions but also involves specific mood-elevating properties that are detected with standardized scales of drug-induced changes in mood states (Ciraulo et al. 2001). No classification scheme for these drugs is either scientifically precise or universally accepted. In this chapter, we discuss benzodiazepines, selective γ-aminobutyric acid type A1 ($GABA_{A1}$) (benzodiazepine$_1$) receptor agonists (i.e., zaleplon and zolpidem), barbiturates, and other agents that are used less commonly clinically but are sometimes abused. The role for pharmacotherapy involves selecting therapeutic agents with the lowest abuse potential and managing abstinence syndromes and overdose.

The definitions of abuse, dependence, and misuse subtly influence both research and clinical practice. The DSM-5 criteria for sedative, hypnotic, or anxiolytic use disorder have eliminated the category of abuse, favoring a severity scale based on the number of criterion symptoms met (American Psychiatric Association 2013). When considering use of therapeutic agents that are associated with both a withdrawal syndrome and tolerance, DSM-5 specifically excludes application of these two criteria. Tolerance to many benzodiazepine effects occurs after a single dose and certainly after a few weeks. Fortunately, tolerance to antianxiety effects is uncommon, although tolerance to sedative and euphoric effects does occur. A well-established withdrawal syndrome also occurs with sedative hypnotics. Therefore, specificity of which drug effects contribute to difficulty stopping use is a clinically relevant approach.

In our experience, most patients would prefer to stop taking a medication that is no longer necessary therapeutically. Long-term use is not equivalent to misuse, nor does patient regulation of dosage based on symptom severity represent abuse. Other DSM-5 criterion symptoms, such as spending a great deal of time obtaining sedative, hypnotics, or anxiolytics or giving up important social, occupational, or recreational activities because of use, are extremely rare in clinical populations. On the other hand, a small but clinically significant group of patients has difficulty discontinuing benzodiazepines, and benzodiazepines are frequently misused by individuals who abuse other drugs or alcohol.

Prescription drugs such as benzodiazepines create difficulties for classification systems because they are used for legitimate medical purposes as well as illicitly, usually in combination with other agents. Both circumstances can create problems, but the therapeutic approaches used for these two groups differ dramatically.

Benzodiazepines and Selective GABA$_{A1}$ Agonists

Prevalence of Misuse, Abuse, and Dependence

Clinical Experience

When benzodiazepines were initially introduced, they were not thought to cause dependence. This was heralded as a pharmacological advance, in contradistinction to the barbiturates. It was therefore of considerable interest when Hollister et al. (1961) reported physiological dependence in humans after abrupt discontinuation of therapy of large doses of chlordiazepoxide for many months. This and other work led to the perspective that physiological dependence did occur with benzodiazepines at high doses but not in regular, therapeutic clinical use. As concern grew over the rapid growth in sales of benzodiazepines in the 1960s, attention was paid to the potential of these drugs to be "addicting." As new information became available, the concept of the dose and exposure time needed to produce physiological dependence changed. Busto et al. (1986a, 1986b) identified a withdrawal syndrome following chronic use of several benzodiazepines at therapeutic doses, and an abstinence syndrome was precipitated in cats after a single dose of diazepam with the benzodiazepine antagonist flumazenil (Rosenberg and Chiu 1985). Thus, the presence of a discontinuation or an abstinence syndrome is common following chronic treatment and is not, in itself, a clinically useful concept of substance abuse or dependence (Lader 2012; Nielsen et al. 2012). This distinction is crucial in considering both the literature and the clinical situations in which benzodiazepine use may come under scrutiny.

Survey Data

National Household Survey on Drug Use and Health.   Prevalence of benzodiazepine use and abuse can be estimated by national and cross-national surveys of the general population, medical clinics, psychiatric institutions, and chemical dependency treatment units. In the National Survey on Drug Use and Health (Substance Abuse and Mental Health Services Administration 2012), the definition of *nonmedical use of prescription agents by individuals* was "taking drugs that were not prescribed for them or drugs they took only for the experience or feeling they caused." Lifetime use of these agents was low. In 2011, 2.4% of persons age 12 or older used psychotherapeutic agents for nonmedical purposes, a rate lower than that in 2002 (2.7%), 2009 (2.8%), and 2010 (2.7%). Less than 1% of the population older than 12 reported illicit use of sedatives or tranquilizers in the month before the survey. In 2011, 8 million Americans age 12 and older used illicit therapeutic drugs in the past month, including 4.5 million using pain relievers, 1.8 million using tranquilizers, and 231,000 using sedatives.

Individuals who reported past-year nonmedical use of psychotherapeutic drugs were asked how they obtained the drugs they most recently used nonmedically. From 2009 to 2010, more than half of those age 12 or older who used pain relievers, tranquilizers, stimulants, and sedatives nonmedically had gotten the prescription drugs they most recently used "from a friend or relative for free." In a follow-up question, three-quarters or more of these respondents indicated that their friend or relative had obtained the drugs from one doctor. The nonmedical use of psychotherapeutic agents reported in the latest National Survey on Drug Use and Health is shown in Figures 6–1 through 6–3.

Monitoring the Future.   Monitoring the Future is a survey funded by the National Institute on Drug Abuse and conducted by the University of Michigan Institute for Social Research (Johnston et al. 2012). The latest findings report stable or declining use of illicit drugs in high school students, with annual prevalence rates of 2%, 4.5%, and 5.6% among eighth, tenth, and twelfth graders, respectively. These findings represent modest declines since rates peaked between 1996 and 2003. Among the benzodiazepines, diazepam and alprazolam were most commonly misused. In contrast, 6.6% of twelfth graders reported daily use of marijuana, 11.4% indicated use of synthetic marijuana in the past 12 months, and 22% reported alcohol binge drinking, which suggests that the sedative-hypnotics remain low-preference agents in the high school population.

Drug Abuse Warning Network.   The Drug Abuse Warning Network (DAWN; Substance Abuse and Mental Health Services Administration 2012) is a survey of specific emergency departments that monitors drug "mentions" associated with patients presenting to the emergency department with a variety of medical and psychiatric complications. These data are probably the most difficult to use to make inferences about sedative-hypnotic abuse liability. Emergency department mentions may reflect the availability of a drug, the number of prescriptions of a particular drug, the availability of a drug through illicit sources, and the contributions of the illness (depression, anxiety) to overdose and emergency department presentations. Overwhelming data from DAWN reports indicate that "alcohol alone or in combination with other illicit or prescription drugs" is the leading mention in most emergency department visit categories except for "adverse effects" visits. In the adverse effects category (precipitating emergency department visit), anti-infectives (antibiotics account for the largest category), followed closely by cardiovascular agents, coagulation agents, and metabolic agents, are most fre-

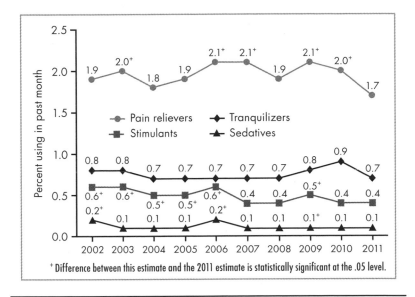

Figure 6–1.   Past-month illicit psychotherapeutic drug use by type in individuals ages 12 years and older, National Survey on Drug Use and Health, 2002–2011 (Substance Abuse and Mental Health Services Administration 2012).

quently cited. The interpretation of DAWN data is complex and open to interpretations that add more heat than light to the issue of the risk of abuse of benzodiazepines. Readers are encouraged to review the DAWN database at www.samhsa.gov/data/DAWN.aspx, in which the strengths and limitations of the survey are outlined.

Treatment Episode Data Set.   The Treatment Episode Data Set (TEDS; http://wwwdasis.samhsa.gov/webt/information.htm) monitors admissions to publicly funded addiction treatment facilities. TEDS has consistently reported that benzodiazepines are rarely primary drugs of abuse that precipitate treatment (Substance Abuse and Mental Health Services Administration 2008). On the other hand, the percentage of benzodiazepines as the primary or secondary agent of abuse has been growing, especially in patients age 55 years or older (Figures 6–4) and among those who also abuse alcohol. Complications from benzodiazepines and Z drugs (zolpidem, zaleplon, and eszop-

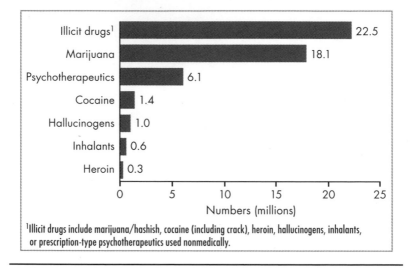

[1]Illicit drugs include marijuana/hashish, cocaine (including crack), heroin, hallucinogens, inhalants, or prescription-type psychotherapeutics used nonmedically.

Figure 6–2.   Past-month illicit drug use among individuals ages 12 and older in 2011 (Substance Abuse and Mental Health Services Administration 2012).

iclone) in this cohort have been largely ignored by researchers, who have focused on the risks of benzodiazepines in elderly patients (usually age 65 years and older). The TEDS findings are consistent with our clinical experience of seeing increasing numbers of high-functioning people between ages 55 and 70 years enter treatment with sedative-hypnotic abuse, both with and without alcohol dependence.

Surveys of medical prescription of benzodiazepines.   Several surveys of medical use of benzodiazepines have been conducted over the last few decades. A national survey of medical use in 1971 showed that 15% (20% of women and 8% of men) had taken at least one dose of a minor tranquilizer in the past year (Parry et al. 1973). A second survey conducted by the same group in 1979 (Mellinger and Balter 1981) reported the use of a "tranquilizer" by 14.1% of women and 7.5% of men (11.1% for both men and women). A multinational survey done in 1981 showed prevalence of 17.6% in Belgium, 12.9% in the United States, and 7.4% in the Netherlands (Balter et al. 1984). Results of these studies are not directly comparable because of differences in

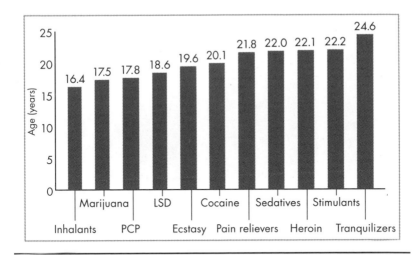

Figure 6–3. Mean age at first use for specific drugs among first-time users ages 12–49 years in 2011, National Survey on Drug Use and Health (Substance Abuse and Mental Health Services Administration 2012).
Note. LSD=lysergic acid diethylamide; PCP=phencyclidine.

how "tranquilizers" were defined. A 1984 survey evaluated chronic anxiolytic use in the United States and found that long-term users were more likely to be older and female and to have high levels of emotional distress and chronic somatic health problems (Mellinger et al. 1984). Although the study concluded that women were more likely than men to use anxiolytics, once men became users, they were at least as likely to become long-term users.

Greenblatt et al. (1975) reported results of the Boston Collaborative Drug Surveillance Program, which showed that of 24,633 consecutive admissions to general medical or surgical wards of 24 Boston, Massachusetts, hospitals, 14% of the patients remembered having taken an antianxiety agent at least once in the preceding 3 months. It is interesting that no cases of physiological withdrawal symptoms were reported.

Marks (1978) reviewed published reports of benzodiazepine dependence in the literature from 1961 to 1977 and estimated that benzodiazepine dependence occurred in one case per 50 million patient-months of use. His assessment of risk has been criticized, however, because published case reports tend to occur less frequently than the phenomenon they describe. Benzodiazepine depen-

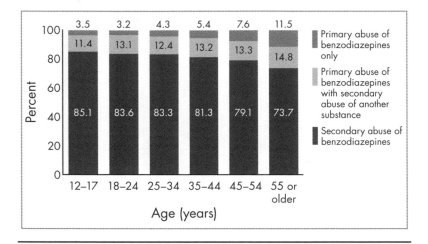

Figure 6–4. Primary and secondary benzodiazepine admissions, 2006, by age: Treatment Episode Data Set.

Note. Percentages may not sum to 100 percent due to rounding.
Source. Substance Abuse and Mental Health Services Administration 2008.

dence case reports peaked between 1969 and 1973, approximately 10 years after the introduction of the drugs (Petursson and Lader 1981a).

In the absence of a diagnosis of substance abuse, most patients taking benzodiazepines continue to benefit from treatment over extended periods, reduce rather than escalate the dose, and do not show evidence of the behaviors associated with addiction to illicit drugs (Apsler and Rothman 1984; Bowden and Fisher 1980; Busto et al. 1986b; Caplan et al. 1985; Dunbar et al. 1989; Olfson et al. 2004; Rickels and Schweizer 1993; Rickels et al. 1991; Romach et al. 1992, 1995; Salinsky and Dore 1987; Svab et al. 2011; Veronese et al. 2007; Zandstra et al 2002). The prevalence of benzodiazepine use among patients with chronic psychiatric disorders is reported to be 17%–36.9% (Cushman and Benzer 1980; Fleischhacker et al. 1986; Garvey and Tollefson 1986; Gottschalk et al. 1971; Hallstrom and Lader 1982; Hoiseth et al. 2013; Manthey et al. 2011; Samarasinghe et al. 1984; Schmidt et al. 1989; Wolf et al. 1989).

In summary, in 2011, 2.7% of the U.S. population older than 12 years reported nonmedical use of a "psychotherapeutic" in the previous month, a rate similar to that in 2002. In 2011, less than 1% reported use of tranquilizers or sedatives. Approximately 7.4%–17.6% of the general population uses a benzodiazepine for medical purposes at least once during any given year, with only about 1% using them daily for 1 year or longer (Piper 1995). This finding can be compared with a 17%–36.9% *usage* rate and less than a 1% *abuse* rate among psychiatric patients. Of patients in treatment for substance dependence, 1.3%–9.2% included benzodiazepines among their multiple substances of abuse, but only a very small number (on the order of 0.2%) were dependent on benzodiazepines only. Studies of benzodiazepine use in alcoholic patients indicate that between 3% and 41% are taking both drugs, with estimated rates of misuse of 10%–20% (Ashley et al. 1978; Bell et al. 1984; Busto et al. 1983; Ciraulo et al. 1988b; Johansson et al. 2003; Kania and Kofoed 1984; Kryspin-Exner 1966; Kryspin-Exner and Demel 1975; Rothstein et al. 1976; Schuckit and Morrissey 1979; Sokolow et al. 1981; Wiseman and Spencer-Peet 1985).

Medical Use

Medical use of benzodiazepines has been declining. Prescribing trends show an overall decline in the number of all benzodiazepine prescriptions written (Table 6–1), with a market shift to increased prescribing of short elimination half-life agents (lorazepam, alprazolam) compared with long elimination half-life agents (diazepam, chlordiazepoxide) (Ciraulo and Sarid-Segal 2005). In 2001, alprazolam was the most widely prescribed benzodiazepine (Ciraulo and Sarid-Segal 2005) and also was the most widely prescribed psychiatric medication in that year for mood and anxiety disorders (Stahl 2002). The approval by the U.S. Food and Drug Administration of selective serotonin reuptake inhibitor (SSRI) antidepressants and some atypical antipsychotics for anxiety has contributed to the shift away from benzodiazepines.

Most medical use is short-term (less than a month), with long-term users more likely to be older and women, with high levels of psychological distress. Psychiatric patients have higher rates of benzodiazepine use than in the general population but still have low rates of misuse. Patients presenting for treatment of benzodiazepine dependence have high rates of psychiatric comorbidity, especially depression and anxiety, as well as polysubstance abuse (Busto et al. 1996; Romach et al. 1995).

Table 6–1. Annual U.S. retail sales of benzodiazepines and Z drugs (2008–2012)[a]

	2008	2009	2010	2011	2012
Anxiolytics					
Alprazolam	$114.2	$119.3	$127.6	$124.1	$113.1
Diazepam	$25.7	$25.8	$42.1	$75.5	$82.6
Lorazepam	$85.7	$83.7	$77.6	$73.3	$68.2
Clonazepam	$51.4	$54.6	$60.7	$63.9	$64.2
Oxazepam	$11.9	$11.1	$10.3	$12.3	$25.5
Chlordiazepoxide	$12.1	$39.8	$30.4	$26.4	$24.7
Hypnotics					
Eszopiclone (Lunesta)	$789.3	$761.9	$806.7	$820.3	$779.4
Zolpidem (Ambien)	$41.5	$47.0	$138.9	$479.9	$373.4
Temazepam (Restoril)	$35.9	$64.9	$63.1	$60.3	$61.6
Zaleplon (Sonata)	$11.7	$6.8	$7.5	$7.9	$7.7
Triazolam (Halcion)	$5.5	$5.5	$5.5	$5.3	$5.2
Grand total (billions)	$1.9	$1.2	$1.4	$1.8	$1.6

[a]Individual drugs are listed in millions (rounded). Grand total is in billions.
Source. Data provided by IMS Health and reproduced with permission.

Prevalence in Special Populations

Substance Abusers

A dramatically different pattern is found in surveys of drug abuse treatment facilities. Substance abuse treatment centers report that more than 20% of patients use benzodiazepines weekly or more frequently, with 30%–90% of opioid abusers reporting illicit use (Iguchi et al. 1993; Stitzer et al. 1981). Methadone clinics report that high proportions of urine samples are positive for benzodiazepines (Darke et al. 2003; Dinwiddie et al. 1996; Ross and Darke 2000; Seivewright 2001; Strain et al. 1991; Williams et al. 1996). The reasons for the high rates of benzodiazepine use in opioid-addicted individuals include self-medication of insomnia, anxiety, and withdrawal symptoms, as well as attempts to "boost" the euphoric effects of opioids.

Some evidence indicates a synergistic effect on reinforcement with concurrent administration of benzodiazepines and opioids (Walker and Ettenberg 2003). Cocaine abusers are less likely than opioid abusers to abuse benzodiazepines, preferring alcohol and opioids as secondary drugs of abuse. The most common pattern of benzodiazepine misuse in these individuals is intermittent use of therapeutic or supratherapeutic doses to counter unwanted effects of cocaine.

Although estimates vary widely, approximately 10%–20% of individuals presenting for treatment of alcohol dependence may be using or abusing benzodiazepines (Ciraulo and Sarid-Segal 2005; Ciraulo et al. 1988b; Johansson et al. 2003; Lejoyeux et al. 1998). Similar to opioid-dependent persons, these individuals report that they use benzodiazepines to self-medicate anxiety, insomnia, and alcohol withdrawal and, less commonly, to enhance the effects of ethanol. Approximately 16%–25% of individuals presenting for treatment of anxiety disorders abuse alcohol (Kushner et al. 1990; Otto et al. 1992). Controversy exists concerning appropriate benzodiazepine prescribing in this population (Ciraulo and Nace 2000; Posternak and Mueller 2001).

The risk of benzodiazepine misuse in people with anxiety and alcoholism varies, depending on the population sampled. A history of alcohol dependence did not predict longer duration of use, higher doses, or more frequent as-needed doses of prescription benzodiazepines in a large outpatient clinical trial (Mueller et al. 1996). Sokolow et al. (1981) reported that over an 8-month period following alcohol detoxification, concurrent benzodiazepine use declined from 12.7% at admission to 8.1% at 8 months, suggesting that even alcoholic patients have a decreasing pattern of use over time. Among individuals entering a benzodiazepine discontinuation program, 40% of those with long-term use (averaging 70 months of daily use) had an alcohol use disorder. Of particular interest is that typical use was at constant or decreasing therapeutic doses, with efforts to discontinue the medication and appropriate use for symptom control (Busto et al. 1996; Romach et al. 1995).

The subjective rewarding effects of alprazolam, and probably of other rapid-onset benzodiazepines, are greater among individuals with alcoholism than among those without alcoholism (Ciraulo et al. 1988a, 1988b). Differences in abuse potential may exist between individual benzodiazepines (Griffiths and Wolf 1990). For example, the onset of positive mood effects for oxazepam and halazepam is slower than for diazepam (Griffiths et al. 1984; Jaffe et al. 1983). The actual risk of benzodiazepine dependence among alcoholic patients is unclear because the methodological deficiencies of existing studies are substantial, but the risk in this group is probably higher than in the general population but lower than among opiate-addicted persons. There is a high likelihood that patients with alcoholism who receive benzodiazepines will take them inappropriately. On the other hand, anxiety disorder patients who are in stable recovery are at much lower risk for benzodiazepine abuse than are nonabstinent or recently abstinent alcoholic patients (Posternak and Mueller 2001).

Elderly Patients

Elderly patients may be at risk for falls (Cumming and Le Couteur 2003; Cumming et al. 1991) and impaired cognition (Barker et al. 2004a; Dealberto et al. 1997; Hanlon et al. 1998; Pat McAndrews et al. 2003) from benzodiazepine toxicity. Little evidence suggests that elderly patients are more likely to misuse these drugs, although they do have higher rates of prescriptions than do younger patients. Although many studies have found an association between benzodiazepines and falls in the elderly (Cumming and Le Couteur 2003), it should be noted that one study found that SSRI antidepressants and narcotics were more likely than benzodiazepines to be associated with non-spine fractures in the elderly (Ensrud et al. 2003). The reader is cautioned that the published literature on the elderly often mistakenly views long-term use as equivalent to dependence or abuse. A study of elderly hospitalized patients older than 70 years who had been taking a benzodiazepine for an average of

3.6 years at a mean diazepam equivalent dose of 11 mg found that they had more severe personality pathology, anxiety, and dysthymia than a similar inpatient group not taking benzodiazepines (Petrovic et al. 2002). Although the most common interpretation of these and similar findings is that they support the position that benzodiazepines are prescribed appropriately in the elderly, others have raised the question of whether chronic prescribing actually induces or worsens anxiety and depression. A study that reviewed insurance claims alleging benzodiazepine-induced behavioral toxicity found that psychiatric symptoms most often represented preexisting psychopathology and were not the result of benzodiazepine use (Mattila-Evenden et al. 2001), but the issue requires further study.

Chronic Pain Patients

Several studies have reported that as many as 40%–60% of chronic pain patients receive benzodiazepines, even though these agents have limited effectiveness for most pain conditions (Fishbain et al. 1992; Hardo and Kennedy 1991; Hendler et al. 1980; King and Strain 1990a, 1990b; Kouyanou et al. 1997). The role of benzodiazepines in pain is not straightforward; no doubt these medications help with sleep, anxiety, and dysphoria secondary to medical illness. Despite high rates of use, rates of misuse in one study were low, ranging from 3.2% to 4.8% (Kouyanou et al. 1997). An intriguing finding is that some novel benzodiazepines may have direct effects on pain, through actions as either bradykinin B_1 antagonists (Wood et al. 2003) or κ receptor agonists (Anzini et al. 2003).

Overview of Neuropharmacology

The term *benzodiazepine* refers to drugs with a structural core consisting of a benzene ring fused to a diazepine ring. All benzodiazepines in clinical use also contain a 5-aryl substituent ring and a 1,4-diazepine ring; and so the term refers to the 5-aryl-1,4-benzodiazepines (Charney et al. 2001; Greenblatt et al. 1983a, 1983b; Harvey 1985). Variations on the benzodiazepine ring structure have produced the triazolo (e.g., alprazolam, triazolam, estazolam), 2-keto (e.g., diazepam), 3-hydroxy (e.g., lorazepam, oxazepam), and imidazo (e.g., midazolam) agents and other agents that produce similar clinical actions: sedative, hypnotic, anxiolytic, muscle relaxant, and anticonvulsant effects. Substantial controversy exists as to whether certain classes of benzodiazepines differ in efficacy (antipanic, antidepressant actions), severity of withdrawal syndromes, or abuse liability.

Three selective $GABA_{A1}$ receptor agonists are currently marketed in the United States: zaleplon (a pyrazolopyrimidine), zolpidem (an imidazopyridine), and eszopiclone (cyclopyrrolone and dextro isomer of zopiclone). The Z drugs—zolpidem, zaleplon, and eszopiclone—serve as positive modulators of $GABA_A$ receptor-channel complex. The Z drugs are approved for the treatment of primary insomnia. The relative abuse liability compared with nonselective benzodiazepines is a matter of some controversy. Acute doses produce similar positive reinforcing effects, but some studies have indicated that rebound insomnia and tolerance are less likely with the Z drugs than with the benzodiazepine hypnotics. Our clinical experience (which may not be representative of a typical population) has found tolerance developing rapidly and little difference between temazepam and the Z drugs. Furthermore, the appearance of complicated nocturnal behaviors, such as eating, cleaning, and hallucinations, is more common with the Z drugs, especially zolpidem.

Benzodiazepines, the Z drugs, barbiturates, and related compounds exert their actions at the $GABA_A$ receptor complex, a pentameric structure composed of alpha (α), beta (β), and gamma (γ) subunits forming a chloride channel (Atack 2003) (Figure 6–5). It is known that these (and other) subunits exist as several subtypes and can combine in many ways; however, comparatively few combinations have physiological relevance. The actions resulting from agonist binding at the $GABA_A$ receptor vary depending on the composition of the subunits. Benzodiazepine-sensitive $GABA_A$ receptors are composed of five subunits: two α, two β, and one γ (Barnard et al. 1998). Benzodiazepines show activity at receptors that contain the α_2 subunit. The benzodiazepine binding site lies at the interface of α and γ subunits (Stephenson et al. 1990). A specific histidine residue (H101) within the α_1 subunit and homologous residues within the α_2, α_3, and α_5 subunits (H101, H126, H125) are essential for benzodiazepine action (Tan et al. 2011). Diazepam has a high affinity for α_1, α_2, α_3, and α_5 subunits in the $GABA_A$ receptor but not for the α_4 or α_6 subunits (Hadingham et al. 1993; Luddens et al. 1990; Wafford et al. 1996). The sedative effects of benzodiazepines are associated with the presence of α_1 subunits in the $GABA_A$ receptor structure (the $GABA_{A1}$ receptor subtype) (McKernan et al. 2000), and the presence of α_2 units in this receptor may be required for the antianxiety effect (Löw et al. 2000). The Z

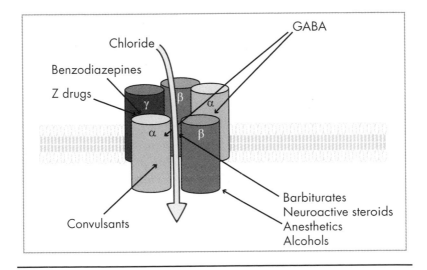

Figure 6–5.   Model γ-aminobutyric acid type A (GABA$_A$) receptor showing drug binding sites.

drugs (Pritchett and Seeburg 1990; Sanna et al. 2002) act on and bind to GABA$_{A1}$ receptors more selectively than do classic benzodiazepines, permitting them to act as hypnotic agents that, when compared with the benzodiazepines, are less likely to produce antianxiety and anticonvulsant effects. Elimination of activity at the α$_1$ receptor alone does not produce an agent free of dependence potential, although when coupled with reduced α$_{2/3}$ efficacy may enhance reduced addictive potential (Ator et al. 2010).

The different α subunits that are contained in GABA$_A$ receptors are distributed in a heterogeneous manner throughout the brain. GABA$_A$ receptors having the α$_1$ subunit are located predominantly in sensorimotor areas, cortical areas, the globus pallidus, ventral thalamic complex, subthalamic nucleus, substantia nigra, and cerebellum in primates (Dennis et al. 1988). Positron emission tomography evidence suggests that high concentrations of GABA$_A$ receptors that contain the α$_5$ subunit exist in human limbic structures, including the hippocampus, septal region, amygdala, and anterior cingulate cortex (Lingford-Hughes et al. 2002).

Although barbiturates, benzodiazepines, and GABA$_{A1}$ selective agonists increase chloride ion flux, the barbiturates both enhance GABA binding and directly activate the channel, whereas the benzodiazepines and $GABA_{A1}$ agonists act only to increase the actions of GABA and other direct GABA agonists such as muscimol (Charney et al. 2001). Benzodiazepines and the $GABA_{A1}$ agonists are allosteric modulators of the GABA binding site in the $GABA_A$ receptor complex. The duration of channel opening is increased by barbiturates, whereas benzodiazepines primarily increase the frequency of openings. Barbiturates also differ from benzodiazepines in that they do not require the γ subunit to produce their effects, and, in addition, they directly inhibit the excitatory α-amino-3-hydroxy-5-methylisoxazole-4-propionate (AMPA) receptor, whereas benzodiazepines indirectly oppose the excitatory actions of glutamate by acting as positive modulators of GABA inhibitory activity (Saunders and Ho et al. 1990). Benzodiazepines also may have effects on adenosine reuptake and the activity of calcium and sodium channels.

The mood-elevating effect of the benzodiazepines and barbiturates is probably mediated not only by acute increases in the actions of GABA but also by neural connections. Depletion of dopamine from the nucleus accumbens may attenuate the rewarding effects of diazepam (Spyraki and Fibiger 1988), as may the administration of AMPA/kainate receptor antagonists (Gray et al. 1999). In addition to $GABA_A$ receptor antagonists, both dopamine and opioid receptor antagonists may block the rewarding actions of pentobarbital (Bossert and Franklin 2001). The precise mechanism through which benzodiazepines and barbiturates produce mood elevation remains to be elucidated. The administration of benzodiazepines (DiChiara and Imperato 1988; Finlay et al. 1992) and higher doses of barbiturates (Pontieri et al. 1995) reduces rather than increases dopamine concentrations in the nucleus accumbens. The rewarding effects of many commonly abused drugs, including morphine and cocaine, are associated with drug-induced increases in dopamine concentrations in the nucleus accumbens (Pontieri et al. 1995).

Several benzodiazepine receptor ligands have been characterized and may have one or more modes of action at the $GABA_A$ receptor (Ator 2003; Braestrup et al. 1983). These include 1) agonist action, in which ligands produce benzodiazepine-like effects, such as diazepam; 2) antagonist action, when the ligands bind to benzodiazepine receptors and block the effects of agonists, as does flumazenil; and 3) inverse agonist actions, characterized by binding to the benzodiazepine receptor, resulting in effects that are opposite those of agonists. Examples of the last group are methyl beta-carboline-3-carboxylate, methyl 6,7-dimethoxy-4-ethyl-beta-carboline-3-carboxylate, Ro 15-4513, and CGS 8216. A classification scheme proposed by Nutt and Linnoila (1988) divides ligands into agonists or inverse agonists and then subclassifies each as full or partial. This classification scheme is not absolute—a given benzodiazepine may have different actions depending on the composition of receptor subunits. For example, replacement of the γ_2 subunit with the γ_1 subunit reduces positive modulation and may result in an inverse agonist acting as a weak agonist (Barnard et al. 1998).

Pharmacodynamic tolerance to the psychomotor effects of benzodiazepines has been confirmed after single or multiple doses (File 1985; Greenblatt and Shader 1978; Rosenberg and Chiu 1985). Pharmacodynamic tolerance to the anxiolytic effect (over a 6-month period) has not been shown (Rickels et al. 1983), and clinical experience suggests that many patients with anxiety disorders require long-term therapy with benzodiazepines or alternative antianxiety agents. An important clinical consequence of tolerance to sedative effects is observed in benzodiazepine overdoses, when patients may initially be somnolent but often wake up and recover while the serum level of the benzodiazepine active metabolite is very high and still rising.

Tolerance to the psychomotor impairment associated with lorazepam has been shown in animal models (Miller et al. 1988a, 1988b), but it is our clinical impression that even though impairment decreases with continued use in patients, it never completely remits. In most cases, it does not persist at levels that cause significant impairment in daily functioning. On the other hand, amnesic effects of benzodiazepines, especially the high-potency agents, seem to be a problem for some individuals whose occupations demand high levels of cognitive function. Using the lowest possible doses of these drugs during periods when cognitive performance is critical (e.g., test taking) is a successful therapeutic strategy.

The extent to which tolerance develops to the actions of the Z drugs is not yet clear. In contrast to triazolam, zolpidem was not associated with the development of behavioral tolerance to impairments of psychological performance produced by repeated administration (Stoops and Rush 2003). Several reports have indicated that tolerance does not develop to the sleep-promoting effects of these agents over a 1-month period (Elie et al. 1999; Fry et al. 2000) and that significant rebound insomnia does not occur with the prolonged administration of these agents (Voderholzer et al. 2001). However, other evidence suggests that rebound insomnia may occur after zolpidem treatment (Elie et al. 1999; Fry et al. 2000). Some data support lower risk for tolerance to hypnotic effects with Z drugs compared with nonselective benzodiazepines, but this has not been our experience. There does seem to be less rebound insomnia with these drugs, but some patients do experience this withdrawal effect. In our experience, the adverse effect of complex nocturnal behavioral toxicity appears more frequently with these agents, especially zolpidem.

Tolerance to benzodiazepines is pharmacodynamic, whereas barbiturates induce their own metabolism (pharmacokinetic tolerance) as well as induce receptor changes (pharmacodynamic tolerance). Receptor changes have been best studied with benzodiazepines; however, the exact mechanisms responsible for benzodiazepine tolerance remain uncertain. Furthermore, although the consensus is that tolerance develops for clinical effects such as sedation and motor impairment, clinical experience suggests that antianxiety effects are long lasting. It is well established that chronic administration of benzodiazepines in experimental models results in decreased GABA-stimulated chloride influx. Several mechanisms have been implicated in the development of tolerance to benzodiazepines. These include downregulation of cortical benzodiazepine binding sites (Fahey et al. 2001), alterations in $GABA_A$ receptor subunit composition (Chen et al. 1999), and increased expression of AMPA (Allison and Pratt 2003; Van Sickle and Tietz 2002) and N-methyl-D-aspartate (NMDA) (Perez et al. 2003) receptor subunits in the hippocampus.

Pharmacokinetics

Absorption of benzodiazepines by the oral route is essentially complete, except for clorazepate, which is decarboxylated in gastric secretions to N-desmethyldiazepam, which is absorbed. Diazepam and N-desmethyldiazepam are rapidly absorbed and will reach a peak in serum soon after ingestion (Greenblatt et al. 1983a, 1983b). Prazepam and halazepam are inactive or only slightly active prodrugs that are converted slowly to the active form. The rate of appearance in serum of N-desmethyldiazepam from prazepam is the slowest among the benzodiazepines. Some researchers believe that this property conveys lower abuse liability, although there is no consensus on this question.

Some patients have reported sublingual use (particularly of lorazepam and alprazolam) to obtain a "high," presumably as a result of faster absorption, although clinicians rarely see either a high or a more rapid onset of action. Although one group has found faster absorption of lorazepam by the sublingual route (Caille et al. 1983), a rigorous kinetic comparison of intravenous, intramuscular, oral, and sublingual routes failed to detect significant differences between sublingual and oral administration in the fasted state (Greenblatt et al. 1982). Sublingual absorption may offer an increased rate of absorption in the postprandial state. Alprazolam and triazolam may reach higher peak levels via the sublingual route. Although benzodiazepines are all highly lipophilic, the lipophilicity varies more than 50-fold among individual benzodiazepines (Harvey 1985). The more lipophilic drugs tend to enter the cerebrospinal fluid most rapidly, but in a study of diazepam, N-desmethyldiazepam, midazolam, lorazepam, alprazolam, flunitrazepam, and clobazam, all attained peak cerebrospinal fluid concentrations within 15 minutes of intravenous administration (Arendt et al. 1983). Benzodiazepines and their active metabolites all bind to plasma proteins, and this binding correlates with lipophilicity—from 70% for alprazolam to 99% for diazepam (Harvey 1985).

Benzodiazepines are metabolized via the hepatic microsomal system. The cytochrome P450 (CYP) 3A4 isoform may mediate the metabolism of several benzodiazepines, including triazolam, alprazolam, and midazolam. The clearance of triazolam can be reduced by the administration of CYP3A4 inhibitors such as ritonavir (Greenblatt et al. 2000). The metabolism of diazepam is catalyzed, in part, by the CYP2C19 isoform. All benzodiazepines ultimately undergo glucuronidation, and some require prior oxidative metabolism, either N-dealkylation or aliphatic hydroxylation. Oxidative metabolism is relatively more susceptible to impairment from certain population characteristics (aging), coadministration of other drugs (cimetidine, disulfiram), or disease states (cirrhosis) than is glucuronidation. The metabolism of those drugs that require only glucuronidation (oxazepam, lorazepam, temazepam) is less susceptible to these influences than that of those drugs that require oxidation (chlordiazepoxide, diazepam, clorazepate, prazepam, halazepam, flurazepam, triazolam, and alprazolam).

Benzodiazepines do not induce their own metabolism, and there is no evidence for the development of pharmacokinetic tolerance (Greenblatt and Shader 1986). The behavioral tolerance seen with chronic dosing is explicable entirely as a result of pharmacodynamic tolerance (as described earlier in the subsection "Overview of Neuropharmacology").

Zolpidem and zaleplon preferentially bind to α_1-containing $GABA_A$ receptors, whereas eszopiclone has a less selective binding profile. The time to maximal concentration (T_{max}) is about 1.5 hours with zolpidem, immediate or extended release, or with eszopiclone. Zolpidem oral spray and sublingual formulations reach T_{max} in a little more than an hour, whereas zaleplon has the shortest T_{max} at 45 minutes postingestion. Clinical sedation occurs within an hour of ingestion, although zolpidem oral spray, zolpidem sublingual, and zaleplon are expected to cause sedation in less than 30 minutes. The elimination half-life of zolpidem (including immediate-release, oral spray, and sublingual formulations) is approximately 2–2.5 hours. The half-life of zolpidem extended release is 3 hours. Zaleplon has the shortest half-life, at 1 hour, and eszopiclone has the longest, at 6 hours. Metabolism of all three Z drugs is primarily hepatic.

Etiological Theories of Misuse, Abuse, and Dependence

Although many factors contribute to drug dependence and misuse, only the pharmacological origins of benzodiazepine dependence are considered here. The capacity of a benzodiazepine to induce dependence is related to its ability to produce a desired effect (a pleasant mood, relief of anxiety or dysphoria, and less commonly a "high") and to attempts to self-medicate an abstinence syndrome (physical dependence) from either the benzodiazepine or another abused substance (e.g., alcohol).

Benzodiazepines and similar agents occupy a position of intermediate abuse potential compared with most other sedative-hypnotics (Griffiths and Weerts 1997). Animal models of abuse liability indicate that the reinforcing effects of benzodiazepines are less pronounced than are those of the barbiturates, opioids, and stimulants. Differences in abuse potential within the class have not been consistently shown, but most clinicians agree that those benzodiazepines with a rapid onset and short duration of action pose the greatest risk in susceptible individuals.

Limited results from clinical laboratory evaluations suggest that the $GABA_{A1}$ agonists zaleplon (Rush et al. 1999b) and zolpidem (Rush et al. 1999a) produce effects that are consistent with abuse potential comparable to that of the benzodiazepine triazolam. The reported incidence of dependence on zolpidem in the medical literature is low compared with that for benzodiazepines and is characterized by use of high doses, often in individuals with histories of substance abuse (Hajak et al. 2003; Vartzopoulos et al. 2000).

Diazepam has a rapid onset of action in producing a euphoric effect, but as the desmethyl metabolite levels increase and the level of the parent compound, diazepam, declines, the mood-elevating effect declines rapidly (Ciraulo et al. 1997; Jaffe et al. 1983). Benzodiazepines that are prodrugs for desmethyldiazepam, such as prazepam or halazepam, produce fewer euphoric effects (Jaffe et al. 1983; Orzack et al. 1982). Other pharmacokinetic factors influence the time course of withdrawal and by extension the proper medical management of the abstinence syndrome; however, no human data clearly establish that the withdrawal syndrome is more severe with agents with a short than with a long elimination half-life. The partial agonists (or, more accurately, *partial positive modulators*) abecarnil and bretazenil consistently showed lower abuse liability in animal models but still produce mood elevation on standardized scales assessing abuse liability in human subjects (D. A. Ciraulo, unpublished data, Boston, MA). Prior exposure to ethanol or sedative-hypnotic drugs may increase the reinforcing properties of benzodiazepines. Flunitrazepam is associated with a particularly disturbing form of abuse—surreptitious combination with beverage alcohol to induce amnesia and increase vulnerability to sexual assaults.

Nonhuman primates will self-administer benzodiazepines and zolpidem (Weerts and Griffiths 1998), indicating that these agents produce moderate positive reinforcing effects (Ator 2002). Both drug-experienced and drug-naïve animals will self-administer benzodiazepines (Griffiths and Weerts 1997), and the self-administration of these agents has been shown to occur over periods lasting several months. Evidence that benzodiazepines produce positive reinforcing effects in humans is mixed and includes results of self-administration and choice studies (Griffiths and Weerts 1997). Benzodiazepines are less efficacious as reinforcers in humans than is pentobarbital (Griffiths et al. 1980), and diazepam may be a more efficacious reinforcer than oxazepam (Griffiths et al. 1984). The degree of reinforcing effects of benzodiazepines in humans appears to be determined by the psychiatric and substance use history of subjects being tested. In several studies involving healthy volunteers, benzodiazepines, including diazepam (Johanson and de Wit 1992), lorazepam (de Wit et al. 1984), and triazolam (Roehrs et al. 1992), were not found to be reinforcers. In contrast, alprazolam (Ciraulo et al. 1988a, 1989, 1990, 1996; Mumford et al. 1995a, 1995b), diazepam and triazolam (Roache and Griffiths 1989), and other agents clearly act as reinforcers in subjects with a history of drug abuse or alcoholism. Benzodiazepines also appear to have reinforcing effects in moderate drinkers (de Wit et al. 1989; Evans et al. 1996) and anxious individuals (Roache et al. 1996, 1997).

Physiological dependence develops with high doses and therapeutic doses of benzodiazepines. Difficulty discontinuing use can be related to the individual's inability to tolerate discontinuation symptoms or the return of the preexisting anxiety disorder. Physical dependence can also develop in primates taking high doses of zolpidem (Ator et al. 2000; Richards and Martin 1998; Weerts and Griffiths 1998) and zaleplon (Ator et al. 2000; Weerts and Griffiths 1998).

Clinical Signs and Symptoms of Intoxication and Abstinence Syndrome

Intoxication

Benzodiazepines produce few pathognomonic signs of intoxication. Sedation, behavioral disinhibition, and occasional paradoxical excitation may all be seen. Toxicity can occur after large single doses (as in some cases of abuse or in deliberate overdose) and by drug accumulation in persons with impaired metabolism. Three cardinal features of benzodiazepine toxicity are ataxia, diplopia, and impaired gag reflex. Level of consciousness may vary from light sedation to obtundation. Unless benzodiazepines are combined with other drugs (such as alcohol), the rate of mortality in persons with benzodiazepine intoxication is low. Tolerance develops rapidly, and it is common following single large doses to see an initial period of sedation followed by apparent recovery while serum levels of active metabolites are still rising (Greenblatt et al. 1979). The competitive benzodiazepine antagonist flumazenil has been used to reverse benzodiazepine-induced sedation following surgery or diagnostic procedures (Brogden and Goa 1988).

Abstinence Syndrome

An abstinence syndrome after prolonged, high-dose administration was reported to occur with chlordiazepoxide (Hollister et al. 1961) and with diazepam (Hollister et al. 1963). This high-dose abstinence syndrome has been repeatedly confirmed and has been categorized by Smith and Wesson (1983) into either a minor withdrawal syndrome consisting of "anxiety, insomnia, and nightmares" or a major withdrawal syndrome consisting of "grand mal seizures, psychosis, hyperpyrexia, and possibly death" (p. 87).

An abstinence syndrome after long-term, low-dose treatment also has been described (Busto et al. 1986b; Covi et al. 1973; Petursson and Lader 1981b; Tyrer et al. 1981). Symptoms reported include muscle twitching, abnormal perception of movement, depersonalization or derealization, anxiety, headache, insomnia, diaphoresis, difficulty concentrating, tremor, fear, fatigue, lowered threshold to perception of sensory stimuli, and dysphoria.

A rebound sleep disturbance has been found after only 7–10 days of treatment with therapeutic doses of triazolam (Greenblatt et al. 1987). A withdrawal syndrome also has been described after substitution of a short-acting benzodiazepine for a long-acting benzodiazepine (Conell and Berlin 1983). Rebound insomnia may occur with zolpidem or other Z drugs but may be less intense and less common than with nonselective benzodiazepines. This issue requires further study, preferably by research funded by entities other than the manufacturers of these agents.

The clinician must be cautious in interpreting some of the above symptoms (especially anxiety) in patients withdrawing from benzodiazepines. Anxiety, fearfulness, and dysphoria may represent symptoms that were treated by the benzodiazepine and unmasked on withdrawal.

Protocols for Detoxification

Indications for Detoxification

Clinical situations in which detoxification is indicated can be grouped into three categories: 1) patients who have been maintained on therapeutic dosages for moderate to long periods and for whom a trial off their medication is warranted; 2) patients taking supratherapeutic doses (usually in the context of benzodiazepine dependence); and 3) patients who use benzodiazepines as part of mixed substance abuse. Detoxification should be approached differently in each category.

Therapeutic doses.   Patients may have been prescribed benzodiazepines for an acute problem that has since resolved, but prescriptions were nonetheless renewed, for ill-defined reasons or for a diagnosed anxiety disorder. The unifying features in this group are that patients have been using benzodiazepines at stable, therapeutic doses; they have been obtaining them from legitimate sources; and they may or may not still be deriving clinical benefit from the medication. Determining continued benefit may be difficult and may require periodic tapering or discontinuation of the benzodiazepine. Return of symptoms during the taper may support continued treatment, but the clinician also should consider the possibility of a discontinuation syndrome.

Detoxification usually can be accomplished by using the same benzodiazepine that the patient is taking. Switching from a benzodiazepine with a short elimination half-life to one with a long elimination half-life may not be necessary if the tapering program is sufficiently long. If difficulty is encountered in tapering one benzodiazepine, however, then switching to one with a longer elimination half-life may be helpful. Substituting a medication with a shorter elimination half-life for one with a longer elimination half-life is not advised (Conell and Berlin 1983). Approximate dosage equivalencies of benzodiazepines are listed in Table 6–2.

We recommend an initial 10%–25% dose reduction, followed by careful observation of the patient for signs of the abstinence syndrome. Patients withdrawing from agents with a shorter elimination half-life (lorazepam, oxazepam) may have an earlier onset of symptoms, and withdrawal from agents with a longer half-life (clonazepam, diazepam) may not occur until several days after reducing the dose. Exceptions to this do occur—some patients seem exquisitely sensitive to the rate of decline of drug levels and may have abstinence symptoms in the presence of therapeutic drug concentrations.

Clinical experience suggests that alprazolam can be particularly difficult to taper when lower doses are reached (e.g., tapering from 1 to 0 mg) (Ciraulo et al. 1990). One possible explanation for this is suggested by data in an animal model showing that alprazolam at doses of 0.02–0.05 mg/kg increases benzodiazepine receptor number above baseline (Miller et al. 1987). When difficulty is encountered in tapering the last 1–2 mg of alprazolam, the rate of dose reduction can be decreased to 0.25 mg/week, and/or adjunctive medication strategies may be used, as described later in this chapter (see subsection "Adjunctive Medication Strategies"). We have not had extensive experience tapering the controlled-release preparation of alprazolam; however, one study (Schweizer et al. 1993) found "moderate but transient levels of distress" in 48% of the patients with panic disorder who were discontinued from the controlled-release formulation of alprazolam compared with 10% of subjects in the placebo group.

There has been some interest in flumazenil as a treatment for benzodiazepine withdrawal (Gerra et al. 2002). Although of theoretical interest, this procedure is not recommended for clinical use. Because there is a body of lit-

Table 6–2. Approximate benzodiazepine dose equivalency

Generic name	Trade name	Dose (mg)
Alprazolam	Xanax	1
Chlordiazepoxide	Librium	25
Clonazepam	Klonopin	0.5–1.0
Clorazepate	Tranxene	15
Diazepam	Valium	10
Eszopiclone	Lunesta	3
Flurazepam	Dalmane	30
Lorazepam	Ativan	2
Oxazepam	Serax	30
Temazepam	Restoril	20
Triazolam	Halcion	0.25
Zaleplon	Sonata	10
Zolpidem	Ambien	10

erature on the topic, clinicians should have some familiarity with the rationale underlying the use of flumazenil in withdrawal. In healthy, nonanxious volunteers who have not been exposed to benzodiazepines, high doses of flumazenil inconsistently produce agonist effects (Darragh et al. 1982; Higgitt et al. 1986; Lupolover et al. 1984; Mintzer et al. 1999). Experimental evidence supports both an antagonist and an agonist action for flumazenil, which may be dependent on dose and subject heterogeneity (Buldakova and Weiss 1997). Administration of flumazenil to benzodiazepine-tolerant individuals resulted in some symptoms of withdrawal (Griffiths et al. 1993), but one study found improvement in symptoms in patients with long-term abstinence (Saxon et al. 1997). Further complicating the interpretation of the data are findings that subjects with panic disorder and generalized anxiety disorder can have different responses to flumazenil (Nutt et al. 1990).

Supratherapeutic doses.   Patients requiring detoxification from high or supratherapeutic doses of benzodiazepines constitute a smaller number of patients than those requiring detoxification from therapeutic doses, but they are at greater risk for life-threatening discontinuation symptoms, such as seizures, delirium, and psychoses. There has been more experience with inpatient detoxification in this group, but outpatient detoxification is possible if conducted slowly (5% reduction per week), with frequent contact, and in the context of a therapeutic alliance with the patient. Often, such an alliance proves unworkable because the patient's impoverished control results in supplementation from outside sources or early exhaustion of prescribed supplies meant to be tapered. In these cases, as in those with a history of seizures, delirium, or psychoses during previous detoxification attempts, inpatient detoxification is indicated.

In high-dose detoxification, the risk of major adverse consequences requires that a smooth decline in plasma benzodiazepine levels be achieved. Here, switching from the substance of abuse to diazepam or another long-acting benzodiazepine is recommended. The patient's medication should be switched to an equivalent dose of long-acting benzodiazepine given in divided daily doses (see Table 6–2), and the patient should be stabilized with this regimen for the first day (some clinicians use a stabilization period of 2–3 days). Following stabilization, a 30% cut is made in the dose on day 2 (or on days 3–4 if a longer stabilization period is used), followed by a 5% cut on each day thereafter. This will result in complete detoxification in about 2 weeks for most patients, but the rate of tapering should be slowed even further in the presence of diaphoresis, tremulousness, or elevated vital sign measurements. Hyperpyrexia is a grave sign and should prompt aggressive management. Supplemental benzodiazepines and supportive medical care are necessary in these instances. This protocol should serve only as a guideline because individual patients will vary in their sensitivity to withdrawal. True withdrawal is best distinguished from recurrence of anxiety by the development of new symptoms and/or the appearance of perceptual disturbance (e.g., ringing in ears, sensitivity to sounds, and dizziness). Whenever possible, doses should be adjusted to keep patients comfortable. Adjunctive medications can be used as described later in this chapter. Close monitoring for the week following detoxification is prudent because some symptoms may not be evident until then, as the desmethyldiazepam and other metabolite levels continue to fall.

Benzodiazepines in mixed substance abuse.   Sporadic use (as in the induction of sleep following a psychostimulant binge) does not require specific detoxification. Sustained use can be treated as described in the previous subsections on detoxification from therapeutic or high doses but with added caution. In mixed opiate and benzodiazepine abuse, the patient should be stabilized with methadone (some clinicians use other oral preparations of opioids) and a benzodiazepine. Buprenorphine should not be administered with benzodiazepines because a pharmacodynamic interaction is possible, and fatalities have been reported with the combination (Ibrahim et al. 2000; Kilicarslan and Sellers 2000; Reynaud et al. 1998). Sedative-hypnotic withdrawal is the more medically serious procedure, and we usually taper the benzodiazepine first. If the doses of the abused drugs are low, simultaneous tapering may be possible. For patients who are misusing several different anxiolytics and hypnotics (e.g., benzodiazepines, barbiturates, ethanol, and propanediols), adequate coverage can be achieved most often by a single medication, and a benzodiazepine is probably the safest choice; however, some experienced clinicians prefer to prescribe barbiturates in these cases.

Adjunctive Medication Strategies

Adjunctive medications that may be of value in the management of benzodiazepine withdrawal are listed in Table 6–3. The two major roles for adjunctive medication are to reduce acute withdrawal symptoms and to maintain long-term discontinuation. Although neither approach is well studied, clinical experience suggests that adjunctive medications are of value in acute withdrawal. Long-term discontinuation depends on many factors, such as psychiatric diagnosis, personality traits, and the efficacy of alternative agents in treating anxiety (e.g., antidepressants).

In acute withdrawal, blockade of β-adrenergic receptors by propranolol (60–120 mg/day) attenuates some withdrawal symptoms (Tyrer et al. 1981), and it or another β-blocker is commonly used. The benzodiazepine still should be gradually tapered, however, because abrupt discontinuation even in the presence of propranolol will lead to severe withdrawal symptoms (Cantopher et al. 1990). Reduction of adrenergic transmission by use of clonidine (an α_2 agonist) also has been used with moderate success (Ashton 1984; Fyer et al. 1988). Clonidine can be started at 0.1 mg twice a day and increased to 0.2 mg three times a day if adequate blood pressure is sustained. The use of a clonidine patch is now common. Some evidence suggested that clonidine is not an effective agent for reducing symptoms of benzodiazepine withdrawal (Goodman

Table 6–3. Adjunctive medications used in the treatment of benzodiazepine withdrawal

Medication Class	Medication
α_2 Receptor agonists	Clonidine
Anticonvulsants	Carbamazepine, pregabalin, baclofen, valproic acid, gabapentin, topiramate
Antidepressants[a]	Trazodone, mirtazapine, paroxetine, other selective serotonin reuptake inhibitors; venlafaxine
β Receptor antagonists	Propranolol, others
Serotonin type 1A receptor (5-HT$_{1A}$) agonists	Buspirone[b]

Note. Efficacy of these agents is not established.
[a]Sedative antidepressants are used in acute withdrawal; antidepressants with antianxiety actions are used for long-term discontinuation.
[b]Not cross-tolerant to benzodiazepines and should not be used for acute withdrawal; high doses may be used to treat anxiety disorders to help maintain long-term discontinuation after abstinence has been achieved.

et al. 1986). It must be stressed that neither propranolol nor clonidine reduces the risk of seizures; therefore, neither agent alone is sufficient to treat benzodiazepine withdrawal. Buspirone is not cross-tolerant to benzodiazepines and is not helpful in relieving withdrawal symptoms (Lader and Olajide 1987).

Other medication strategies have been shown to be of benefit in assisting alprazolam tapering. Clonazepam can be substituted gradually over the course of a week at an alprazolam-to-clonazepam equivalency ratio of 2:1 (Herman et al. 1987) and with the clonazepam tapered as described earlier in this chapter. It is important to note that diazepam may not block alprazolam withdrawal symptoms in some patients, either because of insufficient doses of diazepam or because of different pharmacodynamic actions of alprazolam. Carbamazepine also has been used to facilitate alprazolam withdrawal (Klein et al. 1986). The optimal dose to help with withdrawal has yet to be experimentally verified. In practice, once the alprazolam has been tapered to the lowest level tolerable for the patient, carbamazepine, 200 mg twice a day, can be added. The carbamazepine dose is adjusted to obtain a serum level found to be therapeutic in seizure disorders (4–10 μg/mL), and then the alprazolam is tapered over 1–2 weeks. Carbamazepine can then be rapidly tapered, but while it is being administered, the usual laboratory indices (liver function tests and complete blood count) should be monitored. The use of carbamazepine has been extended to withdrawal from all benzodiazepines.

The use of divalproex in benzodiazepine withdrawal has also become a common clinical strategy. It is usually started at a dosage of 500–1,000 mg taken in two or three divided doses daily and increased to achieve serum levels of 50–120 µg/mL. Some protocols recommend a loading dose of 20 mg/kg. Other anticonvulsants, such as gabapentin and topiramate, are also being used by some clinicians, but controlled trials are lacking.

Antidepressants are commonly used to treat both acute withdrawal and persistent anxiety or insomnia. Evidence suggests that they are effective in relieving some acute abstinence symptoms, but it has been more difficult to establish their effectiveness in long-term discontinuation. Antidepressants with sedative and antianxiety effects are the preferred drugs.

Medical and Psychological Consequences of Abuse

No convincing evidence suggests that long-term benzodiazepine use has adverse medical consequences. In one European study (Piesiur-Strehlow et al. 1986), patients with isolated benzodiazepine dependence showed a mortality rate greater than in the general population but equivalent to that in the control group (nondependent patients with comparable psychiatric illnesses). Virtually all reported medical morbidity and mortality result from the combination of benzodiazepines with other central nervous system (CNS) depressants in individual occurrences; for example, a person chronically abusing diazepam in high doses who then drinks alcohol may encounter severe CNS depression, resulting in respiratory depression or coma.

Anterograde amnesia has been well documented with a variety of benzodiazepines, and decrement in learning probably represents the single most significant drawback to medically indicated chronic use (Barker et al. 2004a; Curran 1986; Lister 1985; Vermeeren and Coenen 2011; Vermeeren et al. 1995). In persons with preexisting deficits in learning or orientation, the effect is magnified and may be a contraindication to use. The mechanism for memory impairment is unclear but may become further elucidated in studies with animal models. Preliminary data suggest that the benzodiazepine inverse agonists may enhance learning and memory (Maubach 2003; Venault et al. 1986), although tolerability has been a problem limiting human studies. The

α_5 subunit of the $GABA_A$ receptor appears to mediate cognitive effects of drugs that act on this receptor.

Studies of cognitive function in long-term benzodiazepine users have yielded contradictory results. A meta-analysis of 13 studies published between 1980 and 2000 found persistent deficits in long-term users compared with control subjects, especially in the areas of sensory processing, verbal reasoning, verbal memory, attention, and concentration (Barker et al. 2004b). One study reported that in a sample of individuals ages 60–70, followed up for 4 years, those taking benzodiazepines had a more rapid decline in cognitive function than did those who were not taking benzodiazepines (Paterniti et al. 2002). Puustinen et al. (2007) found no difference in cognitive function between elderly long-term users of zopiclone, temazepam, and oxazepam and a group of nonusers. Supporting these findings was the study by Leufkens et al. (2009), which found no difference in cognitive performance or driving ability between chronic hypnotic users and control subjects. Most studies have found that discontinuation of benzodiazepines results in gradual improvement in cognitive function, but the extent of recovery and the time required to recover is not consistent in the literature (Barker et al. 2004b; Curran et al. 2003; Pat McAndrews et al. 2003; Salzman et al. 1992).

Several studies have examined brain structure in chronic benzodiazepine users without consistent findings (Busto et al. 2000; Lader 2011; Lader et al. 1984; Moodley et al. 1993; Perera et al. 1987; Schmauss et al. 1987; Uhde and Kellner 1987). Although some authorities have expressed concerns about structural CNS changes occurring with chronic benzodiazepine treatment, no adequately designed studies exist. In particular, alcohol intake and psychiatric comorbidity often have been ignored.

Role of Psychosocial Therapy

In two studies in which benzodiazepines were gradually tapered, concurrent cognitive-behavioral therapy (CBT) did not increase the proportion of patients who were able to successfully discontinue their use of these agents (Vorma et al. 2003; Voshaar et al. 2003). On the other hand, other studies of patients with panic disorder found that CBT facilitated the discontinuation of benzodiazepine use (Otto et al. 1993). Similarly, CBT may be superior to supportive medical management in preventing the reoccurrence of panic attacks in panic disorder patients in whom alprazolam has been tapered (Bruce et al. 1999).

Predictors of Long-Term Discontinuation

Factors that may predict the maintenance of abstinence from benzodiazepines include a low dosage before the discontinuation attempt (Vorma et al. 2003; Voshaar et al. 2003) and high levels of life satisfaction (Vorma et al. 2003). In a 1-year follow-up study of patients with high-dose benzodiazepine dependence (mean of 51.8 diazepam equivalents at baseline) and comorbidity (50% with anxiety disorder, 44% with depressive disorder, 64% with personality disorder, 31% with current and 64% with lifetime alcohol use disorder) who had received benzodiazepine withdrawal treatment with CBT or treatment as usual (Doble et al. 1993), 25% of the entire sample remained benzodiazepine free, independent of treatment (Vorma et al. 2002, 2003). Lower initial benzodiazepine dose, lack of previous withdrawal attempts, and high life satisfaction (which was inversely related to psychopathology) predicted discontinuation. Contrary to studies of patients with less complex clinical characteristics (Bruce et al. 1999), these investigators found equivalent efficacy for CBT and treatment as usual.

Investigators used a standardized scale to assess benzodiazepine dependence in more than 1,000 patients in a primary care setting and found that high dosage, long duration of use, and the concomitant use of antidepressants were associated with dependence (de las Cuevas et al. 2003). The last finding is of particular importance because it may imply that long-term users have more severe or treatment-resistant anxiety that requires combination drug therapy for successful long-term treatment.

In patients with sedative-hypnotic dependence who underwent detoxification in an addiction treatment unit, a significant association was not found between abstinence rate and either gender or psychiatric status (Charney et al. 2000). Patients dependent on benzodiazepines reported decreased anxiety during follow-up, even though their use of these agents had decreased.

Summary of Benzodiazepine Dependence Issues

Anxiety is a normal part of mental life and plays a crucial role in human psychological development and other forms of learning. Although systematic studies are lacking, suppression of normal levels of anxiety could impair the development of adaptive coping mechanisms. On the other hand, disabling anxiety impairs adaptation as well and is associated with significant morbidity and mortality.

Patients with specifically diagnosed anxiety disorders often require psychopharmacological treatment. Data are inadequate to provide absolute guidelines for the optimal length of treatment, but the prudent clinician should periodically assess the need for continued pharmacotherapy. It is well established that the longer the period of therapy and the higher the benzodiazepine dose, the more severe the discontinuation syndrome. Most withdrawal symptoms are easily managed by slow taper or adjunctive therapy with anticonvulsants, such as carbamazepine, valproate, and gabapentin; β-blockers; α-adrenergic blockers; or antidepressants.

In clinical practice, patients are referred for assessment of benzodiazepine dependence in the context of both therapeutic use and drug misuse. For the group of patients taking legitimately prescribed medication, it is necessary to reevaluate the indications for the benzodiazepine, assess for the presence of adverse effects, and determine whether a trial at a lower dose, with alternative agents (an SSRI or buspirone), psychotherapy, or a medication-free period is appropriate. Patients who are using the drugs outside the therapeutic context are rarely dependent on benzodiazepines alone, and these drugs are usually part of a picture of mixed substance dependence. When benzodiazepines are part of mixed substance dependence, the doses tend to be higher and the patients younger than in "pure" benzodiazepine dependence (Busto et al 1986a, 1986b). High-dose use may be correlated with high levels of caffeine use, male sex, and youth (Perera and Jenner 1987).

Benzodiazepines have a low risk for abuse in anxiety disorder patients without a history of alcoholism or drug abuse. Among the benzodiazepines, there may be a spectrum of abuse liability, with drugs that serve as prodrugs for desmethyldiazepam (e.g., clorazepate), slow-onset agents (e.g., oxazepam), and partial agonists (e.g., abecarnil) having the least potential for abuse. However, no currently marketed benzodiazepine or related drug is free of potential for abuse.

Barbiturates

Prevalence of Dependence

Dependence on barbiturates has declined in recent years as physicians have substituted benzodiazepines for the treatment of many conditions for which barbiturates were formerly used. Clinicians will still see cases of abuse and dependence in medical patients receiving barbiturates or barbiturate combination products (e.g., Fiorinal) and in substance abusers (Silberstein and McCrory 2001).

Pharmacology

Charney et al. (2001), Harvey (1985), Matthew (1971), and Wesson and Smith (1977) have discussed the pharmacology of barbiturates. Barbiturates are derived from barbituric acid, which is the product of the fusion of malonic acid and urea. Barbituric acid lacks CNS activity. The two main classes of barbiturates are the highly lipid-soluble *thiobarbiturates,* in which sulfur replaces oxygen at the second carbon atom of the barbituric acid ring, and the less soluble *oxybarbiturates,* with oxygen at the second carbon atom. Lipid-soluble barbiturates have a more rapid onset, a short duration of action, and greater potency than those with lower lipid solubility.

In Table 6–4, barbiturates are listed according to their duration of action. The ultra-short-acting barbiturates include methohexital sodium (Brevital) and thiopental sodium (Pentothal). These are used as anesthetics and are administered intravenously. Barbiturates with short to intermediate duration of action are used for their sedative-hypnotic effect in the treatment of anxiety. These include amobarbital (Amytal), butabarbital (Butisol), sodium pentobarbital (Nembutal), and secobarbital (Seconal). Long-acting barbiturates that are used as sedative-hypnotics and also for their anticonvulsant effects include phenobarbital (Luminal) and mephobarbital (Mebaral).

Although these divisions are of historical interest, duration of action, especially with a single dose, depends more on distribution effects than on elimination half-life. Furthermore, as the dose increases, duration of action is prolonged. In addition, the availability of these drugs in the United States is limited.

Barbiturates produce CNS depression, which ranges from sedation to general anesthesia. Action is through suppression of the mesencephalic reticular activating system. Barbiturates enhance GABA-induced inhibition; the site of inhibition may be presynaptic in the spinal cord or postsynaptic in the cortical and cerebellar pyramidal cells, substantia nigra, and thalamic relay neurons. Studies have shown that barbiturates potentiate GABA-induced increases in chloride ion conductance in spinal neurons while reducing glutamate-induced depolarization. Barbiturates may block the excitatory effects of glutamate by inhibiting the actions of AMPA receptors (Marszalec and Nara-

Table 6–4. Barbiturates

Duration of action	Generic name	Brand name(s)
Ultra-short acting (15 minutes to 3 hours)	Thiopental Methohexital	Pentothal Brevital
Short acting (3–6 hours)	Pentobarbital Secobarbital	Nembutal Seconal, Tuinal (with amobarbital)
Intermediate acting (6–12 hours)	Amobarbital Butabarbital	Amytal, Tuinal (with secobarbital) Butisol
	Butalbital	Many combination products (e.g., Esgic, Fioricet, Fioricet with Codeine, and Fiorinal with Codeine)
Long acting (12–24 hours)	Phenobarbital	Luminal and many combination products, such as antispasmodic drugs, Barbidonna (belladonna alkaloids plus phenobarbital), Bel-Phen-Ergot SR, and Hyosophen
	Mephobarbital	Mebaral

hashi 1993); however, barbiturate inhibition of AMPA receptors may not play a role in either the hypnotic (Kamiya et al. 1999) or the anesthetic (Joo et al. 1999) actions of these agents. In high concentrations, barbiturates depress the activity of voltage-dependent sodium channels (Frenkel et al. 1990). Although barbiturates decrease the frequency of chloride channel openings, this is more than compensated for by their ability to increase the length of time the channels remain open. In addition to the CNS effect, barbiturates depress autonomic ganglia and nicotinic excitation. This effect may explain drops in blood pressure in cases of barbiturate intoxication. The type of α subunit in $GABA_A$ receptors may determine the extent to which pentobarbital can potentiate the effects of GABA (Mehta and Ticku 1999). In contrast to benzodiazepines such as diazepam, pentobarbital can potentiate the action of GABA in receptors containing α_4 and α_6 subunits (Mehta and Ticku 1999).

Psychological Effects

Barbiturates create a sense of relaxation, reduce tensions, and induce euphoria as measured by standardized scales. Concentration is greatly reduced, as is judgment, and irritability often results. Chronic use slurs speech and leads to incoherence, staggered gait, and tremors.

Central Nervous System Effects

The administration of butabarbital to recreational drug users produces significant elevations in drug liking and abuse potential scales (Zawertailo et al. 2003). The abuse potential of butabarbital appears to be significantly greater than that of either triazolam or meprobamate (Zawertailo et al. 2003). As previously described, all barbiturates produce general CNS depression, and they have been used to treat anxiety. Barbiturates with a 5-phenyl substituent (phenobarbital and mephobarbital) have an anticonvulsant effect as well. The effects of barbiturates are largely nonselective, and general CNS depression is required to produce a particular effect, although pain sensitivity is unaffected by barbiturates until the subject loses consciousness.

Barbiturates alter characteristics of sleep. Body movement and the number of awakenings per night are reduced. Rapid eye movement (REM) activity is reduced, although in the last third of the night, some REM compensation occurs. Slow-wave sleep (stages 3 and 4) is shortened, although phenobarbital may increase stage 4 sleep.

Effects on Other Organs

Respiratory drive and rhythm are depressed by barbiturates. Coughing, sneezing, hiccuping, and laryngospasm may occur during anesthesia with barbiturates. Sedative or hypnotic doses of barbiturates reduce heart rate and blood pressure to levels found in normal sleep. Anesthetic doses produce more pronounced effects. Barbiturates cross the placenta; when used in labor, they can cause respiratory depression in neonates. Anesthetic doses decrease force and frequency of uterine contractions among pregnant women.

Pharmacokinetics

The pharmacokinetics of barbiturates have been discussed by Charney et al. (2001) and Harvey (1985). When used as hypnotics or antianxiety agents, barbiturates are administered orally. As anticonvulsants, they may be used either orally or intravenously, although the latter route of administration may be problematic because these drugs are very alkaline, and necrosis and pain occur at the site of injection.

Barbiturates are primarily absorbed in the intestine and bind to plasma albumin in varying degrees based on their lipid solubility (the more lipid soluble, the more highly bound). The most lipid-soluble barbiturates (e.g., thiopental) reach the gray matter of the brain in a flow-limited uptake within 30 seconds, inducing sleep shortly thereafter. Because they are highly vascular, the heart, liver, and kidney also quickly reach their equilibrium concentrations. In contrast, barbiturates with low lipid solubility such as phenobarbital take up to 20 minutes to induce sleep because permeability, and not flow, is the limitation on uptake. In both cases, the drug then redistributes to the less vascular brain areas and to smooth muscle and skin within about 30 minutes and to fat after 60 minutes. With short-acting barbiturates, this redistribution reduces gray matter levels of the drug by up to 90% and is responsible for termination of the drug effect after a single dose.

Elimination of barbiturates depends on their lipid solubility. Lipid-soluble barbiturates are highly bound; these are poorly filtered by the kidneys and reabsorbed from the lumina and tubules. Appreciable amounts (e.g., 25%) of less lipid-soluble barbiturates, such as phenobarbital, may be excreted unchanged in the urine. Both urine alkalinization and osmotic diuresis increase renal excretion of phenobarbital or other less lipid-soluble barbiturates. Oxybarbiturates are metabolized exclusively in the liver; thiobarbiturates are also metabolized in the kidney and brain. Metabolites are more polar than parent compounds and are easily excreted. Because of long elimination half-lives, oral doses of barbiturates will accumulate during chronic administration, requiring dosage adjustment to avoid toxicity. Some evidence indicates that enantiomers of barbiturates have different clinical effects and kinetic characteristics.

Tolerance and Withdrawal

Pharmacodynamic tolerance to barbiturates develops over weeks to months, whereas pharmacokinetic tolerance occurs in a period of days. At maximum tolerance, the dosage of a barbiturate may be six times the original dosage.

Pentobarbital withdrawal may involve a distal region of chromosome 1 in the mouse (Buck et al. 1999). This site may be identical to a site associated with alcohol withdrawal. This finding suggests that common genes may be involved in both ethanol and pentobarbital dependence.

Detoxification

Tolerance to the clinical effects of barbiturates and an abstinence syndrome occurring on abrupt discontinuation of administration are well recognized, and we have previously described the management of barbiturate withdrawal (Ciraulo and Ciraulo 1988). The oxybarbiturates, with short to intermediate elimination half-lives, such as butalbital, amobarbital, secobarbital, and pentobarbital, are most likely to produce a withdrawal syndrome. Figure 6–6 describes the signs and symptoms of the barbiturate abstinence syndrome occurring after the abrupt withdrawal of secobarbital or pentobarbital following chronic intoxication at oral doses of 0.8–2.2 g/day for 6 weeks or more. According to Wikler's classification (Wikler 1968), minor symptoms (apprehension, muscular weakness, tremors, postural hypotension, twitches, insomnia, diaphoresis, paroxysmal discharges in the electroencephalogram, and anorexia) appear within 24 hours of the last barbiturate dose and persist up to 2 weeks. Major abstinence syndrome phenomena include tonic-clonic seizures and delirium. Two-thirds of patients with seizures have more than one, and they may have as many as four. The interictal electroencephalogram shows recurrent 4-per-second spike-wave discharges. The delirium may be accompanied by hyperthermia, which can be fatal. Chronic intoxication with pentobarbital at daily doses of 0.6–0.8 g for periods of 35–57 days produces a clinically significant withdrawal syndrome; daily doses of 0.2–0.4 g for 90 days or more rarely leads to withdrawal symptoms.

There are three common protocols for barbiturate detoxification. In all approaches, the goal is to prevent the occurrence of major symptoms and to minimize the development of intolerable minor symptoms.

The first approach (Table 6–5) is based on protocols described by several authors (Ewing and Bakewell 1967; Isbell 1950; Wikler 1968). The first step is determination of the severity of tolerance. If the patient is intoxicated, no additional barbiturate should be given until these symptoms have resolved. If there is substantial evidence or strong suspicion of chronic barbiturate use, it is not necessary or desirable to wait until withdrawal symptoms appear. A 200-mg oral dose of pentobarbital is given on an empty stomach to a sober patient (i.e., one who is not exhibiting signs of barbiturate intoxication), and the effects are observed at 1 hour. The patient's condition 1 hour after the test is used to determine the daily dose for stabilization.

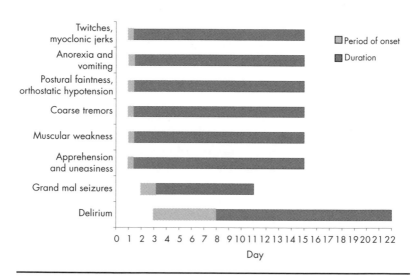

Figure 6–6.   Signs and symptoms of barbiturate withdrawal.

If no physical changes are observed after 1 hour, the test is repeated 3 hours later with 300 mg. If no response is seen after the 300-mg dose, the probable 24-hour requirement is greater than 1,200 mg/day. The daily dose is given every 4–6 hours for a 2- to 3-day stabilization period. Withdrawal regimens must be individualized, but the initial reduction is usually 10% of the daily stabilization dose. Some clinicians recommend the use of phenobarbital for stabilization and withdrawal because it is longer acting and may provide a smoother course of withdrawal. Phenobarbital doses are one-third those suggested for pentobarbital and may be adapted to the schedule described earlier for pentobarbital. The barbiturate withdrawal protocol can also be used for other sedative-hypnotic abstinence syndromes (e.g., those associated with chloral hydrate, glutethimide, and meprobamate).

The second protocol for barbiturate detoxification has been proposed by Sellers (1988). Citing uncertainties regarding dosage, reinforcement of drug-taking behavior by repeated administration, and difficulties assessing the clinical state as shortcomings of the older protocol, he proposed a loading-dose strategy. With this protocol, 120-mg doses of phenobarbital are given every 1–2 hours until three of the five signs—nystagmus, drowsiness, ataxia, dysarthria, and

Table 6–5.   Guidelines for barbiturate detoxification

Symptoms after test dose of 200 mg of oral pentobarbital	Estimated 24-hour oral pentobarbital dose (mg)	Estimated 24-hour oral phenobarbital dose (mg)
Asleep, but can be aroused	0	0
Sedated, drowsy, slurred speech, nystagmus, ataxia, positive Romberg test result	500–600	150–200
Few signs of intoxication, patient is comfortable, may have lateral nystagmus	800	250
No drug effect	1,000–1,200	300–400

Note.   Maximum phenobarbital dose is 600 mg.
Source.   Procedure modified from Ewing and Bakewell 1967.

emotional lability—are present or, if patients are symptomatic, withdrawal signs disappear. Patients are assessed for therapeutic or toxic effects prior to each dose. (It should be emphasized that some clinicians recommend lower individual phenobarbital doses, such as 40 mg). Sellers reported that the total loading dose was 1,440 mg. In some cases, hourly doses are required for 15–20 hours. In medically ill patients, phenobarbital may be infused intravenously (0.3 mg/kg/min). Under this protocol, medical supervision is necessary for 3 days. Those who require less than 7 mg/kg (usually about 480 mg) are not sufficiently dependent to require further detoxification.

The third protocol for barbiturate detoxification is to determine the level of drug use and calculate equivalent doses of phenobarbital (Table 6–6). The patient is stabilized on this dose (divided into administration every 8 hours) for a few days, and then the dose is tapered by 10% daily. Although this method has its proponents, the determination of equivalency is an approximation, drug histories are unreliable, and mixed sedative-hypnotic dependence will complicate the procedure.

Clinical Uses

Although benzodiazepines have largely replaced barbiturates in the treatment of anxiety and insomnia, barbiturates still have many therapeutic uses (Cooper

Table 6–6.   Sedative-hypnotic dose equivalency (equal to 30 mg of phenobarbital)

Generic name	Dose (mg)
Secobarbital	100
Pentobarbital	60
Chloral hydrate	250
Glutethimide	250
Meprobamate	200
Diazepam	5

1977; Harvey 1985). In psychiatry, they are used to treat agitated psychosis that is unresponsive to neuroleptics alone or to neuroleptics with benzodiazepines. Occasionally, patients withdrawing from alcohol will be resistant to benzodiazepines yet be responsive to barbiturates. Barbiturates are also used in catatonia ("Amytal interview") to temporarily relieve symptoms, permitting the patient to eat, bathe, and give historical information to the staff. Butalbital is a component of a commonly used treatment for migraine and tension headaches (Silberstein and McCrory 2001). In other areas of medicine, barbiturates are sometimes used as sedatives for ill children, in seizure disorders, as preanesthetic agents, and to induce anesthesia.

Toxicity

The most common unwanted effects of barbiturates are oversedation and psychomotor impairment, which may persist well into the next day following a hypnotic dose. Paradoxical excitement, hypersensitivity reactions, and muscle or joint pain may occur in rare cases. Drug-drug interactions occur with the CNS sedatives, and several drugs have enhanced metabolism when coadministered with barbiturates (Barnhill et al. 1989).

Death from overdose of barbiturates may occur and is more likely when more than 10 times the hypnotic dose is ingested. The barbiturates with high lipid solubility and short half-lives are the most toxic. Thus, the lethal dose of phenobarbital is 6–10 g, whereas that of secobarbital, pentobarbital, or amobarbital is 2–3 g. Symptoms of barbiturate poisoning include depression of the CNS, coma, depressed reflex activity, a positive Babinski reflex, contracted pupils (with hypoxia, there may be paralytic dilation), altered respiration, hypothermia, depressed cardiac function, hypotension, shock, pulmonary complications, and renal failure.

Glutethimide Dependence

Glutethimide (3-ethyl-3-phenyl-2, 6-piperidinedione) is a sedative-hypnotic drug rarely used therapeutically today because of wide variation in gastrointestinal absorption, fast development of pharmacodynamic tolerance, a fairly severe discontinuation syndrome, and potential for abuse. Reports of glutethimide dependence had declined *pari passu* with a decline in physician prescribing. The drug, when taken along with codeine orally, is reported to be euphorigenic in a manner resembling parenteral opiates (Khajawall et al. 1982; Sramek and Khajawall 1981).

Patients with glutethimide intoxication may present with CNS depression, widely dilated and fixed pupils, less respiratory depression than with barbiturates (although sudden apnea may occur), and a waxing and waning course that may persist for up to 120 hours (Maher et al. 1962). It has been suggested that such fluctuations may actually represent superimposed withdrawal phenomena (Bauer et al. 1988). The abstinence syndrome may include tremulousness, nausea, tachycardia, fever, tonic muscle spasms, and generalized convulsions (Harvey 1985). There has been one report of catatonia-like symptoms and dyskinesias associated with withdrawal (Campbell et al. 1983; Good 1975).

Detoxification may be accomplished with phenobarbital (60 mg of phenobarbital for 500 mg of glutethimide). If concomitant codeine dependency is present (and this should be strongly suspected), then methadone can be used adjunctively (10 mg of methadone for 120 mg of codeine) (Khajawall et al. 1982). Approximate sedative-hypnotic dosage equivalencies are listed in Table 6–6.

Conclusion

The benzodiazepines and selective $GABA_{A1}$ agonists are associated with lower abuse liability and toxicity than are older sedative-hypnotics, including the barbiturates. Their mechanisms of action are similar but not identical, which may influence their efficacy, abuse liability, and abstinence syndrome. Clinically significant differences in abuse liability are seen between and within the drug classes, although patient characteristics strongly influence the potential for misuse. The mechanisms by which tolerance develops to these agents also differ, as does the specific pattern of pharmacological actions that are most affected by tolerance. However, the therapeutic principles of prescribing are similar, requiring accurate diagnosis, appropriate dose and length of treatment, close medical management of the abstinence syndrome, and vigilance concerning misuse, especially in high-risk populations.

Case Examples

All case examples are composites of actual patients who underwent treatment at Boston University Medical Center. No identifiers are included, and cases have been modified to maintain basic teaching points without representing circumstances of specific patients.

Case Example 1: Triple Threat: Combined Methadone, Anabolic Steroids, and Benzodiazepine Dependence

A 24-year-old man who was an executive at an insurance company presented to the Boston University clinic because he had heard of our expertise in treating benzodiazepine withdrawal. He was taking 30 mg/day of clonazepam. After gradual reduction in dosage of the clonazepam to 5 mg/day, the patient was unable to taper further. At that time, he admitted to also using 60 mg/day of methadone, obtained through illicit sources. He was able to discontinue anabolic steroids without medical assistance.

Because sedative-hypnotic withdrawal results in the greatest morbidity, we recommended that he maintain the clonazepam at a dosage of 5 mg/day and focus on withdrawal from the methadone. Very experienced psychiatrists attempted two outpatient and one inpatient withdrawals with Suboxone, but the Suboxone substitution and taper were not well tolerated, and the patient developed lethargy, depression, vomiting, diarrhea, and trouble with his boss because he was not attending work. The methadone dosage was reduced to 30 mg/day, but further reductions were not tolerated. After another inpatient hospitalization that failed to switch him to Suboxone taper, the clinicians decided that the goal of treatment was maintenance Suboxone with the option of future slow withdrawal. He agreed to a slow taper of clonazepam.

We could not identify any underlying anxiety or depressive disorder, although we considered the possibility of drugs masking such symptoms.

Case Example 2: Too Empathic to Be Observant: Clonazepam Prescribed to Woman Who Denied Alcohol Abuse—Yet the Evidence Was in Plain View

A 27-year-old Boston, Massachusetts, police officer was walking her beat and got into an argument with a 60-year-old man who was intoxicated. Although she took standard precautions, before backup arrived the man hit her with a baseball bat. Fortunately, he was so intoxicated that he only grazed her scalp, and then other police officers arrived to arrest him. She was referred to our clinic by her primary care physician because she refused to leave her home, had recurrent thoughts of the event, had sleep disturbance, and felt hopeless about her future. The predominant symptom was avoidance—staying home and not being able to go to work—and she began a process for disability compensation.

She presented as a very sympathetic patient who had performed her job well until this incident. She obsessed about the incident and feared reprisal, especially when she was informed that she had to testify at the perpetrator's trial. The psychiatrist thought that no standard algorithm was available to follow because the patient's main complaint was panic disorder with agoraphobia, comorbid with posttraumatic stress disorder.

After 1 year of treatment that included SSRIs and atypical antipsychotics, in conjunction with psychotherapy, no improvement was seen, and in fact symptoms worsened. At this point, the psychiatrist introduced clonazepam to directly treat panic and agoraphobia. After 4 months, the treating psychiatrist realized that the patient was increasing her clonazepam doses without authorization.

The psychiatrist requested consultation from another psychiatrist experienced in addictions. When the other psychiatrist saw the patient, she immediately recognized signs of alcohol dependence—palmar erythema, Dupuytren contracture, and a ruddy complexion. The consultant ordered a complete blood count and differential and liver enzyme studies, which showed a macrocytic anemia, elevated liver enzyme levels, high levels of high-density lipoprotein cholesterol, and hyperuricemia. The patient was hospitalized and safely withdrawn from medications. She was referred to CBT. She continues to take SSRI and low-dose atypical antipsychotic drugs.

Case Example 3: No Good Deed Goes Unpunished

The on-call psychiatry resident evaluated a relative of a prominent politician and called a senior faculty member for input. The patient had left work that evening and described to the resident classic panic disorder symptoms. Laboratory tests and an interview with the patient's wife verified that a drug was not contributing to his symptoms. After a full discussion with the resident, the faculty member gave the patient an appointment for the following day and thereafter saw him twice weekly for 2 weeks.

After an appropriate evaluation period, the senior faculty member prescribed clonazepam, 0.5 mg three times daily; referred the patient to a specialized group for anxiety disorders; and continued with psychotherapy and clonazepam therapy. After 3 weeks of outpatient treatment, the senior attending was called by the state police, who informed him that the patient had driven off the road, and they determined that he was intoxicated and had psychomotor impairment resulting from the prescribed agent. They were bringing him to our hospital so that his psychiatrist could continue management. That was at 3:00 A.M. Saturday night, and the attending saw him in the hospital at 7:00 A.M. Sunday. As he walked in, the patient's mother yelled: "We are going to sue you for everything you are worth for putting our boy in this hospital." No matter how assiduous this attending had been in diagnosis, consultation, and medication treatment, the verbal confrontation was enough to shake him. He consulted with department leadership, who investigated in greater detail and found that the police had found 200 turquoise tablets, which are 1-mg clonazepam, at the accident and no yellow tablets, the 0.5-mg formulation. Nevertheless, the treating psychiatrist was shaken and transferred care to another psychiatrist. The family was contrite when they realized that their son had obtained illicit clonazepam.

Case Example 4: Did It Really Take Three Automobile Accidents to Realize That Benzodiazepines Impair Psychomotor Performance?

In the Boston area, academic psychiatrists often maintain small, private psychotherapy practices in a home office. A 45-year-old man was receiving treatment for "an anxiety disorder, with components of agoraphobia" according to the referring clinician. At the psychiatrist's home office, the man received a combination of psychotherapy and lorazepam. The patient's pathology was greater than anticipated and included paranoid ideation, but he made great strides during only 1 year. Perhaps the clinical improvement made the psychiatrist lower his vigilance, but after the first month of lorazepam, the patient drove his new luxury vehicle into a tree, which caused minimal damage. A few months later, the patient drove his luxury car over a series of in-ground electrical spotlights lining a 500-foot driveway. However, it was not until the patient backed into another patient's car that the psychiatrist was convinced that persistent psychomotor impairment occurred with benzodiazepine treatment in this patient. He refused to prescribe the drug any longer, and the patient sought other treatment.

Case Example 5: An Alcoholic Patient With 2 Years of Abstinence and Panic Disorder With Agoraphobia: Is There Any Support for a Benzodiazepine?

A 32-year-old woman had 2 years of abstinence from alcohol but was still severely hampered by panic attacks and agoraphobia. She did not respond to CBT by a skilled therapist. Her symptoms also did not respond to antidepressant therapy. The clinician is faced with a decision about whether to institute a trial with a benzodiazepine for panic disorder with agoraphobia.

Case Example 6: Alcohol Withdrawal Syndrome, Haloperidol, and Lorazepam: What Is Causing the Delirium?

A 55-year-old man presented for an outpatient evaluation with the addiction treatment team. As the evaluation progressed, the man developed increasing tremulousness and sweating. In retrospect, he was also developing confusion and disorientation, but he was able to hide it, even from experienced clinicians. The attending missed the level of confusion and sent the patient to the emergency department for evaluation with a hospital assistant. While the assistant was distracted by a page regarding another patient, the man he was escorting to the emergency department wandered off and could not be located. It took 2 hours to find the patient on the perimeter of the medical campus. By then, the man did not know what city he was in and was asking for a cab to drive him to New Hampshire (his home). The patient was admitted to the medical unit, where the alcohol and benzodiazepine detoxification protocol was started. Lorazepam, 1 mg, and haloperidol, 1 mg, were administered every 4 hours, but the patient's condition worsened. The chief medical resident started an increasing dosage of haloperidol and lorazepam. Although the patient was on cardiac telemetry, the cardiology fellow restricted his treatment with haloperidol out of concern for the possible occurrence of torsades de pointes. Increasing doses of lorazepam were administered, but the delirium worsened. Lorazepam was discontinued, and amobarbital was substituted. In 3 days, the delirium resolved, and the patient was discharged.

References

Allison C, Pratt JA: Neuroadaptive processes in GABAergic and glutamatergic systems in benzodiazepine dependence. Pharmacol Ther 98:171–195, 2003

American Psychiatric Association: Diagnostic and Statistical Manual of Mental Disorders, 5th Edition. Arlington, VA, American Psychiatric Association, 2013

Anzini M, Canullo L, Braile C, et al: Synthesis, biological evaluation, and receptor docking simulations of 2-[(acylamino)ethyl]-1,4-benzodiazepines as kappa-opioid receptor agonists endowed with antinociceptive and antiamnesic activity. J Med Chem 46:3853–3864, 2003

Apsler R, Rothman E: Correlates of compliance with psychoactive prescriptions. J Psychoactive Drugs 16:193–199, 1984

Arendt RM, Greenblatt DJ, deJong RH, et al: In vitro correlates of benzodiazepine cerebrospinal fluid uptake, pharmacodynamic action and peripheral distribution. J Pharmacol Exp Ther 227:98–106, 1983

Ashley MJ, le Riche WH, Hatcher J, et al: "Mixed" (drug abusing) and "pure" alcoholics: a socio-medical comparison. Br J Addict Alcohol Other Drugs 73:19–34, 1978

Ashton H: Benzodiazepine withdrawal: an unfinished story. Br Med J (Clin Res Ed) 288:1135–1140, 1984

Atack JR: Anxioselective compounds acting at the GABA(A) receptor benzodiazepine binding site. Curr Drug Target CNS Neurol Disord 2:213–232, 2003

Ator NA: Relation between discriminative and reinforcing effects of midazolam, pentobarbital, chlordiazepoxide, zolpidem, and imidazenil in baboons. Psychopharmacology (Berl) 163:477–487, 2002

Ator NA: Selectivity in generalization to GABAergic drugs in midazolam-trained baboons. Pharmacol Biochem Behav 75:435–445, 2003

Ator NA, Weerts EM, Kaminski BJ, et al: Zaleplon and triazolam physical dependence assessed across increasing doses under a once-daily dosing regimen in baboons. Drug Alcohol Depend 61:69–84, 2000

Ator NA, Atack JR, Hargreaves RJ, et al: Reducing abuse liability of GABAA/benzodiazepine ligands via selective partial agonist efficacy at alpha1 and alpha2/3 subtypes. J Pharmacol Exp Ther 332:4–16, 2010

Balter MB, Manheimer DI, Mellinger GD, et al: A cross-national comparison of antianxiety/sedative drug use. Curr Med Res Opin 8 (suppl 4):5–20, 1984

Barker MJ, Greenwood KM, Jackson M, et al: Cognitive effects of long-term benzodiazepine use: a meta-analysis. CNS Drugs 18:37–48, 2004a

Barker MJ, Greenwood KM, Jackson M, et al: Persistence of cognitive effects after withdrawal from long-term benzodiazepine use: a meta-analysis. Arch Clin Neuropsychol 19:437–454, 2004b

Barnard EA, Skolnick P, Olsen RW, et al: International Union of Pharmacology, XV: subtypes of gamma-aminobutyric acidA receptors: classification on the basis of subunit structure and receptor function. Pharmacol Rev 50:291–313, 1998

Barnhill JG, Ciraulo AM, Ciraulo DA: Interactions of importance in chemical dependence, in Drug Interaction in Psychiatry. Edited by Ciraulo DA, Shader RI, Greenblatt DJ, et al. Baltimore, MD, Williams & Wilkins, 1989, pp 234–237

Bauer MS, Fus AF, Hanich RF, et al: Glutethimide intoxication and withdrawal. Am J Psychiatry 145:530–531, 1988

Bell R, Havlicek PL, Roncek DW: Sex differences in the use of alcohol and tranquilizers: testing a role convergence hypothesis. Am J Drug Alcohol Abuse 10:551–561, 1984

Bossert JM, Franklin KB: Pentobarbital-induced place preference in rats is blocked by GABA, dopamine, and opioid antagonists. Psychopharmacology (Berl) 157:115–122, 2001

Bowden CL, Fisher JG: Safety and efficacy of long-term diazepam therapy. South Med J 73:1581–1584, 1980

Braestrup C, Nielsen M, Honoré T, et al: Benzodiazepine receptor ligands with positive and negative efficacy. Neuropharmacology 22(12B):1451–1457, 1983

Brogden RN, Goa KL: Flumazenil: a preliminary review of its benzodiazepine antagonist properties, intrinsic activity and therapeutic use. Drugs 35:448–467, 1988

Bruce TJ, Spiegel DA, Hegel MT: Cognitive-behavioral therapy helps prevent relapse and recurrence of panic disorder following alprazolam discontinuation: a long-term follow-up of the Peoria and Dartmouth studies. J Consult Clin Psychol 67:151–156, 1999

Buck K, Metten P, Belknap J, et al: Quantitative trait loci affecting risk for pentobarbital withdrawal map near alcohol withdrawal loci on mouse chromosomes 1, 4, and 11. Mamm Genome 10:431–437, 1999

Buldakova S, Weiss M: Electrophysiological evidence for agonist properties of flumazenil, a benzodiazepine receptor antagonist, in rat hippocampus slices. J Neurol Sci 149:121–126, 1997

Busto U, Simpkins J, Sellers EM, et al: Objective determination of benzodiazepine use and abuse in alcoholics. Br J Addict 78:429–435, 1983

Busto U, Sellers EM, Naranjo CA, et al: Patterns of benzodiazepine abuse and dependence. Br J Addict 81:87–94, 1986a

Busto U, Sellers EM, Naranjo CA, et al: Withdrawal reaction after long-term therapeutic use of benzodiazepines. N Engl J Med 315:854–859, 1986b

Busto UE, Romach MK, Sellers EM: Multiple drug use and psychiatric comorbidity in patients admitted to the hospital with severe benzodiazepine dependence. J Clin Psychopharmacol 16:51–57, 1996

Busto UE, Bremner KE, Kinght K, et al: Long-term benzodiazepine therapy does not result in brain abnormalities. J Clin Psychopharmacol 20:2–6, 2000

Caille G, Spénard J, Lacasse Y, et al: Pharmacokinetics of two lorazepam formulations, oral and sublingual, after multiple doses. Biopharm Drug Dispos 4:31–42, 1983

Campbell R, Schaffer CB, Tupin J: Catatonia associated with glutethimide withdrawal. J Clin Psychiatry 44:32–33, 1983

Cantopher T, Oliveri S, Cleave N, et al: Chronic benzodiazepine dependence: a comparative study of abrupt withdrawal under propranolol cover versus gradual withdrawal. Br J Psychiatry 156:406–411, 1990

Caplan RD, Andrews FM, Conway TL, et al: Social effects of diazepam use: a longitudinal field study. Soc Sci Med 21:887–898, 1985

Charney DA, Paraherakis AM, Gill KJ: The treatment of sedative-hypnotic dependence: evaluating clinical predictors of outcome. J Clin Psychiatry 61:190–195, 2000

Charney DA, Paraherakis AM, Gill KJ: Integrated treatment of comorbid depression and substance use disorders. J Clin Psychiatry 62:672–677, 2001

Chen S, Huang X, Zeng XJ, et al: Benzodiazepine-mediated regulation of alpha1, alpha2, beta1–3 and gamma2 GABA(A) receptor subunit proteins in the rat brain hippocampus and cortex. Neuroscience 93:33–44, 1999

Ciraulo DA, Ciraulo AM: Substance abuse, in Handbook of Clinical Psychopharmacology. Edited by Tupin JP, Shader RI, Harnett DS. Northvale, NJ, Jason Aronson, 1988, pp 121–158

Ciraulo DA, Nace EP: Benzodiazepine treatment of anxiety or insomnia in substance abuse patients. Am J Addict 9:276–279; discussion 280–284, 2000

Ciraulo DA, Sarid-Segal O: Sedative-, hypnotic-, or anxiolytic-related abuse, in Comprehensive Textbook of Psychiatry, Vol 1, 8th Edition. Edited by Sadock BJ, Sadock VA. Philadelphia, PA, Lippincott Williams & Wilkins, 2005, pp 1300–1318

Ciraulo DA, Barnhill JG, Greenblatt DJ, et al: Abuse liability and clinical pharmacokinetics of alprazolam in alcoholic men. J Clin Psychiatry 49:333–337, 1988a

Ciraulo DA, Sands BF, Shader RI: Critical review of liability for benzodiazepine abuse among alcoholics. Am J Psychiatry 145:1501–1506, 1988b

Ciraulo DA, Barnhill JG, Ciraulo AM, et al: Parental alcoholism as a risk factor in benzodiazepine abuse: a pilot study. Am J Psychiatry 146:1333–1335, 1989

Ciraulo DA, Antal EJ, Smith RB, et al: The relationship of alprazolam dose to steady-state plasma concentrations. J Clin Psychopharmacol 10:27–32, 1990

Ciraulo DA, Sarid-Segal O, Knapp C, et al: Liability to alprazolam abuse in daughters of alcoholics. Am J Psychiatry 153:956–958, 1996

Ciraulo DA, Barnhill JG, Ciraulo AM, et al: Alterations in pharmacodynamics of anxiolytics in abstinent alcoholic men: subjective responses, abuse liability, and electroencephalographic effects of alprazolam, diazepam, and buspirone. J Clin Pharmacol 37:64–73, 1997

Ciraulo DA, Knapp CM, LoCastro J, et al: A benzodiazepine mood effect scale: reliability and validity determined for alcohol-dependent subjects and adults with a parental history of alcoholism. Am J Drug Alcohol Abuse 27:339–347, 2001

Conell LJ, Berlin RM: Withdrawal after substitution of a short-acting for a long-acting benzodiazepine. JAMA 250:2838–2840, 1983

Cooper JR: Sedative-Hypnotic Drugs: Risks and Benefits (DHEW Publ No ADM-78-592). Rockville, MD, National Institute on Drug Abuse, 1977

Covi L, Lipman RS, Pattison JH, et al: Length of treatment with anxiolytic sedatives and response to their sudden withdrawal. Acta Psychiatr Scand 49:51–64, 1973

Cumming RG, Le Couteur DG: Benzodiazepines and risk of hip fractures in older people: a review of the evidence. CNS Drugs 17:825–837, 2003

Cumming RG, Miller JP, Kelsey JL, et al: Medications and multiple falls in elderly people: the St Louis OASIS study. Age Ageing 20:455–461, 1991

Curran HV: Tranquillising memories: a review of the effects of benzodiazepines on human memory. Biol Psychol 23:179–213, 1986

Curran HV, Collins R, Fletcher S, et al: Older adults and withdrawal from benzodiazepine hypnotics in general practice: effects on cognitive function, sleep, mood and quality of life. Psychol Med 33:1223–1237, 2003

Cushman P, Benzer D: Benzodiazepines and drug abuse: clinical observations in chemically dependent persons before and during abstinence. Drug Alcohol Depend 6:365–371, 1980

Darke S, Ross J, Teesson M, et al: Health service utilization and benzodiazepine use among heroin users: findings from the Australian Treatment Outcome Study (ATOS). Addiction 98:1129–1135, 2003

Darragh A, Lambe R, Kenny M, et al: Tolerance of healthy volunteers to intravenous administration of the benzodiazepine antagonist (letter). Ir J Med Sci 90:151, 1982

de las Cuevas C, Sanz E, de la Fuente J: Benzodiazepines: more "behavioural" addiction than dependence. Psychopharmacology (Berl) 167:297–303, 2003

de Wit H, Johanson CE, Uhlenhuth EH: Reinforcing properties of lorazepam in normal volunteers. Drug Alcohol Depend 13:31–41, 1984

de Wit H, Pierri J, Johanson CE: Reinforcing and subjective effects of diazepam in nondrug-abusing volunteers. Pharmacol Biochem Behav 33:205–213, 1989

Dealberto MJ, Mcavay GJ, Seeman T, et al: Psychotropic drug use and cognitive decline among older men and women. Int J Geriatr Psychiatry 12:567–574, 1997

Dennis T, Dubois A, Benavides J, et al: Distribution of central omega 1 (benzodiazepine1) and omega 2 (benzodiazepine2) receptor subtypes in the monkey and human brain: an autoradiographic study with [3H]flunitrazepam and the omega 1 selective ligand [3H]zolpidem. J Pharmacol Exp Ther 247:309–322, 1988

DiChiara G, Imperato A: Drugs abused by humans preferentially increase synaptic dopamine concentrations in the mesolimbic system of freely moving rats. Proc Natl Acad Sci U S A 85:5274–5278, 1988

Dinwiddie SH, Cottler L, Compton W, et al: Psychopathology and HIV risk behaviors among injection drug users in and out of treatment. Drug Alcohol Depend 43:1–11, 1996

Doble A, Canton T, Dreisler S, et al: RP 59037 and RP 60503: anxiolytic cyclopyrrolone derivatives with low sedative potential. Interaction with the gamma-aminobutyric acidA/benzodiazepine receptor complex and behavioral effects in the rodent. J Pharmacol Exp Ther 266:1213–1226, 1993

Dunbar GC, Perera MD, Jenner FA: Patterns of benzodiazepine use in Great Britain as measured by a general population survey. Br J Psychiatry 155:836–841, 1989

Elie R, Rüther E, Farr I, et al: Sleep latency is shortened during 4 weeks of treatment with zaleplon, a novel nonbenzodiazepine hypnotic. Zaleplon Clinical Study Group. J Clin Psychiatry 60:536–544, 1999

Ensrud KE, Blackwell T, Mangione CM, et al: Central nervous system active medications and risk for fractures in older women. Arch Intern Med 163:949–957, 2003

Evans SM, Griffiths RR, de Wit H: Preference for diazepam, but not buspirone, in moderate drinkers. Psychopharmacology (Berl) 123:154–163, 1996

Ewing JA, Bakewell WE: Diagnosis and management of depressant drug dependence. Am J Psychiatry 123:909–917, 1967

Fahey JM, Pritchard GA, Grassi JM, et al: Pharmacodynamic and receptor binding changes during chronic lorazepam administration. Pharmacol Biochem Behav 69:1–8, 2001

File SE: Tolerance to the behavioral actions of benzodiazepines. Neurosci Biobehav Rev 9:113–121, 1985

Finlay JM, Damsma G, Fibiger HC: Benzodiazepine-induced decreases in extracellular concentrations of dopamine in the nucleus accumbens after acute and repeated administration. Psychopharmacology (Berl) 106:202–208, 1992

Fishbain DA, Rosomoff HL, Rosomoff RS: Drug abuse, dependence, and addiction in chronic pain patients. Clin J Pain 8:77–85, 1992

Fleischhacker WW, Barnas C, Hackenberg B: Epidemiology of benzodiazepine dependence. Acta Psychiatr Scand 74:80–83, 1986

Frenkel C, Duch DS, Urban BW: Molecular actions of pentobarbital isomers on sodium channels from human brain cortex. Anesthesiology 72:640–649, 1990

Fry J, Scharf M, Mangano R, et al: Zaleplon improves sleep without producing rebound effects in outpatients with insomnia. Zaleplon Clinical Study Group. Int Clin Psychopharmacol 15:141–152, 2000

Fyer AJ, Liebowitz MR, Gorman JM, et al: Effects of clonidine on alprazolam discontinuation in panic patients: a pilot study. J Clin Psychopharmacol 8:270–274, 1988

Garvey MJ, Tollefson GD: Prevalence of misuse of prescribed benzodiazepines in patients with primary anxiety disorder or major depression. Am J Psychiatry 143:1601–1603, 1986

Gerra G, Zaimovic A, Gusti F, et al: Intravenous flumazenil versus oxazepam tapering in the treatment of benzodiazepine withdrawal: a randomized, placebo-controlled study. Addict Biol 7:385–395, 2002

Good MI: Catatonia-like symptomatology and withdrawal dyskinesias. Am J Psychiatry 133:1454–1456, 1975

Goodman WK, Charney DS, Price LH, et al: Ineffectiveness of clonidine in the treatment of the benzodiazepine withdrawal syndrome: report of three cases. Am J Psychiatry 143:900–903, 1986

Gottschalk LA, Bates DE, Fox RA, et al: Psychoactive drug use. Patterns found in samples from a mental health clinic and a general medical clinic. Arch Gen Psychiatry 25:395–397, 1971

Gray A, Allison C, Pratt JA: A role for AMPA/kainate receptors in conditioned place preference induced by diazepam in the rat. Neurosci Lett 268:127–130, 1999

Greenblatt DJ, Shader RI: Dependence, tolerance, and addiction to benzodiazepines: clinical and pharmacokinetic considerations. Drug Metab Rev 8:13–28, 1978

Greenblatt DJ, Shader RI: Long-term administration of benzodiazepines: pharmacokinetic versus pharmacodynamic tolerance. Psychopharmacol Bull 22:416–423, 1986

Greenblatt DJ, Shader RI, Koch-Weser J: Psychotropic drug use in the Boston area: a report from the Boston Collaborative Drug Surveillance Program. Arch Gen Psychiatry 32:518–521, 1975

Greenblatt DJ, Shader RI, Harmatz JS, et al: Self-rated sedation and plasma concentrations of desmethyldiazepam following single doses of clorazepate. Psychopharmacology (Berl) 66:289–290, 1979

Greenblatt DJ, Divoll M, Harmatz JS, et al: Pharmacokinetic comparison of sublingual lorazepam with intravenous, intramuscular, and oral lorazepam. J Pharm Sci 71:248–252, 1982

Greenblatt DJ, Shader RI, Abernethy DR: Drug therapy: current status of benzodiazepines. N Engl J Med 309(6):354–358, 1983a

Greenblatt DJ, Shader RI, Abernethy DR: Drug therapy: current status of benzodiazepines. N Engl J Med 309(7):410–416, 1983b

Greenblatt DJ, Harmatz JS, Zinny MA, et al: Effect of gradual withdrawal on the rebound sleep disorder after discontinuation of triazolam. N Engl J Med 317:722–728, 1987

Greenblatt DJ, von Moltke LL, Harmatz JS, et al: Differential impairment of triazolam and zolpidem clearance by ritonavir. J Acquir Immune Defic Syndr 24:129–136, 2000

Griffiths RR, Weerts EM: Benzodiazepine self-administration in humans and laboratory animals—implications for problems of long-term use and abuse. Psychopharmacology (Berl) 134:1–37, 1997

Griffiths RR, Wolf B: Relative abuse liability of different benzodiazepines in drug abusers. J Clin Psychopharmacol 10:237–243, 1990

Griffiths RR, Bigelow GE, Liebson I, et al: Drug preference in humans: double-blind choice comparison of pentobarbital, diazepam and placebo. J Pharmacol Exp Ther 215:649–661, 1980

Griffiths RR, McLeod DR, Bigelow GE, et al: Comparison of diazepam and oxazepam: preference, liking and extent of abuse. J Pharmacol Exp Ther 229:501–508, 1984

Griffiths RR, Evans SM, Guarino JJ, et al: Intravenous flumazenil following acute and repeated exposure to lorazepam in healthy volunteers: antagonism and precipitated withdrawal. J Pharmacol Exp Ther 265:1163–1174, 1993

Hadingham KL, Wingrove P, Le Bourdelles B, et al: Cloning of cDNA sequences encoding human alpha 2 and alpha 3 gamma-aminobutyric acidA receptor subunits and characterization of the benzodiazepine pharmacology of recombinant alpha 1-, alpha 2-, alpha 3-, and alpha 5-containing human gamma-aminobutyric acidA receptors. Mol Pharmacol 43:970–975, 1993

Hajak G, Müller WE, Wittchen HU, et al: Abuse and dependence potential for the non-benzodiazepine hypnotics zolpidem and zopiclone: a review of case reports and epidemiological data. Addiction 98:1371–1378, 2003

Hallstrom C, Lader MH: The incidence of benzodiazepine dependence in long-term users. J Psychiatr Treat Eval 1982:293–296, 1982

Hanlon JT, Horner RD, Schmader KE, et al: Benzodiazepine use and cognitive function among community-dwelling elderly. Clin Pharmacol Ther 64:684–692, 1998

Hardo PG, Kennedy TD: Night sedation and arthritic pain. J R Soc Med 84:73–75, 1991

Harvey SC: Hypnotics and sedatives, in The Pharmacologic Basis of Therapeutics. Edited by Goodman A, Gilman LD. New York, Macmillan, 1985, pp 339–371

Hendler N, Cimini C, Ma T, et al: A comparison of cognitive impairment due to benzodiazepines and to narcotics. Am J Psychiatry 137:828–830, 1980

Herman JB, Rosenbaum JF, Brotman AW: The alprazolam to clonazepam switch for the treatment of panic disorder. J Clin Psychopharmacol 7:175–178, 1987

Higgitt A, Lader M, Fonagy P: The effects of the benzodiazepine antagonist Ro 15–1788 on psychophysiological performance and subjective measures in normal subjects. Psychopharmacology (Berl) 89:395–403, 1986

Hoiseth G, Kristiansen KM, Kvande K, et al: Benzodiazepines in geriatric psychiatry: what doctors report and what patients actually use. Drugs Aging 30:113–118, 2013

Hollister LE, Motzenbecker FP, Degan RO: Withdrawal reactions from chlordiazepoxide ("Librium"). Psychopharmacologia 2:63–68, 1961

Hollister LE, Bennett JL, Kimbell I Jr, et al: Diazepam in newly admitted schizophrenics. Dis Nerv Syst 24:746–750, 1963

Ibrahim RB, Wilson JG, Thorsby ME, et al: Effect of buprenorphine on CYP3A activity in rat and human liver microsomes. Life Sci 66:1293–1298, 2000

Iguchi MY, Handelsman L, Bickel WK, et al: Benzodiazepine and sedative use/abuse by methadone maintenance clients. Drug Alcohol Depend 32:257–266, 1993

Isbell H: Manifestations and treatment of addiction to narcotic drugs and barbiturates. Med Clin North Am 34:425–438, 1950

Jaffe JH, Ciraulo DA, Nies A, et al: Abuse potential of halazepam and of diazepam in patients recently treated for acute alcohol withdrawal. Clin Pharmacol Ther 34:623–630, 1983

Johanson CE, de Wit H: Lack of effect of social context on the reinforcing effects of diazepam in humans. Pharmacol Biochem Behav 43:463–469, 1992

Johansson BA, Berglund M, Hanson M, et al: Dependence on legal psychotropic drugs among alcoholics. Alcohol Alcohol 38:613–618, 2003

Johnston LD, O'Malley PM, Bachman JG, et al: Monitoring the Future National Results on Adolescent Drug Use: Overview of Key Findings, 2011. Ann Arbor, Institute for Social Research, University of Michigan, 2012, p 78

Joo DT, Xiong Z, MacDonald JF, et al: Blockade of glutamate receptors and barbiturate anesthesia: increased sensitivity to pentobarbital-induced anesthesia despite reduced inhibition of AMPA receptors in GluR2 null mutant mice. Anesthesiology 91:1329–1341, 1999

Kamiya Y, Andoh T, Furuya R, et al: Comparison of the effects of convulsant and depressant barbiturate stereoisomers on AMPA-type glutamate receptors. Anesthesiology 90:1704–1713, 1999

Kania J, Kofoed L: Drug use by alcoholics in outpatient treatment. Am J Drug Alcohol Abuse 10:529–534, 1984

Khajawall AM, Sramek JJ Jr, Simpson GM: "Loads" alert. West J Med 137:166–168, 1982

Kilicarslan T, Sellers EM: Lack of interaction of buprenorphine with flunitrazepam metabolism. Am J Psychiatry 157:1164–1166, 2000

King SA, Strain JJ: Benzodiazepines and chronic pain. Pain 41:3–4, 1990a

King SA, Strain JJ: Benzodiazepine use by chronic pain patients. Clin J Pain 6:143–147, 1990b

Klein E, Uhde TW, Post RM: Preliminary evidence for the utility of carbamazepine in alprazolam withdrawal. Am J Psychiatry 143:235–236, 1986

Kouyanou K, Pither CE, Wessely S: Medication misuse, abuse and dependence in chronic pain patients. J Psychosom Res 43:497–504, 1997

Kryspin-Exner K: [Misuse of bezodiazepine derivatives in alcoholics]. Br J Addict Alcohol Other Drugs 61:283–290, 1966

Kryspin-Exner K, Demel I: The use of tranquilizers in the treatment of mixed drug abuse. Int J Clin Pharmacol Biopharm 12:13–18, 1975

Kushner MG, Sher KJ, Beitman BD: The relation between alcohol problems and the anxiety disorders. Am J Psychiatry 147:685–695, 1990

Lader M: Benzodiazepines revisited—will we ever learn? Addiction 106:2086–2109, 2011

Lader M: Dependence and withdrawal: comparison of the benzodiazepines and selective serotonin re-uptake inhibitors. Addiction 107:909–910, 2012

Lader M, Olajide D: A comparison of buspirone and placebo in relieving benzodiazepine withdrawal symptoms. J Clin Psychopharmacol 7:11–15, 1987

Lader MH, Ron M, Petursson H: Computed axial brain tomography in long-term benzodiazepine users. Psychol Med 14:203–206, 1984

Lejoyeux M, Solomon J, Ades J: Benzodiazepine treatment for alcohol-dependent patients. Alcohol Alcohol 33:563–575, 1998

Leufkens TR, Lund JS, Vermeeren A: Highway driving performance and cognitive functioning the morning after bedtime and middle-of-the-night use of gaboxadol, zopiclone and zolpidem. J Sleep Res 18:387–396, 2009

Lingford-Hughes A, Hume SP, Feeney A, et al: Imaging the GABA-benzodiazepine receptor subtype containing the alpha5-subunit in vivo with [11C]Ro15 4513 positron emission tomography. J Cereb Blood Flow Metab 22:878–889, 2002

Lister RG: The amnesic action of benzodiazepines in man. Neurosci Biobehav Rev 9:87–94, 1985

Löw K, Crestani F, Keist R, et al: Molecular and neuronal substrate for the selective attenuation of anxiety. Science 290:131–134, 2000

Luddens H, Prichett DB, Köhler M, et al: Cerebellar GABAA receptor selective for a behavioural alcohol antagonist. Nature 346:648–651, 1990

Lupolover Y, Safran AB, Desangles D, et al: Evaluation of visual function in healthy subjects after administration of Ro 15-1788. Eur J Clin Pharmacol 27:505–507, 1984

Maher JF, Schreiner GE, Westervelt FB Jr: Acute glutethimide intoxication, I: clinical experience (twenty-two patients) compared to acute barbiturate intoxication (sixty-three patients). Am J Med 33:70–82, 1962

Manthey L, van Veen T, Giltay EJ, et al: Correlates of (inappropriate) benzodiazepine use: the Netherlands Study of Depression and Anxiety (NESDA). Br J Clin Pharmacol 71:263–272, 2011

Marks J: Benzodiazepines: Use, Overuse, Misuse, Abuse. Baltimore, MD, University Park Press, 1978

Marszalec W, Narahashi T: Use-dependent pentobarbital block of kainate and quisqualate currents. Brain Res 608:7–15, 1993

Matthew H: Acute Barbiturate Poisoning. Amsterdam, The Netherlands, Excerpta Medica, 1971

Mattila-Evenden M, Bergman U, Franck J: A study of benzodiazepine users claiming drug-induced psychiatric morbidity. Nord J Psychiatry 55:271–278, 2001

Maubach K: GABA(A) receptor subtype selective cognition enhancers. Curr Drug Target CNS Neurol Disord 2:233–239, 2003

McAndrews MP, Weiss RT, Sandor P, et al: Cognitive effects of long-term benzodiazepine use in older adults. Hum Psychopharmacol 18:51–57, 2003

McKernan RM, Rosahl TW, Reynolds DS, et al: Sedative but not anxiolytic properties of benzodiazepines are mediated by the GABA(A) receptor alpha1 subtype. Nat Neurosci 3:587–592, 2000

Mehta AK, Ticku MK: An update on GABAA receptors. Brain Res Brain Res Rev 29:196–217, 1999

Mellinger GD, Balter MB: Prevalence and patterns of use of psychotropic drugs: results from a 1979 national survey of American adults, in Epidemiological Impact of Psychotropic Drugs: Proceedings of the International Seminar on Psychotropic Drugs. Edited by Tognomi G, Bellantuono C, Lader M. Amsterdam, The Netherlands, North Holland Publishing, 1981, pp 117–135

Mellinger GD, Balter MB, Uhlenhuth EH: Prevalence and correlates of the long-term regular use of anxiolytics. JAMA 251:375–379, 1984

Miller LG, Greenblatt DJ, Barnhill JG, et al: Benzodiazepine receptor binding of triazolobenzodiazepines in vivo: increased receptor number with low-dose alprazolam. J Neurochem 49:1595–1601, 1987

Miller LG, Greenblatt DJ, Barnhill JG, et al: Chronic benzodiazepine administration, I: tolerance is associated with benzodiazepine receptor downregulation and decreased gamma-aminobutyric acidA receptor function. J Pharmacol Exp Ther 246:170–176, 1988a

Miller LG, Greenblatt DJ, Roy RB, et al: Chronic benzodiazepine administration, II: discontinuation syndrome is associated with upregulation of gamma-aminobutyric acidA receptor complex binding and function. J Pharmacol Exp Ther 246:177–182, 1988b

Mintzer MZ, Stoller KB, Griffiths RR: A controlled study of flumazenil-precipitated withdrawal in chronic low-dose benzodiazepine users. Psychopharmacology (Berl) 147:200–209, 1999

Moodley P, Golombok S, Shine P, et al: Computed axial brain tomograms in long-term benzodiazepine users. Psychiatry Res 48:135–144, 1993

Mueller TI, Goldenberg IM, Gordon AL, et al: Benzodiazepine use in anxiety disordered patients with and without a history of alcoholism. J Clin Psychiatry 57:83–89, 1996

Mumford GK, Evans SM, Fleishaker JC, et al: Alprazolam absorption kinetics affects abuse liability. Clin Pharmacol Ther 57:356–365, 1995a

Mumford GK, Rush CR, Griffiths RR: Abecarnil and alprazolam in humans: behavioral, subjective and reinforcing effects. J Pharmacol Exp Ther 272:570–580, 1995b

Nielsen M, Hansen EH, Gotzsche PC: What is the difference between dependence and withdrawal reactions? A comparison of benzodiazepines and selective serotonin reuptake inhibitors. Addiction 107:900–908, 2012

Nutt DJ, Linnoila M: Neuroreceptor science: a clarification of terms. J Clin Psychopharmacol 8:387–389, 1988

Nutt DJ, Glue P, Lawson C, et al: Flumazenil provocation of panic attacks: evidence for altered benzodiazepine receptor sensitivity in panic disorder. Arch Gen Psychiatry 47:917–925, 1990

Olfson M, Marcus SC, Wan GJ, Geissler EC: National trends in the outpatient treatment of anxiety disorders. J Clin Psychiatry 65:1166–1173, 2004

Orzack MH, Cole JO, Ionescu-Pioggia M, et al: A comparison of some subjective effects of prazepam, diazepam, and placebo. NIDA Res Monogr 41:309–317, 1982

Otto MW, Pollack MH, Sachs GS, et al: Alcohol dependence in panic disorder patients. J Psychiatr Res 26:29–38, 1992

Otto MW, Pollack MH, Sachs GS, et al: Discontinuation of benzodiazepine treatment: efficacy of cognitive-behavioral therapy for patients with panic disorder. Am J Psychiatry 150:1485–1490, 1993

Parry HJ, Balter MB, Mellinger GD, et al: National patterns of psychotherapeutic drug use. Arch Gen Psychiatry 28:18–74, 1973

Paterniti S, Dufouil C, Alperovitch A: Long-term benzodiazepine use and cognitive decline in the elderly: the Epidemiology of Vascular Aging Study. J Clin Psychopharmacol 22:285–293, 2002

Perera KM, Jenner FA: Some characteristics distinguishing high and low dose users of benzodiazepines. Br J Addict 82:1329–1334, 1987

Perera KM, Powell T, Jenner FA: Computerized axial tomographic studies following long-term use of benzodiazepines. Psychol Med 17:775–777, 1987

Perez MF, Salmiron R, Ramirez OA: NMDA-NR1 and -NR2B subunits mRNA expression in the hippocampus of rats tolerant to diazepam. Behav Brain Res 144:119–124, 2003

Petrovic M, Vandierendonck A, Mariman A, et al: Personality traits and socio-epidemiological status of hospitalised elderly benzodiazepine users. Int J Geriatr Psychiatry 17:733–738, 2002

Petursson H, Lader MH: Benzodiazepine dependence. Br J Addict 76:133–145, 1981a

Petursson H, Lader MH: Withdrawal from long-term benzodiazepine treatment. Br Med J (Clin Res Ed) 283:643–645, 1981b

Piesiur-Strehlow B, Strehlow U, Poser W: Mortality of patients dependent on benzodiazepines. Acta Psychiatr Scand 73:330–335, 1986

Piper A Jr: Addiction to benzodiazepines—how common? Arch Fam Med 4:964–970, 1995

Pontieri FE, Tanda G, Di Chiara G: Intravenous cocaine, morphine, and amphetamine preferentially increase extracellular dopamine in the "shell" as compared with the "core" of the rat nucleus accumbens. Proc Natl Acad Sci USA 92:12304–12308, 1995

Posternak MA, Mueller TI: Assessing the risks and benefits of benzodiazepines for anxiety disorders in patients with a history of substance abuse or dependence. Am J Addict 10:48–68, 2001

Pritchett DB, Seeburg PH: Gamma-aminobutyric acidA receptor alpha5-subunit creates novel type II benzodiazepine receptor pharmacology. J Neurochem 54:1802–1804, 1990

Puustinen J, Nurminen J, Kukola M, et al: Associations between use of benzodiazepines or related drugs and health, physical abilities and cognitive function: a nonrandomised clinical study in the elderly. Drugs Aging 24:1045–1059, 2007

Reynaud M, Petit G, Potard D, et al: Six deaths linked to concomitant use of buprenorphine and benzodiazepines. Addiction 93:1385–1392, 1998

Richards JG, Martin JR: Binding profiles and physical dependence liabilities of selected benzodiazepine receptor ligands. Brain Res Bull 45:381–387, 1998

Rickels K, Schweizer E: Anxiolytics: indications, benefits, and risks of short- and long-term benzodiazepine therapy: current research data. NIDA Res Monogr 131:51–67, 1993

Rickels K, Case WG, Downing RW, et al: Long-term diazepam therapy and clinical outcome. JAMA 250:767–771, 1983

Rickels K, Case WG, Schweizer E, et al: Long-term benzodiazepine users 3 years after participation in a discontinuation program. Am J Psychiatry 148:757–761, 1991

Roache JD, Griffiths RR: Diazepam and triazolam self-administration in sedative abusers: concordance of subject ratings, performance and drug self-administration. Psychopharmacology (Berl) 99:309–315, 1989

Roache JD, Stanley MA, Creson DR, et al: Diazepam reinforcement in anxious patients. Exp Clin Psychopharmacol 4:308–314, 1996

Roache JD, Stanley MA, Creson DR, et al: Alprazolam-reinforced medication use in outpatients with anxiety. Drug Alcohol Depend 45:143–155, 1997

Roehrs T, Merlotti L, Zorick F, et al: Rebound insomnia and hypnotic self administration. Psychopharmacology (Berl) 107:480–484, 1992

Romach MK, Somer GR, Sobell LC, et al: Characteristics of long-term alprazolam users in the community. J Clin Psychopharmacol 12:316–321, 1992

Romach M, Busto U, Somer G, et al: Clinical aspects of chronic use of alprazolam and lorazepam. Am J Psychiatry 152:1161–1167, 1995

Rosenberg HC, Chiu TH: Time course for development of benzodiazepine tolerance and physical dependence. Neurosci Biobehav Rev 9:123–131, 1985

Ross J, Darke S: The nature of benzodiazepine dependence among heroin users in Sydney, Australia. Addiction 95:1785–1793, 2000

Rothstein E, Cobble JC, Sampson N: Chlordiazepoxide: long-term use in alcoholism. Ann NY Acad Sci 273:381–384, 1976

Rush CR, Baker RW, Wright K: Acute behavioral effects and abuse potential of trazodone, zolpidem and triazolam in humans. Psychopharmacology (Berl) 144:220–233, 1999a

Rush CR, Frey JM, Griffiths RR: Zaleplon and triazolam in humans: acute behavioral effects and abuse potential. Psychopharmacology (Berl) 145:39–51, 1999b

Salinsky JV, Dore CJ: Characteristics of long term benzodiazepine users in general practice. J R Coll Gen Pract 37:202–204, 1987

Salzman C, Fisher J, Nobel K, et al: Cognitive improvement following benzodiazepine discontinuation in elderly nursing home residents. Int J Geriatr Psychiatry 7:89–93, 1992

Samarasinghe DS, Tilley S, Marks IM: Alcohol and sedative drug use in neurotic outpatients. Br J Psychiatry 145:45–48, 1984

Sanna E, Busonero F, Talani G, et al: Comparison of the effects of zaleplom, zolpidem, and triazolam at various GABA(A) receptor subtypes. Eur J Pharmacol 451:103–110, 2002

Saunders PA, Ho IK: Barbiturates and the GABAA receptor complex. Prog Drug Res 34:261–286, 1990

Saxon L, Hjemdahl P, Hiltunen AJ, et al: Effects of flumazenil in the treatment of benzodiazepine withdrawal—a double-blind pilot study. Psychopharmacology (Berl) 131:153–160, 1997

Schmauss C, Apelt S, Emrich HM: Characterization of benzodiazepine withdrawal in high- and low-dose dependent psychiatric inpatients. Brain Res Bull 19:393–400, 1987

Schmidt LG, Grohmann R, Müller-Oerlinghausen B, et al: Prevalence of benzodiazepine abuse and dependence in psychiatric in-patients with different nosology: an assessment of hospital-based drug surveillance data. Br J Psychiatry 154:839–843, 1989

Schuckit MA, Morrissey ER: Drug abuse among alcoholic women. Am J Psychiatry 136:607–611, 1979

Schweizer E, Patterson W, Rickels K, et al: Double-blind, placebo-controlled study of a once-a-day, sustained-release preparation of alprazolam for the treatment of panic disorder. Am J Psychiatry 150:1210–1215, 1993

Seivewright N: Benzodiazepine misuse by illicit drug misusers. Addiction 96:333–334, 2001

Sellers EM: Alcohol, barbiturate and benzodiazepine withdrawal syndromes: clinical management. CMAJ 139:113–120, 1988

Silberstein SD, McCrory DC: Butalbital in the treatment of headache: history, pharmacology, and efficacy. Headache 41:953–967, 2001

Smith DE, Wesson DR: Benzodiazepine dependency syndromes. J Psychoactive Drugs 15:85–95, 1983

Sokolow L, Welte J, Hynes G, et al: Multiple substance use by alcoholics. Br J Addict 76:147–158, 1981

Spyraki C, Fibiger HC: A role for the mesolimbic dopamine system in the reinforcing properties of diazepam. Psychopharmacology (Berl) 94:133–137, 1988

Sramek JJ, Khajawall A: "Loads." N Engl J Med 305:231, 1981

Stahl SM: Don't ask, don't tell, but benzodiazepines are still the leading treatments for anxiety disorder. J Clin Psychiatry 63:756–757, 2002

Stephenson FA, Duggan MJ, Pollard S: The gamma 2 subunit is an integral component of the gamma-aminobutyric acidA receptor but the alpha 1 polypeptide is the principal site of the agonist benzodiazepine photoaffinity labeling reaction. J Biol Chem 265:21160–21165, 1990

Stitzer ML, Griffiths RR, McLellan AT, et al: Diazepam use among methadone maintenance patients: patterns and dosages. Drug Alcohol Depend 8:189–199, 1981

Stoops WW, Rush CR: Differential effects in humans after repeated administrations of zolpidem and triazolam. Am J Drug Alcohol Abuse 29:281–299, 2003

Strain EC, Brooner RK, Bigelow GE: Clustering of multiple substance use and psychiatric diagnoses in opiate addicts. Drug Alcohol Depend 27:127–134, 1991

Substance Abuse and Mental Health Services Administration: Overview of Findings From the 2002 National Survey on Drug Use and Health (Office of Applied Studies, NHSDA Series H-21, DHHS Publ No SMA-03-3774). Rockville, MD, Substance Abuse and Mental Health Services Administration, 2003. Available at: http://www.samhsa.gov/data/nhsda/overview/2k2Overview.htm. Accessed November 21, 2012.

Substance Abuse and Mental Health Services Administration, Office of Applied Studies: Treatment Episode Data Set (TEDS): 1996–2006. National Admissions to Substance Abuse Treatment Services, DASIS Series: S-43, DHHS Publ No SMA 08-4347. Rockville, MD, Substance Abuse and Mental Health Services Administration, 2008. Available at: http://wwwdasis.samhsa.gov/teds06/teds2k6aweb508.pdf. Accessed August 6, 2013.

Substance Abuse and Mental Health Services Administration: Drug Abuse Warning Network, 2009: National Estimates of Drug-Related Emergency Department Visits (HHS Publ No SMA-11-4659), DAWN Series D-35. Rockville, MD, Substance Abuse and Mental Health Services Administration, 2011. Available at: http://www.samhsa.gov/data/2k11/dawn/2k9dawned/html/dawn2k9ed.htm. Accessed November 21, 2012.

Substance Abuse and Mental Health Services Administration: Results from the 2011 National Survey on Drug Use and Health: Summary of National Findings, NSDUH Series H-44, Publ No SMA 12-4713, Rockville MD, Substance Abuse and Mental Health Services Administration, 2012. Available at: http://www.samhsa.gov/data/nsduh/2k11results/nsduhresults2011.htm. Accessed July 29, 2013.

Svab V, Subelj M, Vidmar G: Prescribing changes in anxiolytics and antidepressants in Slovenia. Psychiatry Danub 23:178–182, 2011

Tan KR, Rudolph U, Luscher C: Hooked on benzodiazepines: GABAA receptor subtypes and addiction. Trends Neurosci 34:188–197, 2011

Tyrer P, Rutherford D, Huggett T: Benzodiazepine withdrawal symptoms and propranolol. Lancet 1:520–522, 1981

Uhde TW, Kellner CH: Cerebral ventricular size in panic disorder. J Affect Disord 12:175–178, 1987

Van Sickle BJ, Tietz EI: Selective enhancement of AMPA receptor-mediated function in hippocampal CA1 neurons from chronic benzodiazepine-treated rats. Neuropharmacology 43:11–27, 2002

Vartzopoulos D, Bozikas V, Phocas C, et al: Dependence on zolpidem in high dose. Int Clin Psychopharmacol 15:181–182, 2000

Venault P, Chapouthier G, de Carvalho LP, et al: Benzodiazepine impairs and beta-carboline enhances performance in learning and memory tasks. Nature 321:864–866, 1986

Vermeeren A, Coenen AM: Effects of the use of hypnotics on cognition. Prog Brain Res 190:89–103, 2011

Vermeeren A, Jackson JL, Muntjewerff ND, et al: Comparison of acute alprazolam (0.25, 0.50 and 1.0 mg) effects versus those of lorazepam 2 mg and placebo on memory in healthy volunteers using laboratory and telephone tests. Psychopharmacology (Berl) 118:1–9, 1995

Veronese A, Graatti M, Cipriani A, Barbuti C: Benzodiazepine use in the real world of psychiatric practice: low-does, long-term drug taking and low rates of treatment discontinuation. Eur J Clin Pharmacol 63:867–873, 2007

Voderholzer U, Reimann D, Hornyak M, et al: A double-blind, randomized and placebo-controlled study on the polysomnographic withdrawal effects of zopiclone, zolpidem and triazolam in healthy subjects. Eur Arch Psychiatry Clin Neurosci 251:117–123, 2001

Vorma H, Naukkatinen H, Sarna S, et al: Treatment of out-patients with complicated benzodiazepine dependence: comparison of two approaches. Addiction 97:851–859, 2002

Vorma H, Naukkarinen H, Sarna S, et al: Long-term outcome after benzodiazepine withdrawal treatment in subjects with complicated dependence. Drug Alcohol Depend 70:309–314, 2003

Voshaar RC, Gorgels WJ, Mol AJ, et al: Tapering off long-term benzodiazepine use with or without group cognitive-behavioural therapy: three-condition, randomised controlled trial. Br J Psychiatry 182:498–504, 2003

Wafford KA, Thompson SA, Thomas D, et al: Functional characterization of human gamma-aminobutyric acidA receptors containing the alpha 4 subunit. Mol Pharmacol 50:670–678, 1996

Walker BM, Ettenberg A: The effects of alprazolam on conditioned place preferences produced by intravenous heroin. Pharmacol Biochem Behav 75:75–80, 2003

Weerts EM, Griffiths RR: Zolpidem self-injection with concurrent physical dependence under conditions of long-term continuous availability in baboons. Behav Pharmacol 9:285–297, 1998

Wesson DR, Smith DE: Barbiturates: Their Use, Misuse, and Abuse. New York, Human Sciences Press, 1977

Wikler A: Diagnosis and treatment of drug dependence of the barbiturate type. Am J Psychiatry 125:758–765, 1968

Williams H, Oyefeso A, Ghodse AH: Benzodiazepine misuse and dependence among opiate addicts in treatment. Ir J Psychol Med 13:62–64, 1996

Wiseman SM, Spencer-Peet J: Prescribing for alcoholics: a survey of drugs taken prior to admission to an alcoholism unit. Practitioner 229:88–89, 1985

Wolf B, Grohmann R, Biber D, et al: Benzodiazepine abuse and dependence in psychiatric inpatients. Pharmacopsychiatry 22:54–60, 1989

Wood MR, Kim JJ, Han W, et al: Benzodiazepines as potent and selective bradykinin B1 antagonists. J Med Chem 46:1803–1806, 2003

Zandstra SM, Furer JW, van de Lisdonk EH, et al: Different study criteria affect the prevalence of benzodiazepine use. Soc Psychiatry Psychiatr Epidemiol 37:139–144, 2002

Zawertailo LA, Busto UE, Kaplan HL, et al: Comparative abuse liability and pharmacological effects of meprobamate, triazolam, and butabarbital. J Clin Psychopharmacol 23:269–280, 2003

7

Hallucinogens and Related Drugs

Torsten Passie, M.D., M.A.

John H. Halpern, M.D.

Hallucinogens are chemically divergent psychoactive substances primarily used for their potential to alter profoundly the processing of cognitive, perceptual, and emotional understanding of self and reality. Revered in many cultures, hallucinogens historically have been tools of sacrament and direct communion (Schultes and Hofmann 1980). Even into the present, hallucinogens are central to the expression of faith for the estimated 500,000 members of the pan-tribal Native American Church, the various ayahuasca-using Native and syncretic faiths that originated in the Amazon, and the continuing iboga faith in African populations. Peyote is officially protected for Native peoples throughout North America, including the United States. The government of Peru declared the traditional knowledge and use of ayahuasca to be a "national cultural patrimony," and Brazil and Columbia have similar accommodations. The Bwiti spiritual practice with iboga is one of the official recognized religions of the Republic of Gabon. In the United States, religious freedom extends now to American members of the Santo Daime and União do Vegetal churches first founded in Brazil with their ayahuasca sacraments.

Hallucinogens entered the Western model of scientific experiment when Albert Hofmann, a medicinal chemist at Sandoz Pharmaceuticals, accidentally intoxicated himself in 1943 with lysergic acid diethylamide (LSD). From 1949 to 1969, Hofmann's discovery was investigated as a putative treatment for alcoholism, drug addiction, pain control, or mental illness and as a psychotherapy tool. More than 10,000 subjects received LSD (and other hallucinogens) in controlled research settings in studies published from 1951 to the late 1960s, resulting in more than 5,000 clinical papers, dozens of books, and six international conferences on therapeutic application (Hintzen and Passie 2010). LSD's potent ability to produce depersonalization and derealization creates doubt within the user about all varieties of understandings assumed as fact, and by the 1960s, it was considered useful for reasons beyond research within the laboratory. By the early 1970s, most controlled human research with LSD ended. By then, tighter drug control laws had been enacted, government funding had ceased, and the medical utility of LSD had failed to materialize.

Use and Abuse of Hallucinogens

Abusive consumption of hallucinogens in Western culture started in the mid-1960s, and by the end of the decade, hallucinogen use (see DSM-5 criteria for other hallucinogen use disorder and Table 7–1 for a list of physical and psychological effects) was widespread, in part because these drugs were linked to antiauthoritarian and antiwar movements. Especially because of user inexperience with these drugs, a mass wave of complications resulted, which then established their new image as dangerous drugs.

Discussing hallucinogen abuse with patients requires an understanding of the rewarding properties of these drugs as well as their potential risks. It will ultimately prove ineffective to offer only a one-sided discussion about psychiatric comorbidity without expressing awareness of what the user values within his or her experiences, whether rooted in spiritual-religious importance or

Table 7–1. Physical and psychological effects of hallucinogen[a] intoxication

Physical effects[b]	Psychological effects
Slight to moderate	**Usual**
Diaphoresis	Acute cognitive alterations with loosening of
Hyperreflexia	association, inability for goal-directed
Hypertension or hypotension	thinking, and memory disturbance
Hyperthermia	Altered experience of time and space
Motor incoordination	Altered body image
Neuroendocrine alteration	Dreamlike state
Palpitation	Increased suggestibility
Tachycardia	Intensification and lability of affect with
Tremor	euphoria, anxiety, depression, and/or cathartic
Moderate to strong	expressions
Arousal	Lassitude/indifference/detachment
Insomnia	Sensory activation with illusion,
Mydriasis	pseudohallucination, hallucination, and/or
	synesthesia
Occasional	**"Positive"**
Blurred vision	Delight in novelty
Diarrhea	Mystical experience
Nausea/vomiting	Sense of perceiving deeper layers of the world,
Nystagmus	oneself, and others ("consciousness expansion")
Piloerection	Sense of profound discovery/healing
Salivation	
	"Negative"
	Depersonalization
	Derealization
	Hysteria
	Impaired judgment
	Impulsivity
	Megalomania
	Odd behavior
	Panic
	Paranoid ideation
	Psychosomatic complaint
	Suicidal ideation

[a]Indolealkylamine and phenylalkylamine hallucinogens only.
[b]Some effects are reactions to psychological content (e.g., increased heart rate and nausea due to anxiety), and complaints can be dependent on factors such as mind-set, setting, dose, and supervision. Intoxicated individuals may also deny physical impairment and/or claim increased energy, sharpened mental acuity, and improved sensory perception.

"recreational" pursuit for novelty. Complicating the evaluation of abuse is that most hallucinogens are not habit forming, and acute tolerance precludes daily intoxication. Hallucinogens do not primarily induce hallucinations, in the strict definitions of the term, but rather pseudohallucinations and illusions (the user is well aware that changes of perception are drug mediated and can discern them from reality, as opposed to those experiencing true hallucinations fully experienced as "real").

The 2010 National Survey on Drug Use and Health (NSDUH) estimated that almost 37.5 million Americans (14.8%) older than 12 have ingested a hallucinogen at least once in their lifetime (Substance Abuse and Mental Health Services Administration 2011b). The NSDUH estimates of the number of users in 2009 combined with the 2009 data from the National Estimates of Drug-Related Emergency Department Visits from the Drug Abuse Warning Network (Substance Abuse and Mental Health Services Administration 2011a) show how rarely emergency medical attention is sought as a percentage of active users for hallucinogens compared with other illicit substances (Table 7–2). Quite importantly, Table 7–2 shows that medical attention for hallucinogen use is disproportionately a result of ingestion of phencyclidine (PCP). Without inclusion of data on PCP, fewer than 1% of hallucinogen users had an emergency department visit related to their hallucinogen use in 2009 compared with 5.5% of methamphetamine users, 8.8% of cocaine users, and 35.2% of heroin users.

Several substances have been categorized as hallucinogens or hallucinogen-like: 1) the classic hallucinogens (e.g., mescaline, psilocybin, LSD, dimethyltryptamine [DMT]); 2) the phenethylamines (3,4-methylendioxyamphetamine [MDA], 3,4-methylenedioxymethamphetamine [MDMA], 3,4-methylenedioxyethylamphetamine [MDE], 1,3-benzodioxolyl-N-methylbutanamine [MBDB]), which are known as entactogens because they have distinctive emotional and social effects; 3) the anticholinergic dissociatives (atropine, hyoscyamine, scopolamine); and 4) the dissociative anesthetics/miscellaneous (PCP, ketamine, salvinorin A). Table 7–3 presents a partial list of these compounds.

Table 7–2. 2009 National Survey on Drug Use and Health and Drug Abuse Warning Network data on number of users, emergency department (ED) visits for that drug use, and maximum estimated percentage of users seeking emergency medical attention related to their drug use

Drug	Estimated number of users in 2009	Estimated number of ED visits in 2009	Percentage of users with ED visits in 2009[a]
All hallucinogens including phencyclidine (PCP)	4,509,000	70,671	1.57
All hallucinogens excluding PCP	4,387,000	33,952	0.77
Lysergic acid diethylamide (LSD)	779,000	4,028	0.52
PCP	122,000	36,719	30.10
3,4-Methylenedioxymethamphetamine (MDMA)	2,799,000	22,816	0.82
Cocaine	4,797,000	422,896	8.82
Methamphetamine	1,165,000	64,117	5.50
Heroin	605,000	213,118	35.23
Marijuana	28,521,000	376,467	1.32

[a]Some users may have sought more than one ED visit in 2009 for complications related to their use of that drug. Such instances will cause an overestimation of the percentage of users with ED visits for that year.

Table 7–3. Major groups of hallucinogens (partial list)

Class	Chemical name	Common or street name	Source	Dosage	Route	Duration of action	Major neurobiological target	Notes
Indolealkyl-amines	Lysergic acid diethylamide	LSD, acid, blotter	Synthesis	50–200 µg	po	8–14 hours	5-HT$_{2A}$ partial agonist	Distributed on small squares of blotting paper, drops of liquid, gelcaps, small pills
	Psilocybin	Magic mushrooms, shrooms	*Psilocybe cubensis, Psilocybe azurescens,* and many other subspecies; synthesis	10–50 mg, 1–5 g dried mushroom; quite variable	po	1–5 hours	5-HT$_{2A}$ partial agonist	Psilocybin is converted in the body to psilocin, the actual active hallucinogen; continued shamanic use in Mexico; bruising of mushroom turns it blue
	Dimethyltrypt-amine (DMT)	DMT, Yopo, Cohoba, "business-man's trip"	*Psychotria viridis, Anadenanthera peregrina, Mimosa hostilis,* and many other natural sources; synthesis	5–40 mg	Smoked, inhaled snuff	15–90 minutes	5-HT$_{2A}$ partial agonist	Continued Amazonian shamanic use
	DMT+monoamine oxidase inhibitors (MAOIs) (harmala β-carbolines)	Ayahuasca, Daime, yajé, hoasca, "vine of the soul"	*Psychotria viridis* (DMT) + *Banisteriopsis caapi* (MAOI)	Variable	po	2–4 hours	5-HT$_{2A}$ partial agonist	Brewed as a tea; religious sacrament

Table 7–3. Major groups of hallucinogens (partial list) *(continued)*

Class	Chemical name	Common or street name	Source	Dosage	Route	Duration of action	Major neurobiological target	Notes
Indolealkylamines *(continued)*	Ibogaine	Ibogaine	*Tabernanthe iboga*	200–300 mg	po	≥12 hours	Likely 5-HT$_{2A}$ partial agonist	Religious sacrament; long-acting metabolites may contribute to purported antiopioid withdrawal benefits
Phenylalkylamines	3,4,5-Trimethoxyphenethylamine	Mescaline, peyote, San Pedro	*Lophophora williamsii, Echinopsis pachanoi,* and other cacti; synthesis	200–500 mg, 10–20 g or 5–10 dried peyote buttons, 1 kg fresh *E. pachanoi*	po	6–12 hours	5-HT$_{2A}$ partial agonist	Religious sacrament
Entactogenic phenylalkylamines	3,4-Methylenedioxymethamphetamine	MDMA, Ecstasy, X, XTC, rolls, molly	Synthesis	80–150 mg	po	4–6 hours	5-HT release and depletion	Mildly hallucinogenic at high doses
	3,4-Methylenedioxyamphetamine	MDA, love drug, Adam	Synthesis	75–160 mg	po	4–8 hours	5-HT release and depletion	
	4-Bromo-2,5-dimethoxyphenethylamine	2C-B, Nexus	Synthesis	5–30 mg	po	4–8 hours	Unknown	

Table 7–3. Major groups of hallucinogens (partial list) *(continued)*

Class	Chemical name	Common or street name	Source	Dosage	Route	Duration of action	Major neurobiological target	Notes
Entactogenic phenylalkylamines *(continued)*	2,5-Dimethoxy-4-chloroamphetamine	DOC	Synthesis	1–5 mg	po	4–8 hours	Unknown	Has been found on blotting paper
	2,5-Dimethoxy-4-methylamphetamine	DOM, STP	Synthesis	1–10 mg	po	14–20 hours	Unknown	Higher doses used in the 1960s resulted in many emergency department visits
Dissociative	Ketamine	Ketamine, Special K, vitamin K, K-hole	Synthesis	25–50 mg (im), 75–100 mg (po), 25–60 mg (snorted)	im, po, snorted	1–2 hours (im), 1–4 hours (po), 1–3 hours (snorted)	NMDA antagonist	Subanesthetic dose: lost sense of time, space, verbal skills, balance, and drooling
	Dextromethorphan	DXM, Robo, DM	Synthesis	100–600 mg	po	4–8 hours	NMDA antagonist	
	Phencyclidine	PCP, angel dust	Synthesis	2–10 mg	Smoked, po	8–24 hours	NMDA antagonist	
Other	Salvinorin A	Salvia, Sally D, Diviner's Sage	*Salvia divinorum*	250–750 mg (smoked), 2–10 g dried leaves (po)	Smoked, po	30–60 minutes (smoked), 1–3 hours (po)	κ Opioid selective agonist	Atypical hallucinogen; no longer found in the wild

Table 7–3.   Major groups of hallucinogens (partial list) *(continued)*

Class	Chemical name	Common or street name	Source	Dosage	Route	Duration of action	Major neurobio-logical target	Notes
Other *(continued)*	Scopolamine and atropine	Datura, jimsonweed, locoweed, thorn apple, Angel's trumpet, belladonna, deadly nightshade	*Datura stramonium, Atropa belladonna,* and many related species	Highly variable	po	12–48 hours	Competitive muscarinic acetylcholine antagonist	Plants of the Solanaceae family contain various ratios of scopolamine to atropine; blurred vision
	Muscimol (5-[aminomethyl]-isoxazol-3-ol)	Fly agaric, Amanita	*Amanita muscaria, Amanita pantherina*	1–30 g dried mushrooms	po	5–10 hours	GABA$_A$ agonist; glutamate	Shamanic use in eastern Siberia; more than 600 species of agarics—easy to misidentify. Some are extremely poisonous such as "death cap" *Amanita phalloides*; mushrooms also contain ibotenic acid—as it dries/ages, decarboxylation of ibotenic acid creates muscimol.

Note.   GABA=γ-aminobutyric acid; 5-HT=serotonin; im=intramuscular; NMDA=N-methyl-D-aspartate; po=oral.

Lysergic Acid Diethylamide

History and Prevalence of Use

LSD was synthesized in 1938, and its psychoactive effects were discovered in 1943. It was used during the 1950s and 1960s as an experimental drug in psychiatric research for producing so-called experimental psychosis and in psychotherapeutic procedures ("psycholytic" and "psychedelic therapy"). From the mid-1960s onward, it became an illegal drug of abuse. Pharmacological research on LSD was extensive and produced nearly 10,000 scientific papers (Passie et al. 2008). Currently, there is renewed interest in LSD as an experimental tool for elucidating neural mechanisms of (states of) consciousness, in treating cluster headache, and in psychotherapy with the terminally ill, where it intensifies affect and activates mental imagery—effects that may accelerate the psychotherapeutic process (Winkelman and Roberts 2007).

LSD is still a major hallucinogen used worldwide. Although no physical damage results from the use of LSD, many psychiatric complications have been reported, with a peak occurring at the end of the 1960s (Henderson and Glass 1994; Strassman 1984). Toward the end of the 1960s, people began using LSD for recreational and spiritual purposes (Lee and Shlain 1985). Extent of use has remained essentially constant since the 1970s. Data show a more constant pattern of use in the industrialized Western countries, especially the United States and central Europe (Henderson and Glass 1994). A renewed interest in the substance was registered at the end of the 1990s and remains a significant part of youth movements in the United States and central Europe (Reynolds 2012). Although the typical dose (150–250 µg) appeared to be unchanged during the 1970s to the 1980s (Lee and Shlain 1985), it was later used in smaller doses (30–80 µg), mainly for its stimulant properties and often in combination with MDMA ("candy-flipping"). Interestingly, the number of complications has declined since the late 1960s and early 1970s because today there may be better-informed users, better mental preparation and attention to surrounding conditions, and a reduction in the per-unit dosage (now more commonly encountered in units of 50–100 µg).

Today, LSD is still the most widely used hallucinogenic drug. In 2010, an estimated 23.3 million Americans age 12 or older used LSD at least once in their lifetime (Substance Abuse and Mental Health Services Administration 2011b). In both its somatic and its psychological effects, LSD is representative of most of the other hallucinogenic drugs, making it the primary focus of this chapter.

Pharmacology

LSD is a semisynthetic substance derived from lysergic acid as found in the parasitic rye fungus *Claviceps purpurea*. The molecule consists of an indole with a tetracyclic ring ($C_{20}H_{25}N_3O$) (Figure 7–1). The pharmacology of LSD is complex, and its mechanisms of action are still not completely understood (Hintzen and Passie 2010; Nichols 2004).

Pharmacokinetics

Following oral administration, LSD is completely absorbed in the digestive tract (Rothlin 1957; Rothlin and Cerletti 1956). The threshold oral dose for measurable sympathomimetic effects in humans is 0.5–1.0 µg/kg (Greiner et al. 1958). After 100–250 µg LSD, psychological and sympathomimetic effects persist for 30–45 minutes, reaching their peak after 1.5–2.5 hours (Figure 7–2) (Hoch 1956). The distribution of LSD across tissue and organ systems is yet to be quantified for humans. In cats parenterally administered 1 mg/kg, the highest concentrations were detected in the gallbladder and blood plasma (Axelrod et al. 1957; Boyd 1959). The presence of considerable amounts in the brain and cerebrospinal fluid of rats and cats indicates that LSD may easily pass the blood-brain barrier (Axelrod et al. 1957). In two studies (Metzler 1969; Wagner et al. 1968) evaluating a two-compartment model, the authors concluded that the relation between the neuropsychological effects of LSD and tissue concentrations could be linear, logarithmic-linear, or neither.

In humans, a plasma level of 6–7 ng/mL is achieved about 30 minutes following an intravenous dose of 2 µg/kg. Over the course of the next 8 hours, plasma levels gradually fall until only a small amount of LSD is present (Aghajanian and Bing 1964). The half-life of LSD in humans is 175 minutes (Aghajanian and Bing 1964; Upshall and Wailling 1972).

Tolerance to the effects of LSD occurs in humans and animals. Tolerance to autonomic and psychological effects of LSD occurs in humans after a few moderate daily doses (Abramson et al. 1956; Cholden et al. 1955; Isbell et al. 1956). Reduction in receptor density is a possible mechanism for the development of tolerance to LSD.

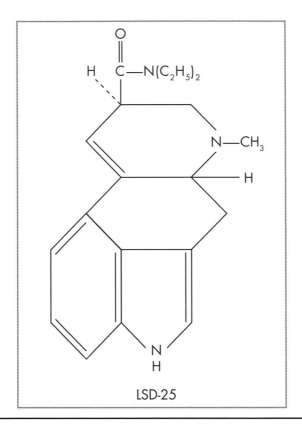

Figure 7–1. Molecular structure of lysergic acid diethylamide (LSD).

No human deaths from an LSD overdose due to toxicity have been documented (Hintzen and Passie 2010), but death may result from drug-induced unrealistic behavior. In 1967, a report gave evidence for LSD-induced chromosomal damage (Cohen et al. 1967), but it could not stand up to meticulous scientific examination (for review, see Grof 1980). Empirical studies showed no evidence of teratogenic or mutagenic effects from use of LSD in humans (Leuner 1981; Robinson et al. 1974; Smart and Bateman 1968). Harm, including death, from LSD appears primarily driven then by impaired judgment and behaviors while intoxicated, often in an "unsafe" setting.

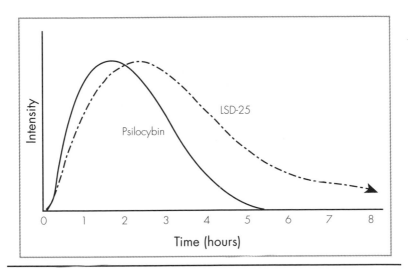

Figure 7–2. Time course of psychopharmacologic effects of medium-range doses of lysergic acid diethylamide (LSD) and psilocybin.

Source. Copyright © 2013 Torsten Passie, M.D., M.A.

Pharmacodynamics

The interaction of LSD with neurotransmitter receptors is complex and not completely understood. LSD acts as a serotonin (5-HT) autoreceptor agonist on 5-HT$_{1A}$ receptors in the locus coeruleus, the raphe nuclei, and the cortex. It inhibits firing and serotonin release by these cells. It also acts as a partial agonist on the postsynaptic 5-HT$_{1A}$ site. LSD has high affinity for other 5-HT$_1$ subtypes, including 5-HT$_{1B}$, 5-HT$_{1D}$, and 5-HT$_{1E}$. Effects of LSD on 5-HT$_{2C}$, 5-HT$_{5A}$, 5-HT$_6$, and 5-HT$_7$ receptors have been described (Erlander et al. 1993; Lovenberg et al. 1993; Monsma et al. 1993), but their significance remains uncertain. The hallucinogenic effect of LSD has been linked to its affinity for the 5-HT$_2$ receptor, where it acts as an agonist. LSD is probably best called a mixed 5-HT$_2$/5-HT$_1$ receptor partial agonist (Pierce and Peroutka 1989; Sanders-Bush et al. 1988). Activation of 5-HT$_{2A}$ also leads to increased cortical glutamate levels (Martin-Ruiz et al. 2001; Winter et al. 2004), probably mediated by thalamic afferents (Nichols 2004), which may lead to an alteration in corticocortical and corticosubcortical transmission. Evidence indicates that LSD interacts with central dopamine D_1 and D_2 receptors (von Hungen et al. 1974; Watts et al. 1995), but it is not known how these changes are involved in its psychoactive effects.

Sokoloff et al. (1957) investigated the effects of LSD on cerebral circulation and metabolism. At peak LSD effects ($n=13$; 120 µg intravenously), general cerebral blood flow (measured with the still valid nitrous oxide method), cerebral vascular resistance, cerebral oxygen consumption, and glucose utilization were not significantly altered. The electroencephalogram (EEG) showed mild specific signs of activation after LSD ingestion. Most common is an increase in alpha mean frequency (Anderson and Rawnsley 1954; Bradley et al. 1953; Elkes et al. 1954). Other researchers have described a progressive desynchronization due to a quantitative decrement of the slow component after LSD (Itil 1969; Were 1964). Goldstein et al. (1963) reported a decrease of EEG variability of 33% after LSD (0.3–1.0 µg/kg orally). Goldstein and Stoltzfus (1973) found in most subjects that lateralization was reversed by LSD.

No studies of the neurometabolic actions of LSD have been reported. However, neurometabolic studies have been published for related hallucinogens such as psilocybin (Gouzoulis-Mayfrank et al. 1999a; Vollenweider et al. 1997b), DMT (Riba et al. 2003), and mescaline (Hermle et al. 1992). Inconsistent study results limit the plausibility of hypotheses developed to explain neurofunctional alterations during hallucinogen effects (Vollenweider and Geyer 2001). The major congruent results show an activation of the right hemisphere, altered thalamic functioning, and increased metabolism in paralimbic structures and the frontal cortex. Some investigators found an increase in global brain metabolism (Hermle et al. 1992; Vollenweider et al. 1997b), but others found no change (Gouzoulis-Mayfrank et al. 1999a; Riba et al. 2006). One functional magnetic resonance imaging (fMRI)/blood-oxygen-level dependent (BOLD) study showed decreased neuronal activity and cerebral blood flow in the anterior and posterior cingulate cortex and thalamus after administration of psilocybin (Carhart-Harris et al. 2012).

Acute and Chronic Effects

LSD-induced sympathetic stimulation is evidenced by pupillary dilation and slight increases in heart rate and blood pressure (DiMascio et al. 1957; Forrer and Goldner 1951); other more inconsistent signs are slight blood glucose elevation (Hollister and Sjoberg 1964; Liddell and Weil-Malherbe 1953), and rarely, an increase in body temperature. Respiration remains generally unchanged. Initial nausea, decreased appetite, temporary mild headache, dizziness, and inner trembling may occur in some subjects. The most consistent neurological effect is an exaggeration of the patellar (and other deep tendon) reflexes (Isbell et al. 1956). More unusual signs include slight unsteadiness of gait to full ataxia.

Psychological Effects

A moderate oral dose (75–150 μg) of LSD will significantly alter the state of consciousness, including stimulation of affect, enhanced capacity for introspection, and altered psychological functioning in the direction of hypnagogia and dreams (Farthing 1992). Typical perceptual changes include illusions, pseudohallucinations, synesthesias, and alterations of thinking and time experience (Table 7–4). Changes of body image and ego function also often occur (Katz et al. 1968; Savage 1955). Religious and mystical experiences may occur.

The acute psychological effects of LSD last between 6 and 10 hours, depending on the dose applied. Traumatic experiences (called "bad trips") can have long-lasting effects, including mood swings and, more rarely, flashback phenomena (Strassman 1984). Conversely, it has been shown that under controlled and supportive conditions, the LSD experience may have lasting positive effects on attitude and personality in healthy humans (Griffiths et al. 2006, 2008; McGlothlin et al. 1967).

LSD decreases performance on tests of attention and concentration and recognition and recall of various stimuli (Jarvik et al. 1955a, 1955b; Wapner and Krus 1960). Thinking processes are more resistant but can also be affected when higher doses of LSD are given (Isbell et al. 1956; Silverstein and Klee 1958). Under the influence of LSD, subjects will overestimate time intervals (Aronson et al. 1959). Lienert (1959, 1961) systematically examined intellectual functioning under the influence of LSD and interpreted his results as a regression of intellectual functions to an ontogenetically earlier state of development (i.e., age 12–14 years). Regarding chronic neurocognitive aftereffects from LSD exposure, a review by Halpern and Pope (1999) indicated no evidence for lasting impairments in performance.

Psychiatric Complications of LSD

Major surveys indicate that LSD is safe when administered in medically supervised settings (Cohen 1960; Malleson 1971). Many reports exist about psychi-

Table 7–4. Typical sensory and psychological effects under the influence of a medium dose of lysergic acid diethylamide (LSD; 100–200 µg orally), mescaline (300–500 mg orally), or psilocybin (15–25 mg orally)

Sensory alterations (visual, auditory, taste, olfactory, kinesthetic)	Illusion
	Pseudohallucination
	Intensification of color perception
	Metamorphosis-like change in objects and faces
	Intense (kaleidoscopic or scenic) visual imagery with transforming content
Alterations of affectivity	Intensification of emotional experience: euphoria, dysphoria, anxiety, mood swings
	Mystical-type experiences
Alterations of thinking	Less abstract and more imaginative thought
	Broader and unusual association
	Attention span shortened
	Delusions
Alterations of body perceptions	Change in body image
	Unusual inner perception of bodily processes
	Metamorphic alteration of body contours
Memory changes	Reexperiencing significant biographical memories
	Hypermnesia
	Age regression

atric complications following LSD ingestion outside the research setting. The most common unpleasant reaction is an episode of anxiety or panic—severe, terrifying thoughts and feelings, fear of losing control, fear of insanity or death, and despair—the so-called bad trip (Strassman 1984). In these cases, unrealistic behavior is a dangerous possibility. Treatment includes providing a comfortable and quiet environment in which empathic communication is used to "talk down" the patient. In some cases, administration of a benzodi-azepine (e.g., 5–10 mg diazepam intravenously) may be indicated. Neurolep-tics do not have an immediate effect and are therefore indicated only in the rare instance of severe, long-lasting LSD reactions with psychotic features. Other complicated reactions include temporary paranoid ideation, unrealistic behavior, and temporary depressive mood swings or increase of psychic labil-ity in the days following the LSD use (Grof 1975; Leuner 1981).

Flashbacks are characterized in ICD-10 (World Health Organization 1992) as of an episodic nature with a very short duration (seconds or minutes) and by their replication of elements of previous drug-related experiences. These reexperiences of previous drug intoxications occur mainly following in-tense negative experiences with hallucinogens but can sometimes also be self-induced by will for positive reexperiences and are in this case sometimes re-ferred to as "free trips" (for review, see Holland and Passie 2011). Possible per-sisting perceptual phenomena are reviewed later in this chapter (see section "Flashback Phenomena and Hallucinogen Persisting Perception Disorder").

Detection of LSD in Body Fluids and Hair

LSD content of blood and urine may be detected by radioimmunoassay and en-zyme immunoassay down to at least 0.5 ng/mL (McCarron et al. 1990) or with enzyme-linked immunosorbent assay (ELISA) down to 1 pg of total drug in 25 μL of blood (Kerrigan and Brooks 1999). The average time over which LSD can be detected is estimated to be 6–12 hours in blood specimens and 2–4 days in urine specimens (Papac and Foltz 1990; Taunton-Rigby et al. 1973; van Bocxlaer et al. 2000). Immunoaffinity chromatography can detect low and sin-gle doses of LSD in hair specimens (Nakahara et al. 1996; Röhrich et al. 2000).

Psilocybin

History and Prevalence of Use

Synthetic psilocybin is very complicated to produce and consequently never ap-peared on the illegal drug market but was used in psychotherapy during the 1960s (Passie 2004) and is again being evaluated in experimental studies for induction of mystical-type experiences (Griffiths et al. 2006), for treatment of advanced-stage cancer anxiety (Grob et al. 2011), and in experimental psychopathology (Stude-rus et al. 2011; Vollenweider 2001; Vollenweider and Kometer 2010).

Mushrooms containing psilocybin are found in many regions of the world, including the United States (Stamets 1996). They continue to be used as sacraments by some Native tribes of Mexico (Heim and Wasson 1958). Psychoactive mushroom availability was not significant until the mid-1970s, when drug aficionados produced guides for collecting wild mushrooms (Pollock 1975) and pamphlets on methods of cultivation (Oss and Oeric 1976).

Data on psilocybin use prevalence are limited, which may be partially a result of the "decentralized" availability of psilocybin through the collection of wild specimens and use of private grow kits. According to the NSDUH, in 2004 and 2005 the most common hallucinogen consumed in the previous year among new hallucinogen users ages 12 and older was *Psilocybe* mushrooms (Substance Abuse and Mental Health Services Administration 2007).

Pharmacology

Psilocybin (4-phosphoryloxy-*N,N*-dimethyltryptamine) and its active metabolite psilocin (4-hydroxy-*N,N*-dimethyltryptamine) are substituted hallucinogenic indolealkylamines. Total content of psilocybin varies with mushroom, subspecies, and preparation, but the most commonly used mushroom, *Psilocybe cubensis,* contains 5–11 mg of psilocybin per gram of dried mushroom. Ingestion of *Psilocybe* mushrooms can in some cases cause nausea and vomiting, but serious toxicity has not been reported in humans. Peak intoxication occurs approximately within the first 2 hours, diminishing over the subsequent 3–4 hours (see Figure 7–2).

Pharmacokinetics

Psilocybin is readily absorbed following oral administration and is widely distributed throughout the body (Hopf and Eckert 1974; Passie et al. 2002). Holzmann (1995) and Hasler (1997) identified four metabolites of psilocybin, including its active metabolite psilocin. Psilocybin/psilocin is detectable in plasma within 20–40 minutes following ingestion. Psychological effects occur with plasma levels of 4–6 μg/mL (Hasler 1997; Holzmann 1995). The full effects occur within 70–90 minutes following oral doses of 8–25 mg. A significant first-pass effect can be assumed (Hasler et al. 1997). After a rapid increase of psilocin plasma levels, a plateau follows for about 50 minutes, after which there is a relatively slow decline of the curve, ending at about 360 minutes.

The half-life of psilocybin is 163.3±63.5 minutes (Hasler et al. 1997). The mean elimination half-life of psilocin is 50 minutes (Holzmann 1995). The time curves indicate highly variable plasma concentrations in different individuals. However, the maximum plasma concentration occurs at approximately 80 minutes (Hasler 1997). The elimination of the glucuronidated metabolites as well as unaltered psilocybin (3%–10%) occurs through the kidneys. Approximately two-thirds of the renal excretion of psilocin is completed after 3 hours (Hasler 1997).

Cerletti (1958) reported a median lethal dose for mice of 280 mg/kg. The predicted human lethal dose of psilocybin is 6 g, which is equivalent to 4 kg of dried mushrooms, an amount unlikely to be consumed (Gable 2004).

Pharmacodynamics

Psilocybin interacts mainly with serotonergic (5-HT$_{1A}$, 5-HT$_{1D}$, 5-HT$_{2A}$, and 5-HT$_{2C}$ receptor subtypes) neurotransmission. It binds with high affinity at 5-HT$_{2A}$ and to a lesser extent at 5-HT$_{1A}$ receptors (McKenna et al. 1990). It should be noted that unlike LSD, psilocybin and its active metabolite psilocin have no affinity for D$_2$ receptors (Creese et al. 1975). A double-blind, placebo-controlled study with ketanserin (a reference standard 5-HT$_{2A}$ receptor antagonist) showed a complete blocking of effects of psilocybin (Vollenweider et al. 1998b).

Positron emission tomography (PET) studies of psilocybin in humans have detected increased glucose metabolism in frontal areas and anterior cingulate cortex, with possibly greater right hemisphere activity (Gouzoulis-Mayfrank et al. 1999a; Vollenweider et al. 1997b). A more recent fMRI/BOLD study showed decreased neuronal activity and cerebral blood flow in the anterior and posterior cingulate cortex and thalamus after psilocybin administration (Carhart-Harris et al. 2012).

Despite significant tolerance that occurs with repeated use of psilocybin, neither physical dependence nor a withdrawal syndrome develops (Abramson et al. 1956; Balestrieri 1967).

Acute and Chronic Effects

Neurovegetative effects within the usual dose range (10–25 mg orally) include mydriasis, slight changes in heart and breathing rate, and discrete hyperglycemic and hypertonic effects (Cerletti 1958; Passie et al. 2002). Electrolyte levels, liver enzyme activity, and blood glucose levels are unaffected (Delay et al. 1958; Hidalgo 1960; Hollister 1961), as are endocrine cortisol, prolactin, and growth hormone levels (Gouzoulis-Mayfrank et al. 1999b). There is no evidence of mutagenic or teratogenic effects (cf. Passie et al. 2002).

The psychopathological phenomena induced by psilocybin are virtually identical to those of LSD (see subsection "Psychological Effects" in the section "Lysergic Acid Diethylamide" earlier in this chapter). At a moderate dose (12–20 mg orally), psilocybin was found to produce an altered state of consciousness marked by stimulation of affect, enhanced ability for introspection, and altered psychological functioning (Studerus et al. 2011). Especially noteworthy are perceptual changes such as illusions, synesthesias, affective activation, and alterations of thought, time sense, and body experience.

Most psilocybin users have an erratic pattern of use. The intense and consciousness-altering/expanding (i.e., psychologically irritating) effects of psilocybin appear to limit frequency of its use. Daily consumption of psilocybin results in acute tolerance, and such users are virtually unknown in the scientific literature (cf. Riley and Blackman 2008).

Complications arising from use and abuse of psilocybin (e.g., emergency department visits) occur with less frequency than with most other hallucinogens (Barbee et al. 2009). This may be partially related to psilocybin's short duration of action: troubled individuals may find the intoxication resolving before arriving or being evaluated in crisis at a hospital. Complications may consist of overarousal with severe panic reactions ("bad trips") and can be treated by transferring the person to a quiet environment and offering empathic supportive reassurances. In clinical situations, the use of an intravenous benzodiazepine, such as diazepam (5–10 mg) or lorazepam (1–2 mg), may be indicated. Somatic effects of psilocybin do not present any danger, but one has to be attentive for the potential ingestion of other, more poisonous mushrooms at the same occasion.

Dimethyltryptamine

DMT is a major hallucinogen with unusual psychological effects (Strassman et al. 1994). It is derived from different plant sources and animal venoms and is also produced endogenously by humans (Barker et al. 2012). Despite much conjecture (Callaway 1988; Strassman 2001), its physiological functions are still unknown, although it has been found to be an endogenous σ_1 receptor regulator agonist (Fontanila et al. 2009).

Many Native peoples of Latin America, especially of Brazil, Colombia, and Peru, have used DMT for spiritual purposes for hundreds of years to the present. It is prepared as a powdered snuff from the seeds of *Anadenanthera peregrina* or the bark of *Virola* species trees. Ayahuasca is another DMT concoction, but ayahuasca is orally active because it also contains natural, reversible monoamine oxidase inhibitors (MAOIs) from the vine *Banisteriopsis caapi* (Schultes and Hofmann 1980), which prevent degradation of DMT by gut-lined monoamine oxidase enzymes (Naranjo 1979).

Ayahuasca is also the sacrament of two religions recognized by the Brazilian government: the Santo Daime and the União do Vegetal, which are syncretic faiths that blend traditional Native beliefs with Christianity. American members of the Santo Daime appear to not have psychiatric sequelae from the use of the drug in a religious setting (Halpern et al. 2008). The ayahuasca preparation of DMT intoxicates for 3–4 hours, peaking within the first hour, and is typically associated with a considerable amount of nausea and vomiting (Riba et al. 2001).

In the United States, illicit DMT usually appears as a synthetic or an extracted powder. DMT is found in and can be extracted from common plants growing in much of the United States, including the root part of the Illinois bundleflower (*Desmanthus illinoensis*) (Halpern 2004). When a small amount (10–20 mg) is smoked alone or on a substrate of tobacco, parsley, or marijuana, DMT intoxicates within seconds, achieving peak effects within 2–3 minutes, and then clears over the next 15 minutes (Cakic et al. 2010). The psychological effects of DMT, especially when they appear very rapidly as with smoking or intranasal insufflation, can be very frightening and may lead to severe nonintentional injuries because of disorientation, motor incoordination, and unrealistic thoughts and behaviors. Severe complications appear to be very rare, especially when the oral route is used, and also may not show up in clinical settings because of the very short duration of action of DMT (15–90 minutes).

The somatic effects of DMT consist of a dose-dependent rise in blood pressure and pulse rate and a sympathomimetic excitation syndrome with hallucinations and overarousal. In some cases, high doses or overdoses may lead to epileptic seizures. The psychological effects of DMT are milder with orally ingested ayahuasca and are very similar to those of LSD and psilocybin (see

Table 7–1). Most people in religious ayahuasca prayer services report significant "spiritual," "cleansing," and "mystical" experiences. In the higher dose
range, some very unusual experiences (such as contact with "alien creatures,"
elves, and gnomes; experiences of tunnels, lights, and even "encounters with
godlike entities") were reported (Strassman 2001).

No deaths have been reported from ayahuasca or other DMT/MAOI combinations so far. If panic reactions and "bad trips" are seen in emergency department settings, they may be treated by 5–10 mg of intravenous diazepam.

Salvia Divinorum and Salvinorin A

History and Prevalence of Use

Salvinorin A is a neoclerodane diterpine alkaloid structurally unrelated to any
other hallucinogen and is a potent and selective agonist at the κ opioid receptor (Roth et al. 2002). It is found in the mint *Salvia divinorum,* a plant initially
cultivated only in Oaxaca, Mexico, where it has been used for spiritual and
divinatory purposes.

Use of salvinorin A, although illegal in more than 13 nations and 15 U.S.
states, is still legal in much of the United States. It has an image of being relatively safe and cannot be detected by established drug tests, leading to its
widespread use. In an NSDUH 2006 survey, an estimated 1.8 million people
age 12 or older in the United States had tried this plant (Substance Abuse and
Mental Health Services Administration 2008). Lifetime prevalence of its use
increased from 0.7% in 2006 to 1.3% in 2008 (an 83% increase). Data suggest that the state of Florida's classification of *S. divinorum* as a Schedule I drug
was followed by a substantial reduction in recreational use (Stogner et al.
2012). Use of *S. divinorum* was shown to be associated with ages 18–25 years,
male gender, residence in large cities, and depression (Wu et al. 2011). The
2011 Monitoring the Future Survey reported an increasing trend in tenth and
twelfth graders with past-year use rates of 1.6% among eighth graders, 3.9%
among tenth graders, 5.9% among twelfth graders, 3.2% for college students,
and 2.5% for young adults (Johnston et al. 2012).

Pharmacology

Early studies isolated salvinorin A as the principal psychoactive constituent responsible for the plant's hallucinogenic effects. It exerts its potent psychotropic

actions through the specific activation of κ opioid receptors: it is the only known nonnitrogenous opioid receptor agonist, and its effects are not mediated by the 5-HT$_{2A}$ receptor, the classic target of hallucinogens (Listos et al. 2011). Its mechanism of action is not fully understood (Cunningham et al. 2011).

A recent survey (Sumnall et al. 2011) found that use of *S. divinorum* was not categorized as a disorder according to the Severity of Dependence Scale (Gossop et al. 1995). This is congruent with preclinical data suggesting that κ opioid receptor agonists are less reinforcing than other opioid receptor agonists (Shippenberg et al. 2001). There are no reports of a withdrawal syndrome from salvinorin A.

Acute and Chronic Effects

The first anecdotal reports of the effect of salvinorin A in humans were described in the mid-1990s (Ott 1995; Siebert 1994). Inhalation of *S. divinorum* is most commonly done by smoking the dried leaves or (sometimes much concentrated) leaf extracts. Other ways of administration include inhalation via volatilization or use of tinctures for buccal absorption (Babu et al. 2008). If taken orally, leaves or extracts containing salvinorin A have a mild effect, often compared with that of cannabis. Salvinorin A is only minimally absorbed through the mouth, and most is degraded in the gastrointestinal tract. When salvinorin A is smoked, its effects can be much more pronounced. The psychological effects consist of mood changes and hallucinations, which appear very suddenly within seconds and may last from 30 minutes to more than 2 hours depending on dose (and extract concentration) (Gonzalez et al. 2006). Intense hallucinatory effects typically last between 10 and 15 minutes (Gonzalez et al. 2006). A double-blind study with smoked salvinorin A in healthy volunteers reported peak drug effects after 2 minutes that continued for about 20 minutes. Hallucinogenic effects appeared similar to those produced by intravenous DMT (Strassman et al. 1994) and higher oral doses of psilocybin (Griffiths et al. 2006). Salvinorin A does not significantly increase heart rate or blood pressure (Johnson et al. 2011).

Unpleasant aftereffects include reports of tiredness, heaviness of head, dizziness, physical exhaustion, and slowed mental function. Loss of consciousness and unrealistic, partially dangerous, and potentially self-destructive behavior have regularly been reported. Dangerous behaviors with this substance may result from disorientation, incoordination, unrealistic thinking, and hallucinations.

No substances are known to antagonize the effects of salvinorin A. No serious physiological symptoms seem to occur with moderate to high doses of this drug, although users become less aware of their surroundings as dose increases. Should an intoxicated individual present to an emergency department, treatment is to protect the individual from serious injury and potentially self-destructive behavior because of disorientation. Diazepam (5–10 mg intravenously) or other benzodiazepines for treatment of panic and excitation may be indicated in more severe cases. Usually the intoxication lasts no longer than 2 hours, even with higher doses.

Mescaline

The principal hallucinogenic compound of the peyote cactus *Lophophora williamsii* is mescaline (β-3,4,5-trimethoxyphenethylamine), although more than 60 other alkaloids are found as well (mostly other β-phenethylamines and also tetrahydroisoquinolines) (Anderson 1996). Mescaline has never been commonly synthesized and distributed for illicit purposes in the United States on a significant scale. Peyote use is protected by the American Indian Religious Freedom Act of 1994 and is almost solely consumed in religious ceremonies of the Native American Church.

Peyote has a bitter, acrid taste, often inducing nausea and vomiting. Peyote contains at most 1.5% mescaline sulfate. A potent mescaline intoxication occurs at approximately 5 mg/kg or more. Peak intoxication occurs within 2–4 hours, wearing off over the subsequent 4–6 hours. Several reports asserted that peyote consumption, as part of the rituals of the Native American Church, offers a culturally sensitive treatment for alcoholism and other addictions, but efficacy has yet to be validated in double-blind clinical studies (Calabrese 1997; Halpern 1996). Evaluation of neurocognitive competence and psychological health of members of the Native American Church has shown them to perform as well as (and in some domains of mental health better than) nonusing, healthy comparators (Halpern et al. 2004). Panic reactions and "bad trips," if they ever occur, may be treated with diazepam (5–10 mg intravenously). No serious physical complications or dependency syndromes from peyote or mescaline have been documented in the scientific literature.

Although mescaline is regularly mentioned as a "classic hallucinogen" in the scientific literature, its use as a recreational drug is rather limited. There have been virtually no seizures of significant amounts of synthetic mescaline, and it is also not mentioned in statistics of emergency department visits.

Natural Anticholinergics

History and Prevalence of Use

The alkaloids atropine, hyoscyamine, and scopolamine are found in jimsonweed (*Datura stramonium*) and members of the nightshade family, including belladona (*Atropa belladonna*), mandrake (*Mandragora officinarum*), and henbane (*Hyoscyamus niger*) (Emboden 1980). Some of these and related subspecies are all popularly grown as ornamental flowers. In overdose, these plants induce a toxic delirium that lasts hours to days. Recreational use is uncommon because of the frightening adverse side-effect profile and is usually limited to teenagers who are not sufficiently aware of these dangers.

The seeds are the most potent part of the plants, followed by the roots, stems, leaves, and flowers; as few as 10 seeds are sufficient to intoxicate. All parts of the plants contain significant amounts of the three major alkaloids (Fodor 1971; Gyermek 1997). These substances (or a combination of them) in relevant dosages for inducing psychopathological effects typically produce a toxic delirium. Therefore, these substances have also been called *deliriants* and may constitute a distinct subclass of hallucinogenic drugs (Brimblecombe and Pinder 1975).

Recreational use of plant-based anticholinergics is rare. Illegal synthesis and distribution have never occurred. The literature shows more than 100 case presentations, but no systematic study has ever been done on the abuse of these plants or their alkaloids. Virtually all cases are one-time users (Caksen et al. 2003). In most cases, these are adolescents trying to experiment with a nonillegal and easily available mind-altering drug (Spina and Taddei 2007). Because these individuals usually have virtually no knowledge about these plants and their effects, they often ingest a very high dose. Compounding their danger, the plants may contain a wide range in their alkaloid content (even from year to year at the same place), and therefore reliable estimates are impossible.

Pharmacology

Pharmacokinetics

Tropane alkaloids are absorbed rapidly from the gastrointestinal tract (Grynkiewicz and Gadzikowska 2008) after oral consumption and have limited bioavailability because of first-pass metabolism, which results in only 2.6% of the nonmetabolized alkaloids being excreted in urine. Enzymatic hydrolysis of metabolites, glucuronide conjugation, and their renal elimination could be the relevant pathway (Grynkiewicz and Gadzikowska 2008). However, the metabolism of tropane alkaloids in humans has not been completely elucidated (Renner et al. 2005).

The onset of effects of these substances is much later than that for other psychoactive drugs. Initial effects may be perceived 1.5–4 hours after ingestion rather than the typical 30–60 minutes or less for all other psychoactive drugs. Effects in the medium and higher dose range may persist for 24–48 hours. These pharmacokinetic parameters may lead to the observed severity of adverse reactions; the delayed onset may lead to the ingestion of more drug, and the persistence of adverse effects contributes to greater confusion and disorientation.

Pharmacodynamics

Tropane alkaloids, such as atropine, hyoscyamine, and scopolamine, are related chemically and in their key effects. In a comparative study, atropine, scopolamine, and ditran were found "virtually identical" in psychophysical reactions (Ketchum et al. 1973). Scopolamine may be different in that it has more sedative effects (Grynkiewicz and Gadzikowska 2008). These substances act as central nervous system (CNS) depressants and competitively antagonize muscarinic cholinergic receptors. Their peripheral action is to oppose the effects of transmitters at muscarinergic, acetylcholinergic, and nicotinergic receptors. This applies to virtually all cholinergic-affected organs. Tropane alkaloids are competitive antagonists of acetylcholine and inhibit or suppress the effects of cholinergic postganglionergic fibers on the receptors or cells of the affected organs. Younger individuals are more sensitive to anticholinergic effects than are older ones (Unna et al. 1950).

Despite no direct evidence for a relation between anticholinergic activity and hallucinogenic potency, behavioral effects of anticholinergics can be antagonized by anticholinesterase drugs (e.g., physostigmine). In animal experiments, awake animals showed an EEG pattern normally associated with sleep EEG, which points to an EEG-behavior dissociation (Wikler 1952). These results were interpreted as reflecting a cholinergic connection chain in the mesodiencephalic activation system. In conclusion, it is most probable that the psychosis-generating effects are mediated through central competitive antagonism of these substances with acetylcholine at muscarinergic receptors. The mechanism by which pharmacological effects result in psychopathology is not fully understood. An imbalance between acetylcholine and dopamine systems induced by tropane alkaloids has been proposed as the mechanism of tropane-induced delirium (Trzepacz 2000; Yokota et al. 2003).

Acute and Chronic Effects

Significant intoxications show the following vegetative effects: dilation of pupils with inability to accommodate, dryness of mouth, difficulty swallowing, urinary retention, hyperreflexia, and muscle weakness (Inch and Brimblecombe 1974). With higher doses, seizures and coma may occur (Diker et al. 2007). Paralysis of breathing is extremely rare, and the lethal dose therefore is unknown. Typical psychological effects are clouding of consciousness, euphoria, dysphoria, excitation, confusion, depersonalization, sensory illusions and hallucinations (mainly visual), somnolence, memory disorders and amnesia, sudden outbursts of anger, anxiety, paranoid ideation, delusions, bizarre and disorganized speech, and talking to imaginary people (Ketchum et al. 1973; Longo 1966). Although some cases of accidental chronic use have been reported from the use of atropine and hyoscyamine as medications, regular recreational use has not been reported.

Treatment of Intoxication

Treatment of acute intoxications is mainly aimed at removing plant material from the gastrointestinal tract, keeping the patient safe, and reversing severe anticholinergic sequelae. When the symptoms are mild, gastric lavage and leaving active charcoal in the stomach afterward will suffice. More severe intoxications require the administration of a benzodiazepine such as diazepam (5–10 mg intravenously). As an antidote to antagonize the major physiological effects, intravenous physostigmine (0.02 mg/kg) is indicated and may be repeated, if necessary. Neostigmine is not indicated because it does not pass the blood-brain barrier. Usually symptoms are very much reduced with treatment, but some milder symptoms may persist for hours or even days (e.g., inability to accommodate).

3,4-Methylenedioxymethamphetamine ("Ecstasy")

History and Prevalence of Use

MDMA (street name "Ecstasy") was first synthesized by the German pharmaceutical company Merck in 1914 as an intermediary product of synthesis while searching for new styptic substances. It was toxicologically tested by the military in a search for "truth drugs" in 1953 (Hardman et al. 1973). During the mid-1960s, the American chemist Alexander Shulgin synthesized MDMA in the search for a psychotherapeutic drug (Benzenhöfer and Passie 2010) but did not realize the full spectrum of its psychoactive effects. After he discovered its unique effects during the 1970s, he distributed it in psychotherapeutic circles (Adamson and Metzner 1988). By the early 1980s, MDMA use rapidly expanded in popularity before the U.S. Drug Enforcement Administration (DEA) became aware of its hedonistic use and abuse potential. Unexpectedly, the DEA was confronted during its scheduling process by several psychotherapists who had quietly been using the substance and were convinced of its therapeutic potential (Eisner 1989). MDMA was listed in 1985 as a Schedule I drug on an international level, but the appropriate committee of the World Health Organization (WHO) recommended research into the "therapeutic potential of this interesting substance" (WHO Expert Committee on Drug Dependence 1985). Major trafficking and use of MDMA are global.

According to the NSDUH, some 15.9 million Americans age 12 or older have tried MDMA at least once in their life, with 2.6 million trying it for the first time in 2010 (Substance Abuse and Mental Health Services Administration 2011b). MDMA-related emergency department visits expanded 114% in the United States between 2004 and 2010 (from 10,227 to 21,836), which represents approximately 12.9 visits per 100,000 population age 20 or younger and 4.7 visits per 100,000 population age 21 or older (Substance Abuse and Mental Health Services Administration 2012).

Studies of the psychotherapeutic utility of MDMA have been conducted during the last few years, with initial reports of significant clinical improvement for patients with posttraumatic stress disorder (PTSD) (Mithoefer et al. 2011; Passie 2012). Mithoefer and colleagues (2011) performed a double-blind, placebo-controlled pilot study of MDMA-assisted psychotherapy in 20 patients with chronic, treatment-resistant PTSD. Standard measures of PTSD symptoms (the Clinician-Administered PTSD Scale was the primary measure) indicated that after 2 months of treatment, the MDMA group had statistically significant clinical improvement compared with the placebo group, which had received the same psychotherapy.

Pharmacology

The precursor of entactogens, MDA, has properties of both hallucinogens and amphetamines (Nozaki et al. 1977). Compared with the classic hallucinogens (LSD, mescaline, psilocybin), MDA produces only minimal sensory effects (e.g., pseudohallucinations) but consistently increases feelings of elation. MDMA is the N-methyl derivative of MDA. The relatively minimal chemical modification of N-methylation has a significant effect on pharmacological activity: it virtually eliminates hallucinogenic activity (Nichols 1986).

Pharmacokinetics

The first effects of MDMA are usually experienced within 30 minutes after an oral dose of 80–150 mg. Most individuals claim peak effects between 30 and 60 minutes after intake. Metabolites of MDMA identified in humans include MDA, 4-hydroxy-3-methoxy-methamphetamine (HMMA), 4-hydroxy-3-methoxyamphetamine (HMA), 3,4-dihydroxyamphetamine (DHA), and N-hydroxy-3,4-methylenedioxyamphetamine (MDOH).

The enzymes involved in the metabolism of MDMA are cytochrome P450 (CYP), CYP2D6, and catechol O-methyltransferase. Complex, nonlinear pharmacokinetics result from autoinhibition of CYP2D6 and CYP2D8 and can result in higher concentrations if the user takes consecutive doses. MDMA and metabolites are primarily excreted as conjugates through the kidneys. More than 50% of MDMA is excreted unchanged in urine, and 7% is metabolized into MDA. Of the two enantiomers of MDMA, the plasma half-life of (R)-MDMA is much longer than that of the (S)-enantiomer (5.8±2.2

hours vs. 3.6 ± 0.9 hours) (Kraemer and Maurer 2002). The lethal oral dose of MDMA in humans is calculated to be 1,875 mg (Gable 2004).

Mechanism of Action

Amphetamines are potent dopamine-releasing agents (Gunne 1977). MDA, and to a lesser extent MDMA, also increase dopaminergic neurotransmission, but MBDB, the prototype of entactogenic activity (Nichols 1986), has no such effect. The psychoactive effects of entactogens may be, if at all, only minimally transmitted via the dopaminergic system. Also, the blocking of reuptake of noradrenaline may contribute to entactogenesis because all entactogens interact, albeit insignificantly, with this mechanism (Vollenweider 2001). The prevailing theory is that the psychoactive effects of entactogens are mediated by potent synaptic release as well as blockade of resorption of the neurotransmitter serotonin, which results in increased intersynaptic serotonin (Liechti and Vollenweider 2001; Vollenweider 2001). A comprehensive study across multiple parameters found different mechanisms of action for the entactogen MDE, the amphetamine methamphetamine, and the hallucinogen psilocybin (Gouzoulis-Mayfrank et al. 1999a, 1999b).

In a neurometabolic study that used $[^{18}F]$fluorodeoxyglucose (FDG)-PET, MDE caused a metabolic increase in the cerebellum and a reduction of cortical metabolism, particularly in the frontal regions, but the anterior cingulum showed a marked increase in metabolism (Gouzoulis-Mayfrank et al. 1999a). Another FDG-PET study by Gamma et al. (2001), which used MDMA, showed significant bilateral increases in regional cerebral blood flow (rCBF) to the cerebellum, ventromedial prefrontal cortex, ventral anterior cingulum, and inferior temporal and medial occipital lobes. Bilateral decreases of rCBF were observed in the precentral and paracentral lobes, the dorsal and posterior cingulum, and the superior temporal gyrus, insula, and thalamus. The most significant change is a decrease in activity in the left amygdala, which might be the substrate of diminished anxiety and euphoria under MDMA.

Acute and Chronic Effects

Reported adverse effects of MDMA (100–125 mg orally) or MDE (2 mg/kg; 140 mg for a 70-kg adult) include loss of appetite, nonexertion diaphoresis, and bruxism (Gouzoulis et al. 1993; Greer and Tolbert 1986; Liechti and Vollenweider 2000a, 2000b). Increases in blood pressure with MDMA—depending on dosage—were found to be between 20–35 mm Hg systolic and 10–20 mm Hg diastolic (de la Torre et al. 2000; Vollenweider et al. 1998a); with MDE, increases in blood pressure between 30–40 mm Hg systolic and 10–18 mm Hg diastolic have been noted (Gouzoulis et al. 1993). MDMA increases heart rate approximately 10–20 beats/minute (de la Torre et al. 2000; Vollenweider et al. 1998a), and MDE increases heart rate around 30–40 beats/minute (Gouzoulis et al. 1993; Mas et al. 1999). MDMA increases body temperature by 0.3°C–0.4°C (de la Torre et al. 2000; Vollenweider et al. 1998a), and MDE raises temperature by 0.3°C–0.6°C (Gouzoulis et al. 1993). MDMA and MDE also have significant effects on the endocrine system—depending on dosage—with increases in cortisol, prolactin, and growth hormone (Gouzoulis-Mayfrank et al. 1999b; Harris et al. 2002; Mas et al. 1999).

Few studies have reported on the acute effects of MDMA on cognitive functioning. When compared with the typical hallucinogens, MDMA and MDE (in medium-range doses) have minimal acute effects on neuropsychological performance as assessed with different neuropsychological and psychomotor tests (Cami et al. 2000; Lamers et al. 2003; Passie et al. 2005).

Stimulant effects, as noted earlier, occur soon after ingestion, including increased energy and elevated mood. Side effects such as nausea, jaw clenching, muscle tension, and blurred vision are often reported. A "hangover" for some hours or even a day or two can occur with symptoms of insomnia, fatigue, sore muscles, headache, and decreased mood.

Liester et al. (1992) interviewed 20 American psychiatrists who had experimentally ingested between 100 and 200 mg of MDMA to determine the psychic changes induced by the drug. Most of the participants were prepared for MDMA intake and ingested it under quiet and discreet conditions. The results are featured in Table 7–5. Cohen (1995) administered a questionnaire to 500 white American college students ages 18–25 years, who claimed to have taken MDMA at least once in the past; 97% of the participants described experiencing euphoria.

Possible Complications

When medium-range doses of MDMA or MDE are administered to healthy volunteers in a controlled and medically supervised setting, no health risks or significant complications have been reported (de la Torre 2000; Gasser 1997; Mas et al. 1999; Mithoefer et al. 2011; Vollenweider et al. 1998a).

Table 7–5.   Subjective effects of 3,4-methylenedioxymeth-
amphetamine (MDMA)

Altered perception of time	90%
Increased ability to interact with or be open with others	85%
Decreased defensiveness	80%
Decreased anxiety	65%
Decreased sense of separation or alienation from others	60%
Changes in visual perception	55%
Increased awareness of emotions	50%
Decreased aggression	50%
Awareness of previously unconscious memories	40%
Decreased compulsiveness	40%
Decreased restlessness	30%
Decreased impulsivity	25%

Note.   Percentages are subjects with "yes" answers.
Source.   Adapted from Liester et al. 1992.

MDMA ingested recreationally may pose special risks to users (Kiyatkin and Sharma 2012). Heightened empathy and impulsivity may make those who are intoxicated vulnerable to abuse. Intense pleasure and physical stamina may lead to overexertion, increasing body temperature. As dehydration, hyperthermia, and tachycardia continue, individuals can collapse from a potentially life-threatening fever, cardiac arrhythmia, and extreme exhaustion. Fever may eventually lead to rhabdomyolysis (muscle breakdown) and kidney failure (Yamamoto et al. 2010). Data from hospital records report a death rate of 0%–2% from emergency admissions related to Ecstasy. Two major syndromes are most commonly reported as cause of death: hyperthermia and hyponatremia (Rogers et al. 2009). Use of methamphetamine and cocaine in combination with Ecstasy increases the risk of serotonin syndrome (Mohamed et al. 2011).

Case reports have claimed that MDMA use contributed to induction of paranoid psychotic states, anxiety, and depression. In some affected individuals, symptoms persisted, but they soon subsided in others. Most such reports have been subject to bias because of the concomitant use of other drugs, psychiatric symptoms prior to MDMA use, or a pertinent family history of psychiatric disease. Some investigators have pointed out that depressive symptoms in former Ecstasy users are mild and clinically irrelevant. Evidence from studies indicates that users and nonusers do not show differences in depressive symptoms.

Toxicological Implications

Because of preclinical toxicological research with overdose regimens in animals, MDMA is still often viewed as neurotoxic. In fact, the data are much more heterogeneous. In overdose or in combination with other drugs and alcohol, or with a very frequent dosage regimen, MDMA may contribute to acute risk to safety of the individual as well as promote acute or more lasting complications, some of which have rarely proved lethal. Some chronic users report attenuation of drug effects, lack of attention, a feeling of depression, increased extroversion, reduced appetite, insomnia, and increased self-awareness (Karlsen et al. 2007).

The toxic potential of several entactogens has been a subject of heated discussion for some time. MDMA has been successfully and safely investigated. Destructive effects on the serotonergic system have been shown in preclinical studies, usually with very high doses (de la Torre et al. 2004). In studies with chronic users of MDMA, the serotonin transporter density was decreased (McCann et al. 2005) together with other indications of serotonergic neuron impairment, depending on the cumulative doses (Thomasius 2000) and time from last dose. A major study found that people with lifetime self-exposures of 50–100 doses of MDMA had no alteration in any of the diverse parameters used, including neurometabolic and neuropsychological parameters (Thomasius 2000). Detailed reviews (Morton (2005; Gouzoulis-Mayfrank and Daumann (2009) refer to the possible neurotoxic potential of MDMA (mostly combined with other drugs).

Postexposure, in preclinical models, decreased serotonin stores may persist for weeks to months. A "hangover" complaint of decreased mood could be due to serotonin depletion. Neuropsychological studies of MDMA users show that normal functioning is mostly preserved, although difficulties with memory processing also have been reported in MDMA polydrug users. Neurocognitive performance of relatively "pure" (exclusive) moderate and heavy users of

MDMA was not found impaired in comparison to nonusers, who were well matched for sociodemographics, mental health, other drug use, and hours of sleep (Halpern et al. 2011b).

Several investigations to date have reported on the cognitive impairments of chronic users of entactogens, particularly MDMA. These studies relied in all cases on individuals in uncontrolled settings, usually with combined use of other psychoactive substances. Indications of impairments in learning and brain function have been noted, depending on the cumulative dose (Gouzoulis-Mayfrank and Daumann 2009; Halpern et al. 2004). These impairments are proposed to be associated mainly with alterations of the serotonergic system. The question as to the reversibility of these changes is unknown, but some evidence suggests that they may be reversible (Buchert et al. 2006). The Netherlands XTC Toxicity (NeXT) study prospectively tracked youth at risk for MDMA abuse, and then in follow-up, repeated single photon emission computed tomography and other neuroimaging tests compared users with nonusers (de Win et al. 2006, 2007). NeXT study results included no changes in serotonin transporter densities or brain metabolites. The study did find evidence of regional decreased brain perfusion, changes to microvasculature, white matter maturation, and altered axonal expression. Evidence of structural neuronal damage was not observed.

Collectively, in view of the multiple design limitations of most prior investigations, it is unlikely that marked residual cognitive deficits can be attributed to MDMA abuse, although this remains an area of some debate (Halpern et al. 2011a).

Treatment

The primary response to acute intoxication is supportive in nature. If a person is overheated, then the body will need cooling. If timing indicates that an overdose remains in the stomach, emesis can and should be induced. Emotional crisis should first be responded to with supportive reassurances in a quiet, low-light environment. In the rare event that postuse depressed mood is severe enough to elicit concerns for suicide, the patient should be admitted to a locked inpatient psychiatric facility until safety is assured. Some preclinical studies have indicated that ingestion of a selective serotonin reuptake inhibitor (SSRI)–type antidepressant immediately post-MDMA use will diminish/prevent any re-formation of serotonin-rich dendrite pattern in the CNS (Li et al. 2010). Many users do report prevention of postuse dysphoria and other postuse consequences through taking SSRIs and/or herbal supplements, even though they are of questionable benefit (Allott and Redman 2006; Kelly 2009). For additional discussion of treatment, see Chapter 9, "Club Drugs and Synthetic Cannabinoid Agonists."

Phencyclidine and Ketamine

History and Prevalence of Abuse

Phencyclidine (1-[1-phenylcyclohexyl] piperidine) was first tested in humans in 1957. Given in doses of 0.25 mg/kg intravenously, PCP produced anesthesia and was consequently manufactured as an analgesic (Sernyl). Because anesthesia can be achieved without the patient being unconscious or losing autonomic reflexes, PCP was initially thought to have incredible advantages. The paradox of an excited CNS with all reflexes preserved combined with a significant analgesia led to the model that PCP's analgesia is coupled with a dissociative state in which the CNS is disconnected from sensory input from interoception (i.e., the body state: "dissociative anesthesia").

After a short period of use, it became clear that this agent induces alienating trance and dreamlike states, which are invasive and frightening. PCP use ultimately came to a halt for anesthesia. A few years later, the PCP derivative ketamine was tested and found to have more benign side effects and was therefore marketed as a surrogate for PCP.

The use of PCP by drug seekers was first reported in 1967 (Meyers et al. 1967/1968; Perry 1975). During the 1970s, PCP became more popular; the increase in its use coincided with the decline in LSD use. After a period of substantial popularity in the 1980s, PCP abuse declined but still represents a significant drug abuse problem. In 1979, 12.8% of twelfth graders had used PCP, whereas in 1997, only 3.9% had used the drug (National Institute on Drug Abuse 2009). Reasons for its ongoing popularity include its ease of use (i.e., smoking) and its ready availability because of ease of synthesis from available precursor chemicals. PCP may be diverted from veterinary sources or manufactured illegally. In Europe and other countries where the introduction of PCP is recent, there has not been an epidemic of use as there was in the United States during the 1980s.

PCP has appeared on the illicit market as a powder, a tablet, a liquid, or crystals in capsules. PCP may be sprayed on parsley, mint, oregano, or other leaves so that it can be smoked in cigarette form. The primary mode of taking PCP is by smoking, intranasal insufflation, or oral consumption.

Abuse of ketamine started later than that of PCP (Dillon et al. 2003). Its misuse on a broader scale began in the late 1990s (Reynolds 2012) and was never as prevalent as PCP. This may be because of its complicated synthesis and because it cannot be administered as easily (i.e., smoked) (Wolff and Winstock 2006). Its use is significant but has not reached PCP's proportions (Jansen and Darracot-Cankovic 2001). There has yet to be any documentation of illegally manufactured ketamine.

Recently, another PCP-like substance became a drug of abuse. Dextromethorphan (DXM, "Robo") is an easily accessible over-the-counter antitussive. Used in large quantities (more than 2 mg/kg), the drug has been associated with a dissociative effect similar to that of PCP and ketamine. Symptoms of intoxication and treatment are essentially the same as with PCP and ketamine, but the effects are more numbing than with the other two (Romanelli and Smith 2009).

Pharmacology

PCP and ketamine both act on the central and peripheral nervous systems. Animals under the influence of PCP show the following stimulating and depressant effects: tranquilization, excitation, catalepsy, analgesia, and clonic convulsions. Animals will self-administer PCP and, to a lesser degree, ketamine (Marquis and Moreton 1987; Risner 1982; Winter 2009). Both substances cause bronchodilation and moderate stimulation of the sympathetic and cardiovascular system.

Pharmacokinetics

PCP and ketamine are water and lipid soluble, allowing them to be administered conveniently via various routes and providing extensive distribution in the body. PCP and ketamine have complex pharmacokinetics. Both are lipophilic and are stored in fatty tissue, from which they slowly diffuse. The half-life of PCP varies widely, ranging from 10 to 72 hours (after extensive daily use), whereas the half-life of ketamine is less than 2 hours. The drugs are eliminated by hepatic hydroxylation mediated by hepatic microsomal enzymes and subsequent renal excretion. About 10% of total PCP is excreted in the urine and can be detected by suitable screening methods.

The oral dose of PCP in abuse settings is considered to be 2–5 mg. Subjective effects of smoking PCP begin within 1–5 minutes and reach a plateau over 5–30 minutes. Following oral administration, subjects report psychological or physical changes within 45 minutes and maximum effects at 90 minutes (Beech et al. 1961). A more rapid onset of 30 seconds to 1 minute follows insufflation of a street dose in powdered form. Users report staying "high" for 4–6 hours followed by the "comedown" period lasting 6–24 hours. Following a 2- to 3-day binge, the time before the user felt normal again was 2–4 days.

Evidence of hematological, hepatic, or renal toxicity was not found in chronic use of PCP, even for periods greater than 6 months. Lethal doses for PCP are 200 mg orally and for ketamine are 1,300 mg intravenously (Gable 2004).

Pharmacodynamics

PCP and ketamine act as noncompetitive N-methyl-D-aspartate (NMDA) receptor antagonists. PCP and ketamine have a similar spectrum of activity (Chen and Weston 1960). The pharmacological effects of PCP, ketamine, and related arylcyclohexylamines are mediated by NMDA, opioid, muscarinic, and different voltage-gated receptors. The so-called PCP receptor is associated with the NMDA receptor complex (Lodge and Johnson 1990). At substantially higher doses (i.e., those that cause blockade of the NMDA receptor), PCP (but not ketamine) blocks monoamine reuptake, increasing synaptic levels of dopamine and noradrenaline. This action may underpin the stimulatory effects during high-dose PCP intoxication, which can include agitation and violence. There are also effects on cholinergic, opiate, and γ-aminobutyric acid (GABA)/benzodiazepine receptors, and so PCP and ketamine intoxication may result from perturbation of multiple neurotransmitter systems. PCP and ketamine target many of the reward systems in the brain via dopamine reuptake inhibition, NMDA antagonism, and μ opioid affinity (Vignon et al. 1989).

PCP increases firing of dopaminergic neurons (Freedman and Bunney 1987) and may reduce cortical GABAergic function (Grunze et al. 1994) while disinhibiting glutamatergic transmission in the prefrontal cortex (Moghaddam et al. 1997) and the ventral tegmental area (Mathe et al. 1998). This increase in glutamatergic transmission stimulates mesocorticolimbic dopaminergic transmission (Jentsch et al. 1998).

In neurometabolic studies with a dose range typical for drug abuse, ketamine increases frontal cortical blood flow, especially in the anterior cingulate and frontomedial cortical regions (Breier et al. 1997; Vollenweider et al. 1997a). No neurometabolic data about the acute effects of PCP are available. Long-term abuse of PCP leads to reduced frontal lobe blood flow and glucose use (Hertzman et al. 1990; Wu et al. 1991).

Tolerance develops with chronic use of PCP, resulting in consumption of higher doses to achieve the desired subjective effects. Difficulty with discontinuation and resultant craving for reuse may be seen, but a physiological withdrawal syndrome does not appear with the use of PCP (for discussion of ketamine withdrawal, see Chapter 9, "Club Drugs and Synthetic Cannabinoid Agonists"). Tolerance, but not physical dependence, develops to the effects of PCP. Psychological dependence as indicated by craving for the drug has been reported and may lead to a daily consumption of the drug with dangerous consequences. Although withdrawal symptoms have been reported in animals, no clear evidence is seen in humans. A delirious or mental disorganization syndrome lasting 4–6 weeks may follow acute intoxication.

Acute and Chronic Effects

PCP is usually smoked on marijuana or ingested orally. Intoxication occurs within 5 minutes when smoked or 1 hour when ingested, lasting for 4–6 hours and completely resolving after 24 hours. Less than 5 mg, orally ingested, will intoxicate and produce physical symptoms. The typical oral dose is in the range of 2–10 mg, and some individuals take up to three doses a day. Ketamine is rarely smoked, and the typical user will snort it in doses of 25–60 mg, which usually leads to an inebriated state for 30–60 minutes. If taken orally, ketamine undergoes a significant first-pass metabolism, and therefore a dose four to five times higher must be used, which is usually avoided because of "inefficacy." Some users will inject ketamine intramuscularly in doses of 25–50 mg for going on a "voyage" in more quiet and protected private environments for 30–60 minutes (Jansen 2000).

Both substances produce profound mental effects, including changes in body image, loss of ego boundaries, and depersonalization associated with feelings of estrangement, isolation, and dependency. Affectively charged experiences are often evoked, and some subjects show negativism and hostility or apathy. Thinking is slowed with disruption of attention span, inability to sustain organized directed thought, and impairment of learning. Subjects are distractible and perseverate. Time sense is disturbed, with underestimation of time intervals (Pradhan 1984).

PCP intoxication is reported to be very intense. Past users have compared it with LSD but insist that it is different, "in a class by itself" (Feldman et al. 1979). The typical PCP experience is characterized by a feeling of numbness, as if the user no longer possesses a body. This effect is caused by interruption of sensory and proprioceptive input to the brain, from which the brain generates the body image in the usual state of consciousness. Usually PCP induces a change of mood, and a numb kind of euphoria may be experienced. These sensations are relatively stable (i.e., not that sensitive to internal or environmental circumstances) as is true with most hallucinogens. PCP and ketamine users sometimes claim that these drugs are relatively safe because the intoxication is relatively reliable and predictable and because they rarely induce anxiety (Siegel 1978). Other effects include thought disturbance, mainly in the sense of "thinking nothing and flowing around." Mild-to-moderate paranoid ideation is also common, which may lead to omnipotent or magical thinking, thereby fueling unrealistic behavior and sometimes panic. The hallucinatory effects are mainly visual and acoustic and can be very irritating, especially with higher doses. The user of PCP, unlike most other psychedelics, is not always aware that he or she is experiencing drug effects (pseudohallucinations) and therefore may experience real hallucinations, which may promote irrational behaviors.

The typical user of PCP or ketamine tries the drug but a few times or only occasionally; chronic use is much less common. If a pattern of chronic use develops, the dangers of persisting dissociation become more evident. The user may lose contact with reality, thereby creating unrealistic, even violent behaviors as has been reported. PCP is typically used in binges lasting 2–3 days, which are usually followed by periods of hypersomnia, depressed mood, social isolation, and a schizophrenia-like psychotic state. Especially noteworthy are the development of delusional systems and feelings of omnipotence during longer periods of use. Effects of chronic use are listed in Table 7–6.

PCP and ketamine induce nystagmus and ataxia. Dramatic nystagmus may be used to identify intoxication, because no other recreational drugs induce this

Table 7–6. Effects of phencyclidine and ketamine

Regular somatic effects	Increased blood pressure
	Tachycardia
	Nystagmus
	Miosis
	Blurred vision
Rarely observed somatic effects	Nausea, vomiting
	Hypersalivation
	Hyperpyrexia
	Rhabdomyolysis
	Flushing
	Bronchospasm
Acute psychiatric effects	Euphoria/dysphoria
	Agitation
	Hallucinations
	Dissociation from the environment
	Dissociation from the body
	Sensation of floating
	Delusional and omnipotent thinking
	Aggression
	Bizarre behavior
Effects of chronic use	Psychological dependence
	Confusion
	Depression
	Memory disturbances
	Psychosis
	Personality changes
	Flashbacks (rare)

sign. In general, grave impairment of motor and sensory functions makes normal physical activities dangerous during the acute effects of the drugs.

Dangers of PCP ingestion (seemingly much less reported with ketamine), in addition to the somatic side effects mentioned earlier, are typically accidents, jumps from higher places (e.g., cliffs or windows), disorientation, and in some rare cases of chronic use, violent behavior. It may take several days to "come down" after a few days of intake. Most chronic users report that they become depressed when not high on PCP. Memory disturbance may occur after chronic use.

Several chronic PCP users have complained of anxiety or nervousness during and following periods of regular PCP use and have sought psychiatric care. Some individuals become severely depressed and attempt suicide on repeated occasions. Additionally, chronic users report personality change, social withdrawal, social isolation, and divorce resulting from their use of PCP. Users also experience a feeling of strength and endurance. Some thought it was difficult to do rather simple things. Chronic PCP use in some individuals can produce a long-lasting schizophrenia-like psychotic episode. Prolonged and fluctuating effects of PCP have been attributed to the drug's affinity to fatty tissue, its slow release from such tissue, and its subsequent uptake by brain tissue. A newly reported problem resulting from heavy, chronic ketamine abuse is bladder problems, including chronic cystitis with erythematous lesions. Ketamine cessation and intravesical sodium hyaluronate solution provide some symptomatic relief (Lai et al. 2012).

PCP and Ketamine Intoxications

PCP has a wide range of deleterious effects. Drug users may not even know that they have taken PCP because it is so easily disguised. Physicians should look for decreased reality testing, erythema, dry skin, and other manifestations. Often the acute behavioral toxicity is not realized or even felt by the individual because of the anesthetic effects of the drug. The acute toxicity of PCP is often misdiagnosed because of its similarity to schizophrenic episodes.

Ketamine has virtually none of the physical effects described for PCP. It induces significant nystagmus and mild sympathomimetic effects (increased pulse and blood pressure). Complications occur less frequently with ketamine than with PCP, which may be because of ketamine's shorter duration of action, use by individuals with more drug experience, and far broader therapeutic dosage range. In case of a significant anxiety reaction, which occurs very rarely with ketamine, the intravenous use of a benzodiazepine such as diazepam is usually effective.

Most adverse psychological events are associated with PCP at a dose of 5–15 mg and ketamine at a dose of 30–150 mg (snorted or intramuscular) and usually consist of severe numbness, isolation, paralysis, confusion, thought disorder, and transient psychotic behavior and hallucinations. Again, the use of a benzodiazepine appears most appropriate, such as diazepam (5–10 mg intravenously). For severe PCP intoxication, it may be necessary to add an antipsychotic (e.g., haloperidol 5 mg intravenously) to ensure the patient's safety.

Higher doses of PCP produce more sympathomimetic signs such as hypertension, tachycardia, and diaphoresis and cholinergic signs including bronchospasm, salivation, urinary retention, flushing, and miosis. Overdoses of more than 100 mg of PCP (or more than 1,000 mg of ketamine, as virtually never encountered) may result in convulsions, coma, and death from respiratory arrest. There is also a risk of hypertensive crisis and in rare cases intracerebral hemorrhage. In acute PCP intoxication with coma, creatine phosphokinase (CPK) levels greater than 500 U/L are frequently found. In several cases, CPK has been greater than 20,000 U/L, and rhabdomyolysis preceded myoglobinuria and renal failure. PCP also has been shown to be a direct cardiac irritant and may induce arrhythmias and vasospasm. In addition, muscle tone becomes exaggerated, and patients may have hyperreflexia and myoclonic, dystonic, or choreoathetoid movements such as opisthotonos and torticollis. Complications of this hypertonic muscle activity include hyperthermia and rhabdomyolysis (Bey and Patel 2007). Respiratory depression requiring intubation is uncommon in PCP intoxication; however, patients may experience irregular breathing (McCarron et al. 1981). Higher doses of ketamine (80–150 mg intramuscularly or insufflated) are known to be associated with irregular breathing associated with sighing.

Because PCP-induced seizures, myoclonic activity, and trauma may result in rhabdomyolysis, serum potassium, serum urea nitrogen, creatinine, and CPK levels should be measured. Serum CPK level is the preferred screening method for rhabdomyolysis.

Treatment of Intoxication

No known antidote exists for the toxic effects of PCP. The treatment begins just as that for any other intoxication would. First, the patient's airway, breathing, circulation, thermoregulation, and neurological status are stabilized. The patient should then be restrained and sedated. Chemical restraints are preferred over physical restraints, which may induce rhabdomyolysis, the most common cause of morbidity and mortality in these patients (Olmedo 2002). Patients must be on continuous cardiac monitoring because of the frequency and severity of cardiac symptoms with PCP overdoses. Treatment also includes efforts to decrease gastrointestinal absorption of the drug (activated charcoal). Intravenous treatment of hypertension should be administered when appropriate.

Anxiety, agitation, and general excitation can be treated by intravenous use of diazepam (5–10 mg) or lorazepam (2–4 mg). Clinical management includes preventing injury and helping patients cope with disorientation. Sensory stimulation should be minimized, because it increases agitation and hallucinatory effects. Some patients require repeated doses of 10–15 mg of diazepam to control restlessness and agitation during prolonged recovery periods.

In the past, urinary acidification was used to enhance PCP elimination, but this is no longer recommended because acidic urine increases the risk of acute tubular necrosis secondary to myoglobinuria in rhabdomyolysis. Furthermore, only 9% of PCP is excreted in the urine (Bey and Patel 2007).

Intravenous diazepam in doses of 10–15 mg followed by intravenous phenytoin has been effective in the control of seizures. Diazoxide has been used to reduce blood pressure. Hydralazine hydrochloride has been suggested as a possible alternative. Diphenhydramine, 50 mg or 1 mg/kg intravenously, can be used to treat PCP-induced dystonic symptoms. Phenothiazines, like haloperidol, are contraindicated in acute PCP intoxication. They may induce dystonic and anticholinergic reactions and lower the seizure threshold. There is no proof that they reduce or shorten psychotic symptoms in PCP intoxication (Bowers et al. 1990), but in some cases they have produced prolonged, severe hypotension and hyperthermia (Bey and Patel 2007).

Treatment of ketamine intoxication is discussed in Chapter 9, "Club Drugs and Synthetic Cannabinoid Agonists."

Flashback Phenomena and Hallucinogen Persisting Perception Disorder

Hallucinogen aftereffects, also known as flashbacks, are late drug effects that can emerge after the acute effects have worn off. These aftereffects were first described as "a repetition of the acute phase of the experience days or even weeks after the initial doses" (Sandison and Whitelaw 1957). The later-coined term *flashback* is derived from motion picture industry jargon signifying a short cutback from a film's story to an earlier point in time. Because flashbacks appear suddenly and unexpectedly, often at inappropriate times, they are usually associated with foreboding or dread. The person may interpret the strange events as a sign of being out of control or "going mad." In other instances, the response to a flashback may be one of enjoyment and pleasure, perceived as a welcoming "free trip." Some triggers are known to induce flashback phenomena such as being in the same environmental circumstances, listening to the same music, or being in states in which the level of CNS excitation is similar and/or control over the experience is diminished (e.g., experiencing fatigue, hypnagogic states, or cannabis or even alcohol intoxication) (Holland and Passie 2011).

These aftereffects may occur only very rarely under medically controlled conditions, as shown by different surveys about complications in therapeutic and experimental use (Cohen 1960; Malleson 1971; Studerus et al. 2011), but may happen more often in uncontrolled circumstances (Baggott et al. 2011). A diagnostic entity, hallucinogen persisting perception disorder of a postulated permanent visual perceptual disorder type ("HPPD type 2"; Halpern JH, Lerner A, Pope HG Jr, et al: "An exploratory study of subjects reporting symptoms of hallucinogen persisting perception disorder," 2013, unpublished manuscript), was introduced in DSM-III-R (American Psychiatric Association 1987) based primarily on research by Abraham (1983) and Abraham and Duffy (1996, 2001). Abraham and colleagues postulated a permanent disorder of the visual system that may be experienced even by one-time users of a hallucinogen, especially LSD, and may consist of halos around things and "trailing" phenomena. However, no one has endeavored to replicate this research (Holland and Passie 2011).

For patients complaining of HPPD, simple reassurance that the persisting phenomena are not reflective of cognitive damage is important. Atypical antipsychotics have been reported to aggravate the condition (see Halpern and Pope 2003 for review). For some, use of a sedative-hypnotic, such as clonazepam, may be effective, especially for those with chronic complaints that appear to endure in the months since last use and may be associated with anxiety features. Many HPPD patients offer histories of repeating drug use with the very hallucinogenic substances that they believe triggered their condition. As such, it is also important to advise against reexposure to the drug.

Conclusion

Hallucinogens represent a large variety of substances, most of which have been used for millennia to induce trances and religious experiences. Their use has not been dangerous when restricted to traditional ritualistic settings. Use of these substances by laypersons and misuse by some individuals has led to serious problems including addiction, psychotic episodes, and dangerous behaviors. Epidemiological data show consistent levels of use of these substances since the 1970s. Although most of the hallucinogenic substances are physiologically well tolerated, some (e.g., PCP, MDMA, anticholinergics) can have serious toxicological effects.

References

Abraham HD: Visual phenomenology of the LSD flashback. Arch Gen Psychiatry 40:884–889, 1983

Abraham HD, Duffy FH: Stable qEEG differences in post-LSD visual disorder by split half analyses: evidence for disinhibition. Psychiatry Res 67:173–187, 1996

Abraham HD, Duffy FH: EEG coherence in post-LSD visual hallucinations. Psychiatry Res 107:151–163, 2001

Abramson HA, Jarvik ME, Gorin MH, et al: Lysergic acid diethylamide (LSD 25), XVII: tolerance development and its relationship to a theory of psychosis. J Psychol 41:81–86, 1956

Adamson S, Metzner R: The nature of the MDMA experience and its role in healing, psychotherapy, and spiritual practice. ReVision 10:59–72, 1988

Aghajanian GK, Bing OH: Persistence of lysergic acid diethylamide in the plasma of human subjects. Clin Pharmacol Ther 5:611–614, 1964

Allott K, Redman J: Patterns of use and harm reduction practices of ecstasy users in Australia. Drug Alcohol Depend 82:168–176, 2006

American Psychiatric Association: Diagnostic and Statistical Manual of Mental Disorders, 3rd Edition, Revised. Washington, DC, American Psychiatric Association, 1987

Anderson EF: Peyote: The Divine Cactus. Tucson, University of Arizona Press, 1996

Anderson EW, Rawnsley K: Clinical studies of lysergic acid diethylamide. Monatsschr Psychiatr Neurol 128:38–55, 1954

Aronson H, Silverstein AB, Klee MD: Influence of LSD-25 on subjective time. Arch Gen Psychiatry 1:469–472, 1959

Axelrod J, Brady RO, Witkop B, et al: The distribution and metabolism of LSD. Ann NY Acad Sci 66:435–444, 1957

Babu KM, McCurdy CR, Boyer EW: Opioid receptors and legal highs: salvia divinorum and Kratom. Clin Toxicol 46:146–152, 2008

Baggott MJ, Erowid E, Erowid F, et al: Abnormal visual experiences in individuals with histories of hallucinogen use: a Web-based questionnaire. Drug Alcohol Depend 114:61–67, 2011

Balestrieri C: On the action mechanisms of LSD 25, in The Use of LSD in Psychotherapy and Alcoholism. Edited by Abramson HA. New York, Bobbs-Merrill, 1967, pp 653–660

Barbee G, Berry-Cabán C, Barry J, et al: Analysis of mushroom exposures in Texas requiring hospitalization, 2005–2006. J Med Toxicol 5:59–62, 2009

Barker SA, McIlhenny EH, Strassman R: A critical review of reports of endogenous psychedelic N, N-dimethyltryptamines in humans: 1955–2010. Drug Test Anal 4:617–635, 2012

Beech HR, Davies BM, Morgenstern FS: Preliminary investigations of the effects of Sernyl upon cognitive and sensory processes. J Ment Sci 107:509–513, 1961

Benzenhöfer U, Passie T: Rediscovering MDMA (ecstasy): the role of the American chemist Alexander T. Shulgin. Addiction 105:1355–1361, 2010

Bey T, Patel A: Phencyclidine intoxication and adverse effects: a clinical and pharmacological review of an illicit drug. Cal J Emerg Med 8:9–14, 2007

Bowers MB Jr, Mazure CM, Nelson JC, et al: Psychotogenic drug use and neuroleptic response. Schizophr Bull 16:81–85, 1990

Boyd ES: The metabolism of LSD. Arch Int Pharmacodyn Ther 120:292–311, 1959

Bradley PB, Elkes C, Elkes J: On some effects of lysergic acid diethylamide (LSD 25) in normal volunteers. J Physiol 121:50P–51P, 1953

Breier A, Malhotra AK, Pinals DA, et al: Association of ketamine-induced psychosis with focal activation of the prefrontal cortex in healthy volunteers. Am J Psychiatry 154:805–811, 1997

Brimblecombe RW, Pinder R: Hallucinogenic Agents. Bristol, UK, Wright-Scientechnica, 1975

Buchert R, Thomasius R, Petersen K, et al: Reversibility of ecstasy-induced reduction in serotonin transporter availability in polydrug ecstasy users. Eur J Nucl Med Mol Imaging 33:188–199, 2006

Cakic V, Potkonyak J, Marshall A: Dimethyltryptamine (DMT): subjective effects and patterns of use among Australian recreational users. Drug Alcohol Depend 111:30–37, 2010

Caksen H, Odabaş D, Akbayram S, et al: Deadly nightshade (Atropa belladonna) intoxication: an analysis of 49 children. Hum Exp Toxicol 22:665–668, 2003

Calabrese JD: Spiritual healing and human development in the Native American Church: toward a cultural psychiatry of peyote. Psychoanal Rev 84:237–255, 1997

Callaway JC: A proposed mechanism for the visions of dream sleep. Med Hypotheses 26:119–122, 1988

Cami J, Farre M, Mas M, et al: Human pharmacology of 3,4-methylenedioxymethamphetamine ("ecstasy"): psychomotor performance and subjective effects. J Clin Psychopharmacol 20:455–466, 2000

Carhart-Harris RL, Erritzoe D, Williams T, et al: Neural correlates of the psychedelic state as determined by fMRI studies with psilocybin. Proc Natl Acad Sci USA 109:2138–2143, 2012

Cerletti A: Etude pharmacologique de la psilocybine, in Les Champignons Hallucinogenes du Mexique. Edited by Heim R, Wasson RG. Paris, Museum d'Historie Naturelle, 1958, pp 268–271

Chen GM, Weston JK: The analgesic and anesthetic effects of 1-(1-phenyl-cyclohexyl)piperidine HCL on the monkey. Anesth Analg 39:132–137, 1960

Cholden LS, Kurland A, Savage CU: Clinical reactions and tolerance to LSD in chronic schizophrenia. J Nerv Ment Dis 122:211–221, 1955

Cohen MM, Marinello MJ, Back N: Chromosomal damage in human leukocytes induced by lysergic acid diethylamide. Science 155:1417–1419, 1967

Cohen RS: Subjective reports on the effects of the MDMA ("ecstasy") experience in humans. Prog Neuropsychopharmacol Biol Psychiatry 19:1137–1141, 1995

Cohen S: LSD: side effects and complications. J Nerv Ment Dis 130:30–40, 1960

Creese I, Burt DR, Snyder SH: The dopamine receptor: differential binding of d-LSD and related agents to agonist and antagonist states. Life Sci 17:933–1001, 1975

Cunningham CW, Rothman RB, Prisinzano TE: Neuropharmacology of the naturally occurring kappa-opioid hallucinogen salvinorin A. Pharmacol Rev 63:316–347, 2011

de la Torre R, Farré M: Neurotoxicity of MDMA (ecstasy): the limitations of scaling from animals to humans. Trends Pharmacol Sci 25:505–508, 2004

de la Torre R, Farré M, Ortuño J, et al: Non-linear pharmacokinetics of MDMA ("ecstasy") in humans. Br J Clin Pharmacol 49:104–109, 2000

de Win MM, Schilt T, Reneman L, et al: Ecstasy use and self-reported depression, impulsivity, and sensation seeking: a prospective cohort study. J Psychopharmacol 20:226–235, 2006

de Win MM, Reneman L, Jager G, et al: A prospective cohort study on sustained effects of low-dose ecstasy use on the brain in new ecstasy users. Neuropsychopharmacology 32:458–470, 2007

Delay J, Pichot P, Lemperiere T, et al: Etude psycho-physiologique et clinique de la psilocybine, in Les Champignons Hallucinogenes du Mexique. Edited by Heim R, Wasson RG. Paris, Museum d'Historie Naturelle 1958, pp 287–310

Diker D, Markovitz D, Rothman M, et al: Coma as a presenting sign of Datura stramonium seed tea poisoning. Eur J Intern Med 18:336–338, 2007

Dillon P, Copeland J, Jansen K: Patterns of use and harms associated with non-medical ketamine use. Drug Alcohol Depend 69:23–28, 2003

DiMascio A, Greenblatt M, Hyde RW: A study of the effects of LSD: physiologic and psychological changes and their interrelations. Am J Psychiatry 114:309–317, 1957

Eisner B: Ecstasy: The MDMA Story. Berkeley, CA, Ronin, 1989

Elkes J, Elkes C, Bradley PB: The effect of some drugs on the electrical activity of the brain and on behaviour. J Ment Sci 100:125–128, 1954

Emboden W: Narcotic Plants, 2nd Edition. New York, Macmillan, 1980

Erlander MG, Lovenberg TW, Baron BM, et al: Two members of a distinct subfamily of 5-hydroxytryptamine receptors differentially expressed in rat brain. Proc Natl Acad Sci USA 90:3452–3456, 1993

Farthing GW: The Psychology of Consciousness. Englewood Cliffs, NJ, Prentice Hall, 1992

Feldman HW, Agar MH, Beschner GM (eds): Angel Dust. Lexington, MA, Lexington Books, 1979

Fodor G: The tropane alkaloids, in The Alkaloids: Chemistry and Physiology, Vol 13. Edited by Manske RHF. New York, Academic Press, 1971, pp 351–396

Fontanila D, Johannessen M, Hajipour AR, et al: The hallucinogen N,N-dimethyltryptamine (DMT) is an endogenous sigma-1 receptor regulator. Science 323:934–937, 2009

Forrer G, Goldner R: Experimental physiological studies with LSD. AMA Arch Neurol Psychiatry 65:581–588, 1951

Freedman AS, Bunney BS: The effects of phencyclidine and N-allyl-normetazocine on midbrain dopamine neuronal activity. Eur J Pharmacol 104:287–293, 1987

Gable RS: Comparison of acute lethal toxicity of commonly abused psychoactive substances. Addiction 99:686–696, 2004

Gamma A, Buck A, Berthold T, et al: 3,4-Methylenedioxymethamphetamine (MDMA) modulates cortical and limbic brain activity as measured by [H(2)(15)O]-PET in healthy humans. Neuropsychopharmacology 23:388–395, 2001

Gasser P: Die psycholytische Psychotherapie in der Schweiz von 1988–1993: eine katamnestische Erhebung. Schweizer Archiv für Neurologie und Psychiatrie 147:59–65, 1997

Goldstein L, Stoltzfus NW: Psychoactive drug-induced changes of interhemispheric EEG amplitude relationships. Agents Actions 3:124–132, 1973

Goldstein L, Murphree HB, Sugerman AA, et al: Quantitative electroencephalographic analysis of naturally occurring (schizophrenic) and drug-induced psychotic states in human males. Clin Pharmacol Ther 14:10–21, 1963

Gonzalez D, Riba J, Bouso JC, et al: Pattern of use and subjective effects of Salvia divinorum among recreational users. Drug Alcohol Depend 85:157–162, 2006

Gossop M, Darke S, Griffiths P, et al: The Severity of Dependence Scale (SDS): psychometric properties of the SDS in English and Australian samples of heroin, cocaine and amphetamine users. Addiction 90:607–614, 1995

Gouzoulis E, von Bardeleben U, Rupp A, et al: Neuroendocrine and cardiovascular effects of MDE in healthy volunteers. Neuropsychopharmacology 8:187–193, 1993

Gouzoulis-Mayfrank E, Daumann J: Neurotoxicity of drugs of abuse—the case of methylenedioxyamphetamines (MDMA, ecstasy), and amphetamines. Dialogues Clin Neurosci 11:305–317, 2009

Gouzoulis-Mayfrank E, Schreckenberger M, Sabri O, et al: Neurometabolic effects of psilocybin, 3,4-methylenedioxyethylamphetamine (MDE) and d-methamphetamine in healthy volunteers. Neuropsychopharmacology 20:565–581, 1999a

Gouzoulis-Mayfrank E, Thelen B, Habermeyer E, et al: Psychopathological, neuroendocrine and autonomic effects of 3,4-methylenedioxyethylamphetamine (MDE), psilocybin and d-methamphetamine in healthy volunteers. Psychopharmacology (Berl) 142:41–50, 1999b

Greer G, Tolbert R: Subjective reports of the effects of MDMA in a clinical setting. J Psychoactive Drugs 18:319–327, 1986

Greiner TH, Burch NR, Edelberg R: Psychopathology and psychophysiology of minimal LSD-25 dosage. AMA Arch Neurol Psychiatry 79:208–210, 1958

Griffiths RR, Richards WA, McCann U, et al: Psilocybin can occasion mystical-type experiences having substantial and sustained personal meaning and spiritual significance. Psychopharmacology (Berl) 187:268–283, 2006

Griffiths R, Richards W, Johnson M, et al: Mystical type experiences occasioned by psilocybin mediate the attribution of personal meaning and spiritual significance 14 months later. J Psychopharmacol 22:621–632, 2008

Grob CS, Danforth AL, Chopra GS, et al: Pilot study of psilocybin treatment for anxiety in patients with advanced-stage cancer. Arch Gen Psychiatry 68:71–78, 2011

Grof S: Realms of the Human Unconscious: Observations From LSD Research. New York, Viking, 1975

Grof S: The effects of LSD on chromosomes, genetic mutation, fetal development and malignancy, in LSD Psychotherapy. Pomoma, CA, Hunter House, 1980, pp 320–347

Grunze HC, Rainnie DG, Hasselmo ME, et al: NMDA-dependent modulation of CA1 local circuit inhibition. J Neurosci 16:2034–2043, 1994

Grynkiewicz G, Gadzikowska M: Tropane alkaloids as medicinally useful natural products and their synthetic derivatives as new drugs. Pharmacol Rep 60:439–463, 2008

Gunne LM: Effects of amphetamines in humans in, Handbuch der Experimentellen Pharmakologie, Vol 45/II. Edited by Born GVR, Eichler O, Farah A, et al. New York, Springer, 1977, pp 247–266

Gyermek L: Tropane alkaloids, in Pharmacology of Antimuscarinic Agents. Edited by Gyermek L. Boca Raton, FL, CRC Press, 1997, pp 47–160

Halpern JH: The use of hallucinogens in the treatment of addiction. Addiction Research 4:177–189, 1996

Halpern JH: Hallucinogens and dissociative agents naturally growing in the United States. Pharmacol Ther 102:131–138, 2004

Halpern JH, Pope HG Jr: Do hallucinogens cause residual neuropsychological toxicity? Drug Alcohol Depend 53:247–256, 1999

Halpern JH, Pope HG Jr: Hallucinogen persisting perception disorder: what do we know after 50 years? Drug Alcohol Depend 69:109–119, 2003

Halpern JH, Pope HG, Sherwood AR, et al: Residual neuropsychological effects of illicit 3,4-methylenedioxymethamphetamine (MDMA) in individuals with minimal exposure to other drugs. Drug Alcohol Depend 75:135–147, 2004

Halpern JH, Sherwood AR, Passie T, et al: Evidence of health and safety in American members of a religion who use a hallucinogenic sacrament. Med Sci Monit 14:SR15–SR22, 2008

Halpern JH, Sherwood AR, Hudson JI, et al: Reply to Parrott (2011), Fisk et al. (2011), and Rodgers et al. (2011). Addiction 106:1270–1372, 2011a

Halpern JH, Sherwood AR, Hudson JI, et al: Residual neurocognitive features of long-term ecstasy users with minimal exposure to other drugs. Addiction 106:777–786, 2011b

Hardman HF, Haavik CO, Seevers MH: Relationship of the structure of mescaline and seven analogs to toxicity and behavior in five species of laboratory animals. Toxicol Appl Pharmacol 25:299–309, 1973

Harris DS, Baggott M, Mendelson JH, et al: Subjective and hormonal effects of 3,4-methylenedioxymethamphetamine (MDMA) in humans. Psychopharmacology (Berl) 162:396–405, 2002

Hasler F: Untersuchungen zur Humanpharmakokinetik von Psilocybin. Doctoral dissertation. University of Berne, Berne, Switzerland, 1997

Hasler F, Bourquin D, Brenneisen R, et al: Determination of psilocybin and 4-hydroxyindole-3-acetic acid in plasma by HPLC-ECD and pharmacokinetic profiles of oral and intravenous psilocybin in man. Pharm Acta Helv 72:175–184, 1997

Heim A, Wasson RG: Les Champignons Hallucinogenes du Mexique. Paris, Museum d'Historie Naturelles, 1958

Henderson LA, Glass WJ: LSD: Still With Us After All These Years. New York, Macmillan, 1994

Hermle L, Funfgeld M, Oepen G, et al: Mescaline-induced psychopathological, neuropsychological, and neurometabolic effects in normal subjects: experimental psychosis as a tool for psychiatric research. Biol Psychiatry 32:976–991, 1992

Hertzman M, Reba RC, Kotlyarove EV: Single photon emission computerized tomography in phencyclidine and related drug abuse. Am J Psychiatry 147:255–256, 1990

Hidalgo W: Estudio comparativo psicofisiologico de la mescalina, dietilamida del acido D-lysergico y psilocibina. Acta Medica Venezolana 8:56–62, 1960

Hintzen A, Passie T: The Pharmacology of LSD. New York, Oxford University Press, 2010

Hoch PH: Studies in routes of administration and counteracting drugs, in Lysergic Acid Diethylamide and Mescaline in Experimental Psychiatry. Edited by Cholden L. New York, Grune & Stratton, 1956, pp 8–12

Holland D, Passie T: Flashback-Phaenomene als Nachwirkung von Halluzinogeneinnahme. Berlin, VWB Publishers, 2011

Hollister LE: Clinical, biochemical and psychologic effects of psilocybin. Arch Int Pharmacodyn Ther 130:42–52, 1961

Hollister LE, Sjoberg BM: Clinical syndromes and biochemical alterations following mescaline, lysergic acid diethylamide, psilocybin and a combination of the three psychotomimetic drugs. Compr Psychiatry 20:170–178, 1964

Holzmann P: Bestimmung von Psilocybin-Metaboliten im Humanplasma und-urin. Doctoral dissertation. University of Tübingen, Tübingen, Germany, 1995

Hopf A, Eckert H: Distribution patterns of 14C-psilocin in the brains of various animals. Acta Nerv Super (Praha) 16:64–66, 1974

Inch TD, Brimblecombe RW: Antiacetylcholine drugs: chemistry, stereochemistry, and pharmacology. Int Rev Neurobiol 16:67–144, 1974

Isbell H, Belleville RE, Fraser HF, et al: Studies on lysergic acid diethylamide: effects in former morphine addicts and development of tolerance during chronic intoxication. AMA Arch Neurol Psychiatry 76:468–478, 1956

Itil TM: Quantitative EEG and behavior changes after LSD and ditran, in Neurophysiological and Behavioral Aspects of Psychotropic Drugs. Edited by Karczmar AG, Koella WP. Springfield, IL, Charles C Thomas, 1969, pp 72–87

Jansen KL: Ketamine: Dreams and Realities. Sarasota, FL, MAPS, 2000

Jansen KL, Darracot-Cankovic R: The nonmedical use of ketamine, part two: a review of problem use and dependence. J Psychoactive Drugs 33:151–158, 2001

Jarvik ME, Abramson AH, Hirsch MW: Lysergic acid diethylamide: effects on attention and concentration. J Psychol 39:373–383, 1955a

Jarvik ME, Abramson AH, Hirsch MW: Lysergic acid diethylamide: effects upon recall and recognition of various stimuli. J Psychol 39:443–454, 1955b

Jentsch JD, Tran A, Taylor JR, et al: Prefrontal cortical involvement in phencyclidine-induced activation of the mesolimbic dopamine system: behavioral and neurochemical evidence. Psychopharmacology (Berl) 138:89–95, 1998

Johnson MW, MacLean KA, Reissig CJ, et al: Human psychopharmacology and dose-effects of salvinorin A, a kappa opioid agonist hallucinogen present in the plant Salvia divinorum. Drug Alcohol Depend 115:150–155, 2011

Johnston LD, O'Malley PM, Bachman JG, et al: Monitoring the Future National Survey Results on Drug Use, 1975–2011, Vol 1: Secondary School Students. Ann Arbor, Institute for Social Research, University of Michigan, 2012

Karlsen SN, Spigset O, Slørdal L: The dark side of ecstasy: neuropsychiatric symptoms after exposure to 3,4-methylenedioxymethamphetamine. Basic Clin Pharmacol Toxicol 102:15–24, 2007

Katz MM, Waskow IE, Olsson J: Characterizing the psychological state produced by LSD. J Abnorm Psychol 73:1–14, 1968

Kelly BC: Mediating MDMA-related harm: preloading and post-loading among ecstasy-using youth. J Psychoactive Drugs 41:19–26, 2009

Kerrigan S, Brooks DE: Immunochemical extraction and detection of LSD in whole blood. J Immunol Methods 224:11–18, 1999

Ketchum JS, Sidell FR, Crowell EB, et al: Atropine, scopolamine, and ditran: comparative pharmacology and antagonists in man. Psychopharmacologia 28:121–145, 1973

Kiyatkin EA, Sharma HS: Environmental conditions modulate neurotoxic effects of psychomotor stimulant drugs of abuse. Int Rev Neurobiol 102:147–171, 2012

Kraemer T, Maurer HH: Toxicokinetics of amphetamines: metabolism and toxicokinetic data of designer drugs, amphetamine, methamphetamine, and their N-alkyl derivatives. Ther Drug Monit 24:277–289, 2002

Lai Y, Wu S, Ni L, et al: Ketamine-associated urinary tract dysfunction: an underrecognized clinical entity. Urol Int 89:93–96, 2012

Lamers CT, Ramaekers JG, Muntjewerff ND, et al: Dissociable effects of a single dose of ecstasy (MDMA) on psychomotor skills and attentional performance. J Psychopharmacol 17:379–387, 2003

Lee MA, Shlain B: Acid Dreams, the CIA, LSD, and the Sixties Rebellion. New York, Grove Press, 1985

Leuner H: Halluzinogene: Psychische Grenzzustaende in Forschung und Psychotherapie. Bern, Stuttgart, Wien, Huber, 1981

Li IH, Huang WS, Shiue CY, et al: Study on the neuroprotective effect of fluoxetine against MDMA-induced neurotoxicity on the serotonin transporter in rat brain using micro-PET. Neuroimage 49:1259–1270, 2010

Liddell DW, Weil-Malherbe H: The effects of methedrine and of lysergic acid diethylamide on mental processes and on the blood adrenaline level. J Neurochem 16:7–13, 1953

Liechti ME, Vollenweider FX: Acute psychological and physiological effects of MDMA ("ecstasy") after haloperidol pretreatment in healthy humans. Eur Neuropsychopharmacol 10:289–295, 2000a

Liechti ME, Vollenweider FX: The serotonin uptake inhibitor citalopram reduces acute cardiovascular and vegetative effects of 3,4-methylenedioxymethamphetamine ("ecstasy") in healthy volunteers. J Psychopharmacol 14:269–274, 2000b

Liechti ME, Vollenweider FX: Which neuroreceptors mediate the subjective effects of MDMA in humans? A summary of mechanistic studies. Hum Psychopharmacol 16:589–598, 2001

Lienert GA: Changes in the factor structure of intelligence tests produced by d-lysergic acid diethylamide (LSD), in Neuro-Psychopharmacology. Edited by Bradley PB. Amsterdam, Netherlands, Elsevier, 1959, pp 461–465

Lienert GA: Über die Regression psychischer Funktionen als Folge pharmakologischer Belastung durch LSD und Alkohol. Med Exp Int J Exp Med 5:203–208, 1961

Liester MB, Grob CS, Bravo GL, et al: Phenomenology and sequelae of 3,4-methylenedioxymethamphetamine. J Nerv Ment Dis 180:345–352, 1992

Listos J, Merska A, Fidecka S: Pharmacological activity of salvinorin A, the major component of Salvia divinorum. Pharmacol Rep 63:1305–1309, 2011

Lodge D, Johnson KM: Noncompetitive excitatory amino acid receptor antagonists. Trends Pharmacol Sci 11:81–86, 1990

Longo VG: Behavioral and electroencephalographic effects of atropine and related compounds. Pharmacol Rev 18:965–996, 1966

Lovenberg TW, Erlander MG, Baron BM, et al: Molecular cloning and functional expression of 5-HT1E-like rat and human 5-hydroxytryptamine receptor genes. Proc Natl Acad Sci U S A 90:2184–2188, 1993

Malleson N: Acute adverse reactions to LSD in clinical and experimental use in the United Kingdom. Br J Psychiatry 118:229–230, 1971

Marquis KL, Moreton JE: Animal models of intravenous phencyclinoid self-administration. Pharmacol Biochem Behav 27:385–389, 1987

Martin-Ruiz R, Puig MV, Celada P, et al: Control of serotonergic function in medial prefrontal cortex by serotonin2A receptors through a glutamate-dependent mechanism. J Neurosci 21:9856–9866, 2001

Mas M, Farre M, de la Torre R, et al: Cardiovascular and neuroendocrine effects and pharmacokinetics of 3,4-methylenedioxymethamphetamine in humans. J Pharmacol Exp Ther 290:136–145, 1999

Mathe JM, Nomikos GG, Schilstrom B, et al: Non-NMDA excitatory amino acid receptors in the ventral tegmental area mediate systemic dizocilpine (MK-801)-induced hyperlocomotion and dopamine release in the nucleus accumbens. J Neurosci Res 51:583–592, 1998

McCann UD, Szabo Z, Seckin E, et al: Quantitative PET studies of the serotonin transporter in MDMA users and controls using [(11)C]McN5652 and [(11)C]DASB. Neuropsychopharmacology 30:1741–1750, 2005

McCarron MM, Schulze BW, Thompson GA, et al: Acute phencyclidine intoxication: incidence of clinical findings in 1,000 cases. Ann Emerg Med 10:237–242, 1981

McCarron MM, Walberg CB, Baselt RC: Confirmation of LSD intoxication by analysis of serum and urine. J Anal Toxicol 14:165–167, 1990

McGlothlin WH, Cohen S, McGlothlin MS: Long lasting effects of LSD on normals. Arch Gen Psychiatry 17:521–532, 1967

McKenna DJ, Repke DB, Peroutka SJ: Differential interactions of indolealkylamines with 5-hydroxytryptamine receptor subtypes. Neuropsychopharmacology 29:193–198, 1990

Metzler CM: A mathematical model for the pharmacokinetics of LSD effect. Clin Pharmacol Ther 10:737–740, 1969

Meyers FH, Rose AJ, Smith DE, et al: Incidents involving the Haight-Ashbury population and some uncommonly used drugs. J Psychoactive Drugs 1:139–146, 1967/1968

Mithoefer MC, Wagner MT, Mithoefer AT, et al: The safety and efficacy of {+/-}3,4-methylenedioxymethamphetamine-assisted psychotherapy in subjects with chronic, treatment-resistant posttraumatic stress disorder: the first randomized controlled pilot study. J Psychopharmacol 25:439–452, 2011

Moghaddam B, Adams B, Verma A, et al: Activation of glutamatergic neurotransmission by ketamine: a novel step in the pathway from NMDA receptor blockade to dopaminergic and cognitive disruptions associated with the prefrontal cortex. J Neurosci 17:2921–2927, 1997

Mohamed WM, Ben Hamida S, Cassel JC, et al: MDMA: interactions with other psychoactive drugs. Pharmacol Biochem Behav 99:759–774, 2011

Monsma FJ Jr, Shen Y, Ward RP, et al: Cloning and expression of a novel serotonin receptor with high affinity for tricyclic psychotropic drugs. Mol Pharmacol 43:320–327, 1993

Morton J: Ecstasy: pharmacology and neurotoxicity. Curr Opin Pharmacol 5:79–86, 2005

Nakahara Y, Kikura R, Takahashi K, et al: Detection of LSD and metabolite in rat hair and human hair. J Anal Toxicol 20:323–329, 1996

Naranjo P: Hallucinogenic plant use and related indigenous belief systems in the Ecuadorian Amazon. J Ethnopharmacol 1:121–124, 1979

National Institute on Drug Abuse: NIDA InfoFacts. PCP (phencyclidine). June 2009. Available at: http://www.drugabuse.gov/PDF/Infofacts/PCP06.pdf. Accessed November 27, 2012.

Nichols D: Differences between the mechanism of action of MDMA, MBDB and the classic hallucinogens: identification of a new therapeutic class: entactogens. J Psychoactive Drugs 18:305–311, 1986

Nichols DE: Hallucinogens. Pharmacol Ther 101:131–181, 2004

Nozaki M, Vaupel DB, Martin WR: A pharmacologic comparison of 3,4-methylenedioxyamphetamine and LSD in the chronic spinal dog. Eur J Pharmacol 46:339–349, 1977

Olmedo R: Phencyclidine and ketamine, in Goldfrank's Toxicologic Emergencies. Edited by Goldfrank LR. New York, McGraw-Hill, 2002, pp 1034–1045

Oss OT, Oeric OR: Magic Mushroom Growers Guide. Berkeley, CA, And/Or Press, 1976

Ott J: Ethnopharmacognosy and human pharmacology of Salvia divinorum and salvinorin A. Curare 18:103–312, 1995

Papac DI, Foltz RL: Measurement of lysergic acid diethylamide (LSD) in human plasma by gas chromatography/negative ion chemical ionization mass spectrometry. J Anal Toxicol 14:189–190, 1990

Passie T: A history of the use of psilocybin in psychotherapy, in Teonancatl: Sacred Mushroom of Visions. Edited by Metzner R. El Verano, CA, Four Trees Press, 2004, pp 109–134

Passie T: Healing With Entactogens. Santa Cruz, CA, MAPS, 2012

Passie T, Seifert J, Schneider U, et al: The pharmacology of psilocybin. Addict Biol 7:357–364, 2002

Passie T, Hartmann U, Schneider U, et al: What are entactogens? Pharmacological and psychopharmacological aspects of a group of substances [in German]. Suchtmedizin 7:235–245, 2005

Passie T, Halpern JH, Stichtenoth DO, et al: The pharmacology of lysergic acid diethylamide: a review. CNS Neurosci Ther 14:295–314, 2008

Perry DC: PCP revisited. PharmChem Newsletter 4:1–7, 1975

Pierce PA, Peroutka SJ: Hallucinogenic drug interactions with neurotransmitter receptor binding sites in human cortex. Psychopharmacology (Berl) 97:118–122, 1989

Pollock SH: The psilocybin mushroom pandemic. J Psychedelic Drugs 7:73–84, 1975

Pradhan SN: Phencyclidine (PCP): some human studies. Neurosci Biobehav Rev 8:493–501, 1984

Renner UD, Oertel R, Kirch W: Pharmacokinetics and pharmacodynamics in clinical use of scopolamine. Ther Drug Monit 27:655–665, 2005

Reynolds S: Energy Flash. Berkeley, CA, Soft Skull Press, 2012

Riba J, Rodríguez-Fornells A, Urbano G, et al: Subjective effects and tolerability of the South American psychoactive beverage ayahuasca in healthy volunteers. Psychopharmacology (Berl) 154:85–95, 2001

Riba J, Valle M, Urbano G, et al: Human pharmacology of ayahuasca: subjective and cardiovascular effects, monoamine metabolite excretion, and pharmacokinetics. J Pharmacol Exp Ther 306:73–83, 2003

Riba J, Romero S, Grasa E, Mena E, et al: Increased frontal and paralimbic activation following ayahuasca, the pan-Amazonian inebriant. Psychopharmacology (Berl) 186:93–98, 2006

Riley SC, Blackman G: Between prohibitions: patterns and meanings of magic mushroom use in the UK. Subst Use Misuse 43:55–71, 2008

Risner ME: Intravenous self-administration of phencyclidine and related compounds in the dog. J Pharmacol Exp Ther 221:637–644, 1982

Robinson JT, Chitham RG, Greenwood RM, et al: Chromosome aberrations and LSD. Br J Psychiatry 125:238–244, 1974

Rogers G, Elston J, Garside R, et al: The harmful health effects of recreational ecstasy: a systematic review of observational evidence. Health Technol Assess 13:iii–iv, ix–xii, 2009

Röhrich J, Zörntlein S, Becker J: Analysis of LSD in human body fluids and hair samples applying ImmunElute columns. Forensic Sci Int 107:181–190, 2000

Romanelli F, Smith KM: Dextromethorphan abuse: clinical effects and management. J Am Pharm Assoc 49:20–25, 2009

Roth BL, Baner K, Westkaemper R, et al: Salvinorin A: a potent naturally occurring nonnitrogenous kappa opioid selective agonist. Proc Natl Acad Sci USA 99:11934–11939, 2002

Rothlin E: Lysergic acid diethylamide and related substances. Ann NY Acad Sci 66:668–676, 1957

Rothlin E, Cerletti A: Pharmacology of LSD-25, in Lysergic Acid Diethylamide and Mescaline in Experimental Psychiatry. Edited by Cholden L. New York, Grune & Stratton, 1956, pp 1–7

Sanders-Bush E, Burris KD, Knoth K: Lysergic acid diethylamide and 2,5-dimethoxy-4-methylamphetamine and partial agonists at serotonin receptors linked to phosphoinositide hydrolysis. J Pharmacol Exp Ther 246:924–928, 1988

Sandison RW, Whitelaw JD: Further studies in the therapeutic value of lysergic acid diethylamide in mental illness. J Ment Sci 103:332–343, 1957

Savage C: Variations in ego feeling induced by D-lysergic acid diethylamide (LSD-25). Psychoanal Rev 1:1–16, 1955

Schultes RE, Hofmann A: Plants of the Gods: Origins of Hallucinogenic Use. New York, McGraw-Hill, 1980

Shippenberg TS, Chefer VI, Zapata A, et al: Modulation of the behavioral and neurochemical effects of psychostimulants by kappa-opioid receptor systems. Ann NY Acad Sci 937:50–73, 2001

Siebert DJ: Salvia divinorum and salvinorin A: new pharmacologic findings. J Ethnopharmacol 43:53–56, 1994

Siegel RK: Phencyclidine and ketamine intoxication: a study of four populations of recreational users, in Phencyclidine (PCP) Abuse: An Appraisal. Edited by Petersen RC, Stillman RC. Rockville, MD, National Institute on Drug Abuse, 1978, pp 119–147

Silverstein AB, Klee GD: Effects of lysergic acid diethylamide (LSD-25) on intellectual functions. AMA Arch Neurol Psychiatry 80:477–480, 1958

Smart RG, Bateman K: The chromosomal and teratogenic effects of lysergic acid diethylamide: a review of the current literature. Can Med Assoc J 99:805–810, 1968

Sokoloff L, Perlin S, Kornetsky C, et al: The effects of d-lysergic acid diethylamide on cerebral circulation and overall metabolism. Ann NY Acad Sci 66:468–477, 1957

Spina SP, Taddei A: Teenagers with Jimson weed (Datura stramonium) poisoning. CJEM 9:467–468, 2007

Stamets P: Psilocybin Mushrooms of the World. Olympia, WA, Ten Speed Press, 1996

Stogner J, Khey DN, Griffin OH 3rd, et al: Regulating a novel drug: an evaluation of changes in use of Salvia divinorum in the first year of Florida's ban. Int J Drug Policy 23:512–521, 2012

Strassman RJ: Adverse reactions to psychedelic drugs: a review of the literature. J Nerv Ment Dis 172:577–595, 1984

Strassman RJ: DMT: The Spirit Molecule. Rochester, VT, Park Street Press, 2001

Strassman RJ, Qualls CR, Uhlenhuth EH, et al: Dose-response study of N,N-dimethyltryptamine in humans, II: subjective effects and preliminary results of a new rating scale. Arch Gen Psychiatry 51:98–108, 1994

Studerus E, Kometer M, Hasler F, et al: Acute, subacute and long-term subjective effects of psilocybin in healthy humans: a pooled analysis of experimental studies. J Psychopharmacol 25:1434–1452, 2011

Substance Abuse and Mental Health Services Administration: The NSDUH Report: Patterns of Hallucinogen Use and Initiation: 2004 and 2005. July 2007. Available at: http://www.samhsa.gov/data/2k7/hallucinogen/hallucinogen.pdf. Accessed November 27, 2012.

Substance Abuse and Mental Health Services Administration: The NSDUH Report: Use of Specific Hallucinogens: 2006. February 2008. Available at: http://www.samhsa.gov/data/2k8/hallucinogens/hallucinogens.pdf. Accessed November 27, 2012.

Substance Abuse and Mental Health Services Administration: Drug Abuse Warning Network, 2009: National Estimates of Drug-Related Emergency Department Visits (HHS Publ No SMA-11-4618). Rockville, MD, Substance Abuse and Mental Health Services Administration, 2011a. Available at: http://www.samhsa.gov/

data/2k11/dawn/2k9dawned/html/dawn2k9ed.htm. Accessed November 26, 2012.

Substance Abuse and Mental Health Services Administration: Results from the 2010 National Survey on Drug Use and Health: Summary of National Findings (NSDUH Series H-41, HHS Publ No SMA-11-4658). Rockville, MD, Substance Abuse and Mental Health Services Administration, 2011b. Available at: http://www.samhsa.gov/data/nsduh/2k10nsduh/2k10results.htm. Accessed November 26, 2012.

Substance Abuse and Mental Health Services Administration: The DAWN Report: Highlights of the 2010 Drug Abuse Warning Network (DAWN) Findings on Drug-Related Emergency Department Visits. July 2012. Available at: http://www.samhsa.gov/data/2k12/DAWN096/SR096EDHighlights2010.pdf. Accessed November 27, 2012.

Sumnall HR, Measham F, Brandt SD, et al: Salvia divinorum use and phenomenology: results from an online survey. J Psychopharmacol 25:1496–1507, 2011

Taunton-Rigby A, Sher SE, Kelley PR: Lysergic acid diethylamide: radioimmunoassay. Science 181:165–166, 1973

Thomasius R: Ecstasy: Eine Studie zu gesundheitlichen und psychosozialen Folgen des Missbrauchs. Stuttgart, Germany, Akademische Verlagsgesellschaft, 2000

Trzepacz PT: Is there a final common neural pathway in delirium? Focus on acetylcholine and dopamine. Semin Clin Neuropsychiatry 5:132–148, 2000

Unna KR, Glaser K, Lipton E, et al: Dosage of drugs in infants and children, I: atropine. Pediatrics 6:197–207, 1950

Upshall DG, Wailling DG: The determination of LSD in human plasma following oral administration. Clin Chim Acta 36:67–73, 1972

van Bocxlaer JF, Clauwaert KM, Lambert WE, et al: Liquid chromatography-mass spectrometry in forensic toxicology. Mass Spectrom Rev 19:165–214, 2000

Vignon J, Chaudieu I, Allaoua H, et al: Comparison of [3H] phencyclidine ([3H] PCP) and [3H] N-[1-(2-thienyl) cyclohexyl] piperidine ([3H] TCP) binding properties to rat and human brain membranes. Life Sci 45:2547–2555, 1989

Vollenweider FX: Brain mechanisms of hallucinogens and entactogens. Dialogues Clin Neurosci 3:265–279, 2001

Vollenweider FX, Geyer MA: A systems model of altered consciousness: integrating natural and drug-induced psychoses. Brain Res Bull 56:495–507, 2001

Vollenweider FX, Kometer M: The neurobiology of psychedelic drugs: implications for the treatment of mood disorders. Nat Rev Neurosci 11:642–651, 2010

Vollenweider FX, Leenders KL, Scharfetter C, et al: Metabolic hyperfrontality and psychopathology in the ketamine model of psychosis using positron emission tomography (PET) and [18F]fluorodeoxyglucose. Eur Neuropsychopharmacol 7:9–24, 1997a

Vollenweider FX, Leenders KL, Scharfetter C, et al: Positron emission tomography and fluorodeoxyglucose studies of metabolic hyperfrontality and psychopathology in the psilocybin model of psychosis. Neuropsychopharmacology 16:357–372, 1997b

Vollenweider FX, Gamma A, Liechti M, et al: Psychological and cardiovascular effects and short-term sequelae of MDMA ("ecstasy") in MDMA-naive healthy volunteers. Neuropsychopharmacology 19:241–251, 1998a

Vollenweider FX, Vollenweider-Scherpenhuysen MFI, Bäbler A, et al: Psilocybin induces schizophrenia-like psychosis in humans via serotonin-2 agonist action. Neuroreport 9:3897–3902, 1998b

von Hungen K, Roberts S, Hill DF: LSD as an agonist and antagonist at central dopamine receptors. Nature 252:588–589, 1974

Wagner JG, Aghajanian GK, Bing OH: Correlation of performance test scores with "tissue concentration" of lysergic acid diethylamide in human subjects. Clin Pharmacol Ther 9:635–638, 1968

Wapner S, Krus DM: Effects of lysergic acid diethylamide, and differences between normals and schizophrenics on the Stroop Color-Word Test. J Neuropsychiatry 2:76–81, 1960

Watts VJ, Lawler CP, Fox DR, et al: LSD and structural analogs: pharmacological evaluation at D1 dopamine receptors. Psychopharmacology (Berl) 118:401–409, 1995

Were PF: Electroencephalographic effects of LSD, and some psychiatric implications. J Neuropsychiatry 5:516–524, 1964

WHO Expert Committee on Drug Dependence: Twenty-Second Report. Technical Report Series, No 729. Geneva, Switzerland, World Health Organization, 1985

Wikler A: Pharmacologic dissociation of behavior and EEG "sleep patterns" in dogs; morphine, n-allylnormorphine, and atropine. Proc Soc Exp Biol Med 79:261–265, 1952

Winkelman MJ, Roberts TB: Psychedelic Medicine: New Evidence for Hallucinogenic Substances as Treatments. Westport, CT, Praeger, 2007

Winter JC: Hallucinogens as discriminative stimuli in animals: LSD, phenethylamines, and tryptamines. Psychopharmacology (Berl) 203:251–263, 2009

Winter JC, Eckler JR, Rabin RA: Serotonergic/glutamatergic interactions: the effects of mGlu2/3 receptor ligands in rats trained with LSD and PCP as discriminative stimuli. Psychopharmacology (Berl) 172:233–240, 2004

Wolff K, Winstock AR: Ketamine: from medicine to misuse. CNS Drugs 20:199–218, 2006

World Health Organization: International Statistical Classification of Diseases and Related Health Problems, 10th Revision. Geneva, World Health Organization, 1992

Wu JC, Buchsbaum MS, Bunney W Jr: Positron emission tomography study of phencyclidine users as a possible drug model of schizophrenia. Yakubutsu Seishin Kodo 11:47–48, 1991

Wu LT, Woody GE, Yang C, et al: Recent national trends in Salvia divinorum use and substance-use disorders among recent and former Salvia divinorum users compared with nonusers. Subst Abuse Rehabil 2011:53–68, 2011

Yamamoto BK, Moszczynska A, Gudelsky GA: Amphetamine toxicities: classical and emerging mechanisms. Ann NY Acad Sci 1187:101–121, 2010

Yokota H, Ogawa S, Kurokawa A, et al: Regional cerebral blood flow in delirium patients. Psychiatry Clin Neurosci 57:337–339, 2003

8

Inhalants

Carlos Hernandez-Avila, M.D., Ph.D.

History

The first reported psychotropic use of inhalants dates to the ancient Greek world (Carroll 1977). However, it was not until 1772 that the English scientist and clergyman Joseph Priestley discovered the first modern inhalant compound, the anesthetic gas nitrous oxide. Because of its euphorigenic effects, this compound acquired the popular name of "laughing gas" (Sharp 1992). The discovery of ether and chloroform soon followed, increasing the number of anesthetics available by inhalation that were susceptible to abuse. Although the anesthetic properties of ether were not discovered until 1841, by the end of the eighteenth century ether was already known for its ability to induce euphoria and hallucinations (Bird 1881; Delteil et al. 1974; Follin and Rousselot 1980). Similarly, the addictive properties of chloroform were also widely known (Payne 1998). In 1867, Thomas Lauder Brunton discovered amyl nitrite, a vasodilator used to treat symptoms of acute coronary occlusion and with the reported ability to enhance sexual performance (Haverkos et al. 1994).

The current widespread abuse of inhalants likely began in the 1920s as a consequence of the rapid growth of industrial society and the ready availability of substances that can be inhaled, such as gasoline, glues, solvents, and nitrites. Inhalant abuse increased after World War II, with workers in industries with high occupational exposure to inhalants being the first group to be at high risk to develop these problems (Sharp 1992).

Epidemiology

The abuse of inhalants is widespread, particularly among adolescents and children. Approximately 3.0% of U.S. children have used inhalants by the time they reach fourth grade. In 2010, 12.1% of adolescents in the United States reported lifetime use of inhalants, with younger children using these substances more frequently than their older counterparts (Johnston et al. 2011). The prevalence of inhalant use reaches a peak among eighth graders, and rates of use are higher for girls than for boys. However, in grades 10 through 12 and after high school, boys again show a higher rate of inhalant abuse (Johnston et al. 2011). Despite the fact that inhalant use disorders typically affect the young, these problems can become chronic and extend into adulthood.

Inhalant abuse is found in both urban and rural settings. Adverse socioeconomic conditions, rather than racial or cultural factors per se, account for most reported ethnic differences in rates of inhalant abuse. Native American youths living on reservations typically have higher rates of inhalant abuse than do either Native American youths not living on reservations or youths in the general population (Substance Abuse and Mental Health Services Administration 2011).

Types of Inhalants

The range of inhalants abused by humans includes a broad and pharmacologically heterogeneous group of substances that are easily available. These are commonly household and industrial solvents, glues, propellants, lighters, and art and office supplies (Table 8–1). These substances, which share a common route of self-administration by inhalation, can be classified as volatile solvents, nitrites, and anesthetics (Sharp 1992).

Table 8–1. Products that may be used as inhalants

Volatile solvents	Nitrites	Anesthetics
Solvents and gases	**Amyl, butyl, alkyl nitrites**	**Nitrous oxide**
Paint thinner/remover	Air fresheners	Dessert topping sprays[a]
Typing correction fluid	Fuel-injection fluid	Balloons
Lighter fluid	Nitrite products sold by sex	High-pressured containers
Gasoline	shops and on the Internet[b]	
Fuel gas	Prescription drug[c]	**Other anesthetics**
Nail polish remover		Ether
		Chloroform
Adhesives		Halothane
Glue		
Rubber and PVC cement		
Cleaning solvents		
Degreaser		
Spot remover		
Dry cleaning fluid		

Note. PVC=polyvinylchloride.
[a]Whipped cream or "whippets."
[b]For example, "Liquid Gold," "Ram," "Thrust," "poppers," "rush."
[c]Isoamyl nitrite.

Volatile Solvents

Volatile solvents are fluids or gases contained in a wide variety of products (e.g., gasoline, paint thinner, butane gas) that have significant concentrations of aliphatic, aromatic, or halogenated hydrocarbons, which vaporize at room temperature. Because of their rapid absorption in the lungs, volatile solvents exert a rapid intoxicating effect.

Many volatile solvents contain more than one potentially psychoactive ingredient, complicating efforts to identify the specific compounds responsible for the psychotropic effects. To date, the best-studied psychoactive compounds identified in volatile solvents are toluene, 1,1,1-trichloroethane, and trichloroethylene. However, other less-well-studied compounds, such as benzene, acetone, and methanol, also appear to have significant psychoactive effects.

Nitrites

Nitrite compounds are often known as "poppers" because of the popping noise produced when the capsules containing them are crushed between the fingers. Both amyl nitrite and butyl nitrite are yellowish liquids that evaporate at room temperature. These compounds are distributed under a variety of names and are contained in a range of commercial products, such as air fresheners.

Isoamyl nitrite is also available in the United States by prescription. Currently, the primary indication for isoamyl nitrite is to treat cyanide poisoning and for the diagnostic evaluation of mitral regurgitation and ventricular septal defects; occasionally, this compound is also prescribed to treat angina pectoris.

Anesthetics

Nitrous oxide, a colorless and nearly odorless gas, is the most frequently abused of the anesthetics. It is a dissociative anesthetic and the only inhalational anesthetic agent that is a true gas, not a vapor. Nitrous oxide can produce a relatively shallow anesthesia, useful in dentistry and during childbirth, but it can also induce a deeper level of narcosis when combined with other anesthetics during general surgery. Nitrous oxide is also known as laughing gas because it produces a state of euphoria, giggling, and laughter.

Other anesthetics susceptible to abuse, such as ether and chloroform, have received less attention, because they are less commonly abused substances. Nonetheless, when inhaled, ether and chloroform are rapidly absorbed and distributed in the central nervous system (CNS), inducing a rapid euphoria (Delteil et al. 1974).

Pharmacokinetics

Volatile Solvents

Because of their high lipid solubility, the active compounds in volatile solvents readily pass through cellular membranes and are rapidly distributed into all fatty tissues. From a pharmacokinetic perspective, toluene is the best-characterized active compound in volatile solvents. When inhaled, toluene is rapidly absorbed by the lungs, with approximately 50% of toluene vapor mixed with air being taken up through the alveoli (Lof et al. 1993). With continuous exposure, toluene saturates the blood and brain in about 60 minutes (Benignus et al. 1981, 1984). Four hours after inhalation, approximately 65% of the toluene that is absorbed is excreted in urine as hippuric acid; 20 hours later, the cumulative excretion of toluene in urine can be 80% (Lof et al. 1993). Although the concentration of toluene in blood appears to reflect its concentration in the air that is breathed, the toluene level in peripheral blood may not accurately reflect its concentration within the CNS, where levels tend to be higher. This difference may be explained by toluene's high affinity for lipids and its tendency to concentrate and be distributed mainly in the abundant cerebral lipids of the white matter (Gerasimov et al. 2002).

Positron emission tomography studies that used ^{11}C-toluene in nonhuman primates and mice showed a rapid uptake of radioactivity into striatal and frontal brain regions (Gerasimov et al. 2002). Maximal uptake of the radiotracer by these structures occurred 1–4 minutes after intravenous administration. Subsequently, clearance of the radiotracer from the striatal and frontal areas occurred rapidly, with a clearance half-life from peak uptake of 10–20 minutes. Radiotracer clearance from white matter appears to be slower than that from the striatum and frontal regions, a finding that is consistent with toluene's high affinity for the high lipid content of white matter (Gerasimov et al. 2002).

Nitrites

Little is known about the pharmacokinetic properties of volatile nitrites in humans, particularly isobutyl nitrite and its primary metabolite, isobutyl alcohol. In rodents, blood concentrations following intravenous infusion of isobutyl nitrite peaked rapidly and then declined, with a half-life of 1.4 minutes and blood clearance rate of 2.9 L/min/kg (Kielbasa and Fung 2000). Approximately 98% of isobutyl nitrite is metabolized rapidly to isobutyl alcohol, concentrations of which also decline rapidly, with a half-life of 5.3 minutes. Bioavailability of inhaled isobutyl nitrite at a concentration of 300–900 ppm is estimated to be 43%.

Anesthetics

Nitrous oxide is rapidly absorbed through inhalation, and it is distributed predominantly in blood, with a blood/gas partition coefficient of 0.5 (Stenqvist 1994). It is rapidly eliminated through the lungs, with small amounts being eliminated through the skin (Stenqvist 1994).

Following inhalation, ether and chloroform are also rapidly absorbed into the bloodstream and rapidly transferred to fatty tissues and the CNS (Baselt 1997; Harbison 1998; Reynolds 1982). Ether undergoes limited metabolism in humans (Haggart 1924), with carbon dioxide (CO_2) and acetaldehyde believed to be minor metabolites (Aune et al. 1978; Price and Dripps 1975). Approximately 90% of ether is eliminated unchanged in expired air, with the rest excreted in urine and perspiration (Haggart 1924). Similarly, chloroform is eliminated primarily by the lungs (Schroeder 1965), with approximately 43% exhaled unchanged (Baselt 1997) and 4%–5% exhaled as CO_2 (Arena and Drew 1986). Only 2% of inhaled chloroform is excreted in urine (Arena and Drew 1986); the average elimination half-life is 1.5 hours. One of the main metabolites of chloroform, diglutathionyl dithiocarbonate, is associated with glutathione depletion in the liver and kidneys. This reaction is believed to result in severe hepatic and renal necrosis (Laurenzi et al. 1987).

Behavioral Pharmacology of Inhalants in Animals and Humans

Reinforcing Effects

Inhalants are readily self-administered by humans and laboratory animals (Yanagita et al. 1970). Rhesus monkeys trained to deliver a volume of solvent vapors (i.e., lacquer thinner, ether, and chloroform) through an implanted nasal catheter after lever pressing initiated and maintained self-administration in excess of 100 deliveries during a 14- to 25-day period (Yanagita et al. 1970). In these monkeys, the frequency of toluene self-administration was positively correlated with toluene vapor concentrations. Self-administration by monkeys of other inhalants, such as nitrous oxide, also has been reported (Wood et al. 1977).

In a comparative study of the positive reinforcing effects of solvents in inhalant-dependent human subjects, solvents induced a more intense sensation of pleasant feelings than that induced by alcohol and nicotine in subjects addicted to those substances (Kono et al. 2001). Solvent-dependent subjects reported pleasant feelings comparable to those reported by stimulant-dependent subjects after use of methamphetamine. Negative reinforcing effects, measured by reports of feelings of relief after inhalant use, were, however, of comparable intensity to those reported by alcoholic subjects after drinking alcohol (Kono et al. 2001).

The reinforcing effects of nitrite inhalation in humans, although not systematically studied, appear to be significant and associated with feelings of euphoria (Schwartz and Peary 1986). In one study, almost half of the subjects who reported having used isobutyl nitrite once found the experience unpleasant. These findings suggest that a subset of individuals are susceptible to the reinforcing effects of nitrite inhalation.

Inhalation of general anesthetics such as nitrous oxide, ether, and chloroform appears to exert significant reinforcing effects in humans (Delteil et al. 1974; Deniker et al. 1972; Dohrn et al. 1993). In a double-blind, placebo-controlled study of healthy volunteers that compared subjective effects of nitrous oxide and 100% oxygen in a free-choice procedure, individuals who preferred nitrous oxide reported greater ratings of drug liking and wanting to inhale the drug again (Walker and Zacny 2002). Subjects' ratings of the peak effect of nitrous oxide were dose related (Dohrn et al. 1992).

Evidence indicates that the reinforcing effects of nitrous oxide are moderated by a history of alcohol drinking. Individuals with a history of moderate drinking appear to have a greater preference for nitrous oxide inhalation than do individuals with a history of light or no drinking (Cho et al. 1997).

Effects on Motor Activity

Inhalants appear to have a dose-effect curve for motor activity similar to that of alcohol and other CNS depressants. In rodents, toluene has a biphasic dose-effect curve on motor activity (Hinman 1987; Riegel and French 1999). At low concentrations (i.e., 2,000–3,000 ppm), toluene increases spontaneous locomotor activity. At higher concentrations (i.e., 10,000–15,000 ppm), toluene decreases locomotor activity and produces ataxia and loss of the righting reflex (Bushnell et al. 1985; Hinman 1987; Saito and Wada 1993; Yavich and Zvartau 1994). Repeated exposure produces sensitization to toluene-induced enhancement of motor activity (Himnan 1984; Moser and Balster 1981). Repeated exposure to toluene also enhances cocaine-induced increases in the locomotor activity of rodents, suggesting that behavioral and neurochemical cross-sensitization exists between these two drugs (Beyer et al. 2001). A biphasic dose-response curve for motor activity also has been described with the experimental administration of trichloroethane, amyl nitrite, and nitrous oxide (Balon et al. 2003b; Bowen and Balster 1998). The biphasic dose-response curve for motor activity has not been described in humans. However, in a study examining the level of motor activity after solvent inhalation, inhalant-dependent subjects reported hyperactivity comparable to that reported by alcohol-dependent subjects after alcohol ingestion but not of the magnitude described by stimulant-dependent subjects after methamphetamine use (Kono et al. 2001).

Tolerance

Tolerance is characterized by reduced responsiveness to the initial effects of a drug after repeated exposure or reduced responsiveness to a related compound (i.e., cross-tolerance). Animal studies have not provided conclusive evidence of tolerance to the effects of the centrally active inhalants toluene or trichloroethane (Moser and Balster 1981; Moser et al. 1985). Observations in humans, however, have documented pronounced tolerance among subjects who chronically inhale substances with high concentrations of toluene (Glaser and Massengale 1962; Press and Done 1967) and butane (Evans and Raistrick 1987). Kono et al. (2001) showed that tolerance to the reinforcing effects of solvents is comparable to that conditioned by nicotine but less intense than that reported with alcohol or methamphetamine use.

No systematic studies of tolerance to the reinforcing effects of inhaled nitrites have been reported. However, anecdotal observations in workers with high exposure to nitrites have suggested that tolerance to the subjective effects of these compounds occurs after a few days of exposure (Marsh and Marsh 2000). On the other hand, clinical and laboratory studies in humans have reported the development of tolerance to the amnestic and analgesic effects of nitrous oxide and isoflurane (see Arnold et al. 1993; Avramov et al. 1990; Rupreht et al. 1985; Whitwam et al. 1976) and, in the case of ether or chloroform, to its reinforcing effects (Krenz et al. 2003).

Withdrawal

Withdrawal symptoms, including nausea, tremor, diaphoresis, insomnia, body aches, anxiety, irritability, and agitation, have been described among chronic solvent abusers (Evans and Raistrick 1987; Knox and Nelson 1966). Subjective symptoms experienced during solvent withdrawal, such as craving, anxiety, and restlessness, appear to be similar to those reported during nicotine withdrawal but less severe than those reported during alcohol or methamphetamine withdrawal (Kono et al. 2001). Although there are anecdotal reports of severe confusion resembling delirium during the early withdrawal phase from solvents (Merry and Zachariadis 1962; Nylander 1962), it is unclear the degree to which this clinical presentation was secondary to withdrawal from other substances, such as alcohol or sedatives.

Research in rodents has provided evidence of solvent withdrawal. Continuous exposure to toluene for 4 days and subsequent cessation produced an increase in handling-induced convulsions for at least 2 hours after cessation (Wiley et al. 2003). A similar pattern of trichloroethane administration to rodents produced pronounced withdrawal, which was worsened by the administration of the proconvulsant drug pentylenetetrazole and attenuated by reexposure to 2,000 ppm of toluene or the administration of alcohol, pentobarbital, or midazolam (Evans and Balster 1993).

Severe withdrawal symptoms, including insomnia, irritability, agitation, withdrawal seizures, and delirium, have been described in both mice and humans chronically exposed to the anesthetics nitrous oxide, ether, and isoflurane (Arnold et al. 1993; Delteil et al. 1974; Deniker et al. 1972; Harper et al. 1980; Smith et al. 1979; Tobias 2000). These symptoms were controlled with the administration of γ-aminobutyric acid (GABA)–ergic agents such as pentobarbital, midazolam, and diazepam (Arnold et al. 1993; Hughes et al. 1993).

No systematic studies have been conducted to examine withdrawal symptoms resulting from continuous exposure to nitrites. However, anecdotal reports indicate that workers, after continuous exposure to these compounds, experienced a recurrent, generalized malaise called "Monday disease" when they returned to work after weekends during which they were not exposed (Nickerson 1970). Workers with this condition found relief by rubbing these substances on their skin or wearing work clothes impregnated with these substances (Schwartz 1946).

Effects of Inhalants on Specific Neurotransmitter Systems

Dopaminergic System

Evidence that dopaminergic neurotransmission mediates the reinforcing effects of toluene is provided by studies showing that the acute instillation of toluene in the striatum of rodents by microdialysis increases dopamine concentrations (Rea et al. 1984; Stengard et al. 1994). Similar to other drugs of abuse (Di Chiara and Imperato 1988; French et al. 1997; Gessa et al. 1985), toluene, when inhaled, initially stimulated and subsequently attenuated dopaminergic neuronal firing in the ventral tegmental area (VTA) (Riegel and French 1999). Low doses of toluene administered subchronically or chronically reduced dopamine turnover (Fuxe et al. 1982) and produced a persistent increase in D_2 receptor binding in the rat neostriatal complex (Hillefors-Berglund et al. 1993; von Euler et al. 1993). Administration of 6-hydroxydopamine to the nucleus accumbens, producing lesions in dopaminergic neurons, significantly attenuated toluene's locomotor stimulatory effects (Riegel et al. 2003). Consistent with this finding, pretreatment with remoxipride, a dopamine D_2 receptor antagonist that appears to bind preferentially to receptors in the nucleus accumbens, significantly reduced toluene-induced hyperactivity by 57% (Riegel and French 1999).

There are few reports on the effects of nitrous oxide on dopaminergic neurotransmission. A study in mice showed that nitrous oxide inhalation produced a significant increase in locomotor activity that was antagonized in a dose-dependent fashion by the dopamine synthesis inhibitor α-methyl-p-tyrosine (Hynes and Berkowitz 1983). Moreover, administration of the D_2 antagonist haloperidol also reduced the locomotor activity induced by nitrous oxide (Hynes and Berkowitz 1983). These results suggest that excitatory effects induced by nitrous oxide also may be mediated by dopaminergic neurotransmission. However, other studies have reported that exposure to nitrous oxide resulted in decreased dopamine release by neurons in the striatum (Balon et al. 2002; Turle et al. 1998).

To date, no studies have examined the effects of nitrite inhalation on dopaminergic neurotransmission. However, some evidence suggests that nitric oxide (NO), the potent compound that mediates the vasodilatory effects of nitrites, also has important CNS modulatory effects (Bredt and Snyder 1992). If NO is released in the CNS by nitrite inhalation, it is plausible that NO could mediate the euphorigenic and motor effects of nitrites by potently inhibiting dopamine uptake and enhancing dopaminergic neurotransmission in the mesolimbic reward circuit (Lonart and Johnson 1994). This mechanism has been shown to mediate some of the reinforcing effects of other drugs of abuse, such as cocaine (Collins and Kantak 2002; Pudiak and Bozarth 2002) and nicotine (Vleeming et al. 2002).

Glutamate/N-Methyl-D-Aspartate Receptor

The glutamatergic neurotransmitter system may also mediate toluene's reinforcing effects by indirectly activating the mesolimbic dopaminergic reward pathway. It has been suggested that the effects of toluene on dopamine cell activity are similar to those of phencyclidine (PCP), a potent antagonist of N-methyl-D-aspartate (NMDA)–type glutamate receptors that has important hallucinatory and stimulant properties (Balster and Willetts 1996). Cruz et al. (1998) found that toluene abolishes NMDA receptor–stimulated currents in Xenopus oocytes, in a subunit-specific manner. However, toluene was not effective in altering kainate-type glutamate receptor–induced currents.

Other abused solvents, including trichloroethane (Cruz et al.1998), and nitrous oxide (Jevtovic-Todorovic et al. 1998; Mennerick et al. 1998) appear to be effective inhibitors of the NMDA receptor. Nitrous oxide also has neurotoxic effects similar to other NMDA receptor antagonists, such as PCP, ketamine, and MK-801. Nitrous oxide inhibited ionic influx mediated by NMDA receptors in cultured rat hippocampal neurons (Jevtovic-Todorovic et al. 1998; Mennerick et al. 1998). In addition, nitrous oxide reversed the increase in striatal dopamine release induced by NMDA receptor activation in the substantia nigra (Balon et al. 2003a). It has been hypothesized that blockade by toluene or nitrous oxide of NMDA receptors on GABA interneurons in the VTA, and the consequent removal of the inhibitory action of these neurons on dopaminergic neurons, may lead to enhanced dopamine cell firing in the VTA and subsequent activation of the dopaminergic reward pathway (Wang and French 1995).

The effects of inhalation of amyl nitrite or butyl nitrite on glutamatergic neurotransmission have not been studied systematically. However, NO, the potent compound that mediates the peripheral effects of nitrites in blood vessels, could be released into the CNS when nitrites are inhaled. NO has been reported to act directly on the postsynaptic NMDA receptor, where it can increase or decrease NMDA-mediated currents and subsequent calcium influx (Aizenman et al. 1990; Dingledine et al. 1999; Manzoni et al. 1992).

Ligand-Gated Ion Channels

Inhalants appear to have significant effects on a superfamily of ligand-gated ion channels, including the $GABA_A$ receptor, the glycine receptor, the nicotinic acetylcholine receptor, and the serotonin type 3 (5-HT_3) receptor. These receptor complexes are composed of five protein subunits surrounding a central ion pore. Each subunit has four transmembrane-spanning domains and distinct binding sites for a variety of ligands (Ortells and Lunt 1995; Smith and Olsen 1995).

$GABA_A$ Effects

There are similarities between the biological actions of inhalants and those of alcohol and barbiturates (Bowen et al. 1996b). For example, acute administration of inhalants affects motor coordination (Moser and Balster 1981) and induces anxiolysis, whereas chronic administration is associated with physical dependence and withdrawal (Bowen et al. 1996a; Evans and Balster 1991, 1993). In addition, some inhalant drugs have anticonvulsant properties (Wood et al. 1984). Like other CNS depressant agents, inhalants have biphasic effects on spontaneous locomotor activity in rodents, with increased activity seen at lower doses and diminished locomotion seen at higher doses (Gause et al. 1985; Kjellstrand et al. 1985).

The effects produced by administration of alcohol, sedatives, and inhaled drugs of abuse are comparable, suggesting that these compounds may have overlapping mechanisms of action. Previous work has established that neurotransmitter-activated ion channels, particularly the $GABA_A$ receptor, are primary sites of action of alcohol and volatile anesthetic agents. For example, as with alcohol (Mihic 1999), pharmacological concentrations of volatile anesthetic agents potentiate $GABA_A$-mediated currents (Franks and Lieb 1994). Similarly, it is known that toluene treatment alters extracellular concentrations of GABA in the cerebellum, hippocampus (Ikeuchi et al. 1993), and globus pallidus (Stengard and O'Connor 1994). Consistent with the hypothesis that inhalants affect $GABA_A$ receptor function, toluene and trichloroethane enhanced bicuculline-sensitive GABA-mediated synaptic currents in rat CA1 hippocampal neurons (Beckstead et al. 2000; Weiner et al. 1997). Toluene, trichloroethylene, and trichloroethane also increased ligand-gated currents in $GABA_A$ α_1–β_1 receptors expressed in *Xenopus laevis* oocytes (Beckstead et al.

2000) at concentrations that have been reported to occur in vivo (Kishi et al. 1988; Naalsund 1986; You et al. 1994). Because no currents were elicited in the absence of GABA, it appears that inhalants act as allosteric modulators at these ligand-gated ion channels.

In contrast, nitrous oxide appears to have a different, but overlapping, pattern of action on $GABA_A$ receptors, compared with alcohol. Nitrous oxide only weakly potentiates $GABA_A$ receptor activity (Yamakura and Harris 2000). However, as with volatile anesthetics and alcohol, nitrous oxide inhibits ρ_1 $GABA_C$ receptors, suggesting that nitrous oxide has a differential effect on these homologous receptor subunits (Yamakura and Harris 2000). Therefore, although the sensitivity differs between nitrous oxide and volatile anesthetics and alcohol, some mechanisms of action of nitrous oxide on GABA receptors appear to be shared among these substances.

To date, the effects of nitrites on GABA neurotransmission have not been studied systematically. However, when NO, the major mediator of the peripheral effects of nitrites, was administered within the paraventricular nucleus, it increased the concentration of GABA (Horn et al. 1994).

Glycine Receptor Effects

Glycine receptors are responsible for most inhibitory neurotransmission in the brain stem and spinal cord. Inhalants, volatile anesthetics, and alcohol may share a common binding site on this ligand-gated ion channel (Beckstead et al. 2000, 2001, 2002). Active compounds in toluene, trichloroethane, and trichloroethylene appear to potentiate glycine receptor–mediated currents (Beckstead et al. 2000). Mutations in glycine receptors result in enhancement of glycine receptor function when these compounds are present, despite the fact that some of these mutants are insensitive to the effects of alcohol and enflurane. These findings suggest that solvents affect glycine receptor function and that, although they differ, the molecular sites of action overlap with those of alcohol and volatile anesthetics (Beckstead et al. 2000).

Nicotinic Acetylcholine Receptor Effects

The nicotinic acetylcholine receptor also shows sensitivity to inhalants (Bale et al. 2002). To varying degrees, toluene appears to antagonize the function of nicotinic acetylcholine receptors that constitute different subunits. At concentrations of 50 μM–10 mM, toluene produces a reversible, concentration-dependent inhibition of acetylcholine-induced current in *Xenopus* oocytes expressing various nicotinic receptor subtypes, with the α_4–β_2 and α_3–β_2 subunit combinations being more sensitive to inhibition than other receptor subtypes. At these same concentrations, toluene dose-dependently inhibits acetylcholine-mediated responses in the hippocampus. These results suggest that nicotinic acetylcholine receptors, like NMDA receptors, show a subunit-dependent sensitivity to toluene and may represent an important site of action for some of the neurobehavioral effects of this volatile solvent (Bale et al. 2002).

5-HT₃ Receptor Effects

5-HT$_3$ Receptor Effects

Trichoroethane, trichloroethylene, and toluene are similar to alcohol (Lovinger and White 1991) and volatile anesthetics (Machu and Harris 1994) in their ability to enhance 5-HT$_3$ receptor function. All three inhalants significantly and reversibly potentiate, in a dose-dependent manner, 5-HT-activated currents mediated by mouse 5-HT$_{3A}$ receptors expressed in *Xenopus* oocytes. 5-HT$_3$-mediated nausea and vomiting are also common to the acute use of inhalants, alcohol, and volatile anesthetics (Meredith et al. 1989). 5-HT$_3$ receptors located in the area postrema are believed to mediate this action of alcohol and the volatile anesthetics (Aapro 1991).

Opioid Receptors

Exposure to nitrous oxide induces opioid peptide release in the periaqueductal gray area of the midbrain and increases opioid receptor density in the brain stem (Fujinaga and Maze 2002; Saracibar et al. 2001). This increase leads to activation of the descending inhibitory pathways that modulate pain and nociceptive processing in the spinal cord. Thus, the opioid receptor system is implicated in the analgesic properties of nitrous oxide, and these effects on opioid receptor function may represent a mechanism for explaining the reinforcing effects of nitrous oxide. However, no evidence implicates opioidergic neurotransmission in the addictive properties of solvents or nitrites.

Clinical Presentation of Inhalant Use Disorder

Diagnostic criteria for inhalant use disorder in DSM-5 (American Psychiatric Association 2013), as previously in DSM-IV-TR (American Psychiatric Association 2000), include biological, cognitive, and behavioral dimensions. As with other substance use disorders, DSM-5 does not differentiate inhalant abuse from dependence (American Psychiatric Association 2013). However, in contrast to other DSM-5 substance use disorders (e.g., alcohol, stimulant, opioid, and cannabis use disorders) that comprise 11 criteria, inhalant use disorder comprises 10 criteria. These criteria include 6 of the 7 DSM-IV-TR inhalant dependence criteria (omitting physical dependence), 3 DSM-IV-TR inhalant abuse criteria (omitting legal problems due to inhalant use), and craving. Inhalant use disorder is considered mild when two or three criteria are met, moderate when four or five criteria are met, or severe when six or more criteria are met.

Clinical and epidemiological observations suggest that inhalant use in humans occurs along a continuum, with considerable variability in usage patterns among individuals as a function of age, sex, socioeconomic status, ethnicity, availability and type of inhalant, and other clinical variables.

Treatment

Accurate diagnosis of inhalant use disorder may require a variety of methods, including psychiatric history and mental status examination, physical examination, and laboratory testing. Once an individual has received a diagnosis of an inhalant use disorder, the initial decisions involve determining the most appropriate setting for treatment and the intensity of treatment required. Continuous inhalant users may require inpatient treatment. Intermittent users without evidence of serious comorbid psychopathology or acute adverse effects of inhalant use can be managed on an ambulatory basis through psychosocial and pharmacological approaches. Despite the relatively high prevalence of inhalant use disorder, especially among children and adolescents, a paucity of studies have examined treatment intervention in this population. Because of the severe cognitive deterioration and comorbid psychopathology associated with inhalant use disorder, treatment can be challenging, even for the most experienced clinicians. Clinicians assessing and treating patients with these disorders should be prepared to work with them for extended periods.

Psychosocial Treatment

Some general guidelines have been developed to address the specific needs of this population (National Inhalant Prevention Coalition 2003). First, given the significant neurotoxicity of inhalants, it is critical to identify cognitive deficits or disruptive behaviors that may interfere with treatment. A neuropsychiatric evaluation, a developmental history, and an examination of school performance may help in achieving this goal. Second, given that family involvement appears to be highly important in the recovery efforts of inhalant abusers, a comprehensive evaluation of the family structure and dynamics is recommended, and family therapy addressing drug education and parenting and social skills training must be considered. Third, given that inhalant use frequently occurs in groups, examination of peer group dynamics is warranted and should be aimed at assisting the patient to break negative peer bonds and substitute positive ones. Fourth, initial therapeutic interventions with inhalant abuse patients should be brief, informal, and concrete, with the aim of developing rapport and enhancing motivation for treatment.

Pharmacotherapy

Management of Inhalant Withdrawal

The objectives in treating inhalant withdrawal are to relieve discomfort, prevent or treat complications, reduce urges to use inhalants, and prepare the patient for rehabilitation. Successful management of inhalant withdrawal should provide a basis for subsequent efforts at rehabilitation. Pharmacological management may potentially assist clinicians and patients in achieving these goals.

Signs and symptoms of inhalant withdrawal, specifically those related to solvents and anesthetics, appear to resemble those of alcohol and sedative withdrawal. It is likely that most inhalant dependence may be safely managed by using social detoxification similar to that used to treat alcohol withdrawal (Naranjo et al. 1983; Sellers et al. 1983). This consists of frequent reassurance, reality orientation, monitoring of vital signs, personal attention, and supportive medical and nursing care (Naranjo and Sellers 1986). Among severely affected inhalant-dependent patients, especially among those dependent on solvents with a high toluene content, pronounced withdrawal symptoms characterized by intense craving, autonomic hyperactivity, seizures, and/or delirium may occur. The inhalant withdrawal clinical picture may also be complicated by intoxication or withdrawal symptoms caused by other substances of abuse, especially alcohol and sedatives. In consideration of these problems, Brouette and Anton (2001) recommended closely monitoring these patients as if they were being treated for alcohol withdrawal. If symptoms develop—particularly signs of autonomic hyperactivity such as tachycardia, elevated blood pressure, and diaphoresis—benzodiazepines are generally the first-line drugs to treat this condition (Mayo-Smith 1997). Nonetheless, because of the abuse potential of these medications and detrimental effects on cognitive function, they should be prescribed with caution.

The apparent commonalities between the effects of chronic consumption of alcohol and inhalants on GABAergic neurotransmission suggest that pharmacological agents that enhance GABAergic function, such as the anticonvulsants carbamazepine, valproate, gabapentin, vigabatrin, and tiagabine, may ameliorate inhalant withdrawal symptoms without the potential risks associated with benzodiazepines. Clinical trials provide evidence of beneficial effects of these compounds in the treatment of alcohol withdrawal. They are not, however, without their potential adverse reactions and disadvantages. The possibility of liver and bone marrow toxicity, for example, necessitates that blood monitoring be done in conjunction with carbamazepine or valproate treatment. Although excessive sedation and drowsiness are common problems with the use of gabapentin, vigabatrin, and tiagabine, this effect can be advantageous in treating the sleep disturbances and anxiety that are frequently associated with inhalant withdrawal. Controlled clinical trials examining the safety and efficacy of these medications for treatment of inhalant withdrawal are needed.

Relapse Prevention

Despite recent advances in understanding the neuropharmacological basis of inhalant dependence, no published study has examined the effects of agents potentially efficacious in the treatment of this condition. In the following subsections, we discuss psychopharmacological agents that, because of their known effects on neurotransmitter systems that mediate inhalants' reinforcing effects, may help inhalant abusers achieve abstinence.

Atypical antipsychotics. Atypical antipsychotics, including clozapine, risperidone, olanzapine, and quetiapine, have been shown to reduce substance use in animals and among patients with schizophrenia or schizoaffective disorders (Brown et al. 2002; Mechanic et al. 2003; Smelson et al. 2002; Zimmet et al. 2000). In contrast to the typical antipsychotics, which generally are antagonists of the D_2 receptor subtype, atypical antipsychotics have a higher affinity for other dopamine receptor subtypes such as the D_3 and D_4 receptors. In addition, atypical antipsychotics have a high affinity for the 5-HT_2 receptor subtype (Bymaster et al. 1996). This broad receptor-binding profile has been implicated in many of the atypical antipsychotics' clinical characteristics and suggests that the agents work by antagonizing D_1 and D_2, the two dopamine receptor subtypes in the nucleus accumbens believed to mediate drug reward (Arnold et al. 1977). Anecdotal reports by clinicians who have used atypical antipsychotics to treat dual diagnoses (e.g., schizophrenia and cocaine abuse) (Littrell et al. 2001; Zimmet et al. 2000) and several controlled studies (Brown et al. 2002; Smelson et al. 2002) showed that these medications reduce craving for cocaine and other stimulants. Given the stimulant-like effects of inhalants on mesolimbic dopaminergic reward circuitry and the cross-sensitization of stimulant effects with toluene or trichloroethane effects, it is plausible that atypical antipsychotics may reduce inhalant use by dampening inhalant reward. Controlled examination of this hypothesis is warranted.

Anticonvulsants. In addition to their potential utility in the treatment of inhalant withdrawal, anticonvulsant medications such as valproate, topiramate, gabapentin, vigabatrin, and tiagabine may have a role in the rehabilitation of inhalant dependence. These compounds may antagonize the rewarding effects of inhalants by inhibiting mesocorticolimbic dopamine release through the facilitation of GABA activity. Topiramate produces a similar effect by inhibition of glutamatergic activity and has been shown in a placebo-controlled clinical trial to reduce alcohol drinking in alcohol-dependent subjects (Johnson et al. 2003). Given the similarities between the effects on GABAergic neurotransmission of alcohol and inhalants, it is plausible that anticonvulsants with significant effects on this neurotransmitter system may help to reduce inhalant use among inhalant-dependent individuals.

Acamprosate. Acamprosate, an amino acid derivative, affects both GABAergic and glutamatergic neurotransmission. Clinical studies have provided some conflicting evidence of the efficacy of acamprosate in alcoholism rehabilitation (Kranzler and Van Kirk 2001). Acamprosate's effects on both GABAergic and glutamatergic neurotransmission, together with a benign side-effect profile, make this compound a potentially useful one to treat inhalant dependence. In rodents, acamprosate has a protective effect against NMDA-mediated neurotoxicity (Koob et al. 2002), suggesting that it may be of utility in preventing or ameliorating the neurotoxicity associated with inhalant use.

5-HT$_3$ antagonists.   Given that the 5-HT$_{3A}$ receptor may also be involved in the reinforcing effects of inhalants (Lovinger and White 1991), it is plausible that medications that antagonize this receptor complex may reduce or dampen the reward produced by inhalant use. Two medications that selectively block 5-HT$_{3A}$ receptors have been used for their psychopharmacological effects: the antiemetic ondansetron and the antidepressant mirtazapine. Ondansetron has been shown to reduce alcohol consumption among alcoholic patients with early-onset problem drinking (i.e., before age 25 years) (Johnson et al. 2000). Mirtazapine is efficacious in the treatment of major depression (see Benkert et al. 2000), but it has not been evaluated in controlled trials to treat substance dependence. Studies examining the effects of these compounds in the treatment of inhalant use disorders may be warranted.

Pharmacological Treatment of Comorbid Psychiatric Conditions

Comorbid psychiatric disorders have been shown to contribute to the development or maintenance of a variety of substance use disorders (Hasin et al. 2004). Effective treatment of the comorbid disorders may have beneficial effects on substance abuse outcomes. Although no systematic studies have been conducted among inhalant abusers, these patients often manifest persistent anxiety symptoms, insomnia, depression, delusions and hallucinations, cognitive impairment, and general distress. These symptoms may last for weeks or months and are difficult to differentiate from the emergence of primary psychiatric disorders.

Despite the high prevalence and clinical significance of comorbid disorders among inhalant abusers, there is only one published pharmacotherapy study of this comorbidity. In a double-blind study comparing the safety and efficacy of carbamazepine or haloperidol treatment of inhalant-induced psychotic symptoms (Hernandez-Avila et al. 1998), 40 male patients were randomly assigned to receive 5 weeks of treatment with carbamazepine or haloperidol. Both treatment groups improved significantly over time, with approximately one-half of the patients in each group considered treatment responders at the end of the study. Adverse effects, especially extrapyramidal symptoms, were significantly more common and more severe in the haloperidol group. Additional studies are needed to address the effects of pharmacotherapy on mood, anxiety, and cognitive symptoms occurring in the context of inhalant abuse.

Conclusion

Inhalant use is a widespread problem, especially among children and adolescents. Acutely, this heterogeneous group of substances (i.e., solvents, nitrites, general anesthetics) exerts significant reinforcing effects, and continuous use of these drugs appears to induce tolerance and withdrawal symptoms. In addition to rapid absorption, rapid entry into the brain, and high bioavailability, inhalants' effects on dopaminergic, glutamatergic, and GABAergic neurotransmission appear to contribute to their abuse liability. Medications that alter these systems, in conjunction with psychosocial interventions, may reduce inhalant use in addicted patients. Further research on the treatment of inhalant use disorders is warranted.

References

Aapro MS: 5-HT3 receptor antagonists: an overview of their present status and future potential in cancer therapy-induced emesis. Drugs 42:551–568, 1991

Aizenman E, Hartnett KA, Reynolds IJ: Oxygen free radicals regulate NMDA receptor function via a redox modulatory site. Neuron 5:841–846, 1990

American Psychiatric Association: Diagnostic and Statistical Manual of Mental Disorders, 4th Edition, Text Revision. Washington, DC, American Psychiatric Association, 2000

American Psychiatric Association: Diagnostic and Statistical Manual of Mental Disorders, 5th Edition. Arlington, VA, American Psychiatric Association, 2013

Arena JM, Drew RH: Poisoning, 5th Edition. Springfield, IL, Charles C Thomas, 1986, pp 258–259

Arnold JH, Truog RD, Rice SA: Prolonged administration of isoflurane to pediatric patients during mechanical ventilation. Anesth Analg 76:520–526, 1993

Arnold EB, Molinoff PB, Rutledge CO: The release of endogenous norepinephrine and dopamine from cerebral cortex by amphetamine. J Pharmacol Exp Ther 202:544–557, 1977

Aune H, Renck H, Bessen A: Metabolism of diethyl ether to acetaldehyde in man (letter). Lancet 2:97, 1978

Avramov MN, Shingu K, Mori K: Progressive changes in electroencephalographic responses to nitrous oxide in humans: a possible acute drug tolerance. Anesth Analg 70:369–374, 1990

Bale AS, Smothers CT, Woodward JJ: Inhibition of neuronal nicotinic acetylcholine receptors by the abused solvent, toluene. Br J Pharmacol 137:375–383, 2002

Balon N, Kriem B, Dousset E, et al: Opposing effects of narcotic gases and pressure on the striatal dopamine release in rats. Brain Res 947:218–224, 2002

Balon N, Dupenloup L, Blanc F, et al: Nitrous oxide reverses the increase in striatal dopamine release produced by N-methyl-D-aspartate infusion in the substantia nigra pars compacta in rats. Neurosci Lett 343:147–149, 2003a

Balon N, Risso JJ, Blanc F, et al: Striatal dopamine release and biphasic pattern of locomotor and motor activity under gas narcosis. Life Sci 72:2731–2740, 2003b

Balster RL, Willetts J: Phencyclidine: a drug of abuse and a tool for neuroscience research, in Pharmacological Aspects of Drug Dependence: Towards an Integrated Neurobehavioral Approach (Handbook of Experimental Pharmacology, Vol 118). Edited by Schuster CR, Kuhar MJ. Berlin, Springer-Verlag, 1996, pp 233–262

Baselt RC: Biological Monitoring Methods for Industrial Chemicals, 3rd Edition. Littleton, MA, PSG Publishing, 1997

Beckstead MJ, Weiner JL, Eger EI 2nd, et al: Glycine and gamma-aminobutyric acid(A) receptor function is enhanced by inhaled drugs of abuse. Mol Pharmacol 57:1199–1205, 2000

Beckstead MJ, Phelan R, Mihic SJ: Antagonism of inhalant and volatile anesthetic enhancement of glycine receptor function. J Biol Chem 276:24959–24964, 2001

Beckstead MJ, Phelan R, Trudell JR, et al: Anesthetic and ethanol effects on spontaneously opening glycine receptor channels. J Neurochem 82:1343–1351, 2002

Benignus VA, Muller KE, Barton CN, et al: Toluene levels in blood and brain of rats during and after respiratory exposure. Toxicol Appl Pharmacol 61:326–334, 1981

Benignus VA, Muller KE, Graham JA, et al: Toluene levels in blood and brain of rats as a function of toluene level in inspired air. Environ Res 33:39–46, 1984

Benkert O, Szegedi A, Kohnen R: Mirtazapine compared with paroxetine in major depression. J Clin Psychiatry 61:656–663, 2000

Beyer CE, Stafford D, LeSage MG, et al: Repeated exposure to inhaled toluene induces behavioral and neurochemical cross-sensitization to cocaine in rats. Psychopharmacology (Berl) 154:198–204, 2001

Bird T: Revelations under ether. Lancet 118:9, 1881

Bowen SE, Balster RL: A direct comparison of inhalant effects on locomotor activity and schedule-controlled behavior in mice. Exp Clin Psychopharmacol 6:235–247, 1998

Bowen SE, Wiley JL, Balster RL: The effects of abused inhalants on mouse behavior in an elevated plus-maze. Eur J Pharmacol 312:131–136, 1996a

Bowen SE, Wiley JL, Evans EB, et al: Functional observational battery comparing effects of ethanol, 1,1,1-trichloroethane, ether, and flurothyl. Neurotoxicol Teratol 18:577–585, 1996b

Bredt DS, Snyder SH: Nitric oxide, a novel neuronal messenger. Neuron 8:3–11, 1992

Brouette T, Anton R: Clinical review of inhalants. Am J Addict 10:79–94, 2001

Brown ES, Nejtek VA, Perantie DC, et al: Quetiapine in bipolar disorder and cocaine dependence. Bipolar Disord 4:406–411, 2002

Bushnell PJ, Evans HL, Palmes ED: Effects of toluene inhalation on carbon dioxide production and locomotor activity in mice. Fundam Appl Toxicol 5:971–977, 1985

Bymaster FP, Hemrick-Luecke SK, Perry KW, et al: Neurochemical evidence for antagonism by olanzapine of dopamine, serotonin, alpha 1-adrenergic and muscarinic receptors in vivo in rats. Psychopharmacology (Berl) 124:87–94, 1996

Carroll E: Notes on the epidemiology of inhalants. NIDA Res Monogr 15:14–24, 1977

Cho AM, Coalson DW, Klock PA, et al: The effects of alcohol history on the reinforcing, subjective and psychomotor effects of nitrous oxide in healthy volunteers. Drug Alcohol Depend 45:63–70, 1997

Collins SL, Kantak KM: Neuronal nitric oxide synthase inhibition decreases cocaine self-administration behavior in rats. Psychopharmacology (Berl) 159:361–369, 2002

Cruz SL, Mirshahi T, Thomas B, et al: Effects of the abused solvent toluene on recombinant N-methyl-D-aspartate and non-N-methyl-D-aspartate receptors expressed in Xenopus oocytes. J Pharmacol Exp Ther 286:334–340, 1998

Delteil P, Stoesser F, Stoesser R: L'Žtheromanie. Ann Med Psychol (Paris) 1:329–340, 1974

Deniker P, Cottereau MJ, Loo H, et al: L'usage de l'Žther dans les toxicomanies actuelles. Ann Med Psychol (Paris) 1:674–683, 1972

Di Chiara G, Imperato A: Drugs abused by humans preferentially increase synaptic dopamine concentrations in the mesolimbic system of freely moving rats. Proc Natl Acad Sci USA 85:5274–5278, 1988

Dingledine R, Borges K, Bowie D, et al: The glutamate receptor ion channels. Pharmacol Rev 51:7–61, 1999

Dohrn CS, Lichtor JL, Finn RS, et al: Subjective and psychomotor effects of nitrous oxide in healthy volunteers. Behav Pharmacol 3:19–30, 1992

Dohrn CS, Lichtor JL, Coalson DW, et al: Reinforcing effects of extended inhalation of nitrous oxide in humans. Drug Alcohol Depend 31:265–280, 1993

Evans AC, Raistrick D: Phenomenology of intoxication with toluene-based adhesives and butane gas. Br J Psychiatry 150:769–773, 1987

Evans EB, Balster RL: CNS depressant effects of volatile organic solvents. Neurosci Biobehav Rev 15:233–241, 1991

Evans EB, Balster RL: Inhaled 1,1,1-trichloroethane-produced physical dependence in mice: effects of drugs and vapors on withdrawal. J Pharmacol Exp Ther 264:726–733, 1993

Follin S, Rousselot Y: [Analysis of the ether addiction behavior of a schizophrenic patient] [in French]. Ann Med Psychol (Paris) 138:405–419, 1980

Franks NP, Lieb WR: Molecular and cellular mechanisms of general anaesthesia. Nature 367:607–614, 1994

French ED, Dillon K, Wu X: Cannabinoids excite dopamine neurons in the ventral tegmentum and substantia nigra. Neuroreport 8:649–652, 1997

Fujinaga M, Maze M: Neurobiology of nitrous oxide-induced antinociceptive effects. Mol Neurobiol 25:167–189, 2002

Fuxe K, Andersson K, Nilsen OG, et al: Toluene and telencephalic dopamine: selective reduction of amine turnover in discrete DA nerve terminal systems of the anterior caudate nucleus by low concentrations of toluene. Toxicol Lett 12:115–123, 1982

Gause EM, Mendez V, Geller I: Exploratory studies of a rodent model for inhalant abuse. Neurobehav Toxicol Teratol 7:143–148, 1985

Gerasimov MR, Ferrieri RA, Schiffer WK, et al: Study of brain uptake and biodistribution of [11C]toluene in non-human primates and mice. Life Sci 70:2811–2828, 2002

Gessa GL, Muntoni F, Collu M, et al: Low doses of ethanol activate dopaminergic neurons in the ventral tegmental area. Brain Res 348:201–203, 1985

Glaser HH, Massengale ON: Glue-sniffing in children: deliberate inhalation of vaporized plastic cements. JAMA 181:300–303, 1962

Haggart HW: The absorption, distribution and elimination of ethyl ether. J Biol Chem 59:737–802, 1924

Harbison RM: Hamilton and Hardy's Industrial Toxicology, 5th Edition. St. Louis, MO, Mosby, 1998

Harper MH, Winter PM, Johnson BH, et al: Withdrawal convulsions in mice following nitrous oxide. Anesth Analg 59:19–21, 1980

Hasin D, Nunes E, Meydan J: Comorbidity of alcohol, drug, and psychiatric disorders: epidemiology, in Dual Diagnosis and Psychiatric Treatment: Substance Abuse and Comorbid Disorders, 2nd Edition. Edited by Kranzler HR, Tinsley JA. New York, Marcel Dekker, 2004, pp 1–34

Haverkos HW, Kopstein AN, Wilson H, et al: Nitrite inhalants: history, epidemiology, and possible links to AIDS. Environ Health Perspect 102:858–861, 1994

Hernandez-Avila CA, Ortega-Soto HA, Jasso A, et al: Treatment of inhalant-induced psychotic disorder with carbamazepine versus haloperidol. Psychiatr Serv 49:812–815, 1998

Hillefors-Berglund M, Liu Y, von Euler G: Persistent, specific and dose-dependent effects of toluene exposure on dopamine D2 agonist binding in the rat caudate-putamen. Toxicology 77:223–232, 1993

Himnan DJ: Tolerance and reverse tolerance to toluene inhalation: effects on open-field behavior. Pharmacol Biochem Behav 21:625–631, 1984

Hinman DJ: Biphasic dose-response relationship for effects of toluene inhalation on locomotor activity. Pharmacol Biochem Behav 26:65–69, 1987

Horn T, Smith PM, McLaughlin BE, et al: Nitric oxide actions in paraventricular nucleus: cardiovascular and neurochemical implications. Am J Physiol 266:R306–R313, 1994

Hughes J, Leach HJ, Choonara I: Hallucinations on withdrawal of isoflurane used as sedation. Acta Paediatr 82:885–886, 1993

Hynes MD, Berkowitz BA: Catecholamine mechanisms in the stimulation of mouse locomotor activity by nitrous oxide and morphine. Eur J Pharmacol 90:109–114, 1983

Ikeuchi Y, Hirai H, Okada Y, et al: Excitatory and inhibitory effects of toluene on neural activity in guinea pig hippocampal slices. Neurosci Lett 158:63–66, 1993

Jevtovic-Todorovic V, Todorovic SM, Mennerick S, et al: Nitrous oxide (laughing gas) is an NMDA antagonist, neuroprotectant and neurotoxin. Nat Med 4:460–463, 1998

Johnson BA, Roache JD, Javors MA, et al: Ondansetron for reduction of drinking among biologically predisposed alcoholic patients: a randomized controlled trial. JAMA 284:963–971, 2000

Johnson BA, Ait-Daoud N, Bowden CL, et al: Oral topiramate for treatment of alcohol dependence: a randomised controlled trial. Lancet 361:1677–1685, 2003

Johnston LD, O'Malley PM, Bachman JG, et al: Monitoring the Future National Results on Adolescent Drug Use: Overview of Key Findings, 2010. Ann Arbor, MI, Institute for Social Research, University of Michigan, 2011

Kielbasa W, Fung HL: Pharmacokinetics of a model organic nitrite inhalant and its alcohol metabolite in rats. Drug Metab Dispos 28:386–391, 2000

Kishi R, Harabuchi I, Ikeda T, et al: Neurobehavioural effects and pharmacokinetics of toluene in rats and their relevance to man. Br J Ind Med 45:396–408, 1988

Kjellstrand P, Holmquist B, Jonsson I, et al: Effects of organic solvents on motor activity in mice. Toxicology 35:35–46, 1985

Knox JW, Nelson JR: Permanent encephalopathy from toluene inhalation. N Engl J Med 275:1494–1496, 1966

Kono J, Miyata H, Ushijima S, et al: Nicotine, alcohol, methamphetamine, and inhalant dependence: a comparison of clinical features with the use of a new clinical evaluation form. Alcohol 24:99–106, 2001

Koob GF, Mason BJ, De Witte P, et al: Potential neuroprotective effects of acamprosate. Alcohol Clin Exp Res 26:586–592, 2002

Kranzler HR, Van Kirk J: Efficacy of naltrexone and acamprosate for alcoholism treatment: a meta-analysis. Alcohol Clin Exp Res 25:1335–1341, 2001

Krenz S, Zimmermann G, Kolly S, et al: Ether: a forgotten addiction. Addiction 98:1167–1168, 2003

Laurenzi RG, Locatelli C, Brucato A: N-Acetylcysteine: a proposal for therapy in acute poisoning due to highly hepatotoxic organic solvents. Vet Human Toxicol 29:95, 1987

Littrell KH, Petty RG, Hilligoss NM, et al: Olanzapine treatment for patients with schizophrenia and substance abuse. J Subst Abuse Treat 21:217–221, 2001

Lof A, Wigaeus Hjelm E, Colmsjo A, et al: Toxicokinetics of toluene and urinary excretion of hippuric acid after human exposure to 2H8-toluene. Br J Ind Med 50:55–59, 1993

Lonart G, Johnson KM: Inhibitory effects of nitric oxide on the uptake of [3H]dopamine and [3H]glutamate by striatal synaptosomes. J Neurochem 63:2108–2117, 1994

Lovinger DM, White G: Ethanol potentiation of 5-hydroxytryptamine3 receptor-mediated ion current in neuroblastoma cells and isolated adult mammalian neurons. Mol Pharmacol 40:263–270, 1991

Machu TK, Harris RA: Alcohols and anesthetics enhance the function of 5-hydroxytryptamine$_3$ receptors expressed in Xenopus laevis oocytes. J Pharmacol Exp Ther 271:898–905, 1994

Manzoni O, Prezeau L, Marin P, et al: Nitric oxide-induced blockade of NMDA receptors. Neuron 8:653–662, 1992

Marsh N, Marsh A: A short history of nitroglycerine and nitric oxide in pharmacology and physiology. Clin Exp Pharmacol Physiol 27:313–319, 2000

Mayo-Smith MF: Pharmacological management of alcohol withdrawal: a meta-analysis and evidence-based practice guideline. American Society of Addiction Medicine Working Group on Pharmacological Management of Alcohol Withdrawal. JAMA 278:144–151, 1997

Mechanic JA, Maynard BT, Holloway FA: Treatment with the atypical antipsychotic, olanzapine, prevents the expression of amphetamine-induced place conditioning in the rat. Prog Neuropsychopharmacol Biol Psychiatry 27:43–54, 2003

Mennerick S, Jevtovic-Todorovic V, Todorovic SM, et al: Effect of nitrous oxide on excitatory and inhibitory synaptic transmission in hippocampal cultures. J Neurosci 18:9716–9726, 1998

Meredith TJ, Ruprah M, Liddle A, et al: Diagnosis and treatment of acute poisoning with volatile substances. Hum Toxicol 8:277–286, 1989

Merry J, Zachariadis N: Addiction to glue sniffing. Br Med J 5317:1448, 1962

Mihic SJ: Acute effects of ethanol on GABAA and glycine receptor function. Neurochem Int 35:115–123, 1999

Moser VC, Balster RL: The effects of acute and repeated toluene exposure on operant behavior in mice. Neurobehav Toxicol Teratol 3:471–475, 1981

Moser VC, Scimeca JA, Balster RL: Minimal tolerance to the effects of 1,1,1-trichloroethane on fixed-ratio responding in mice. Neurotoxicology 6:35–42, 1985

Naalsund LU: Hippocampal EEG in rats after chronic toluene inhalation. Acta Pharmacol Toxicol (Copenh) 59:325–331, 1986

Naranjo CA, Sellers EM: Clinical assessment and pharmacotherapy of the alcohol withdrawal syndrome, in Recent Developments in Alcoholism, Vol 4. Edited by Galanter M. New York, Plenum, 1986, pp 265–281

Naranjo CA, Sellers EM, Chater K, et al: Nonpharmacologic interventions in acute alcohol withdrawal. Clin Pharmacol Ther 34:214–219, 1983

National Inhalant Prevention Coalition: Inhalant Treatment Guidelines. Austin, TX, National Inhalant Prevention Coalition, 2003

Nickerson M: Vasodilator drugs, in The Pharmacological Basis of Therapeutics, 4th Edition. Edited by Goodman LS, Gilman A. New York, Macmillan, 1970, pp 745–763

Nylander I: "Thinner" addiction in children and adolescents. Acta Paedopsychiatr 29:273–283, 1962

Ortells MO, Lunt GG: Evolutionary history of the ligand-gated ion-channel superfamily of receptors. Trends Neurosci 18:121–127, 1995

Payne JP: The criminal use of chloroform. Anaesthesia 53:685–690, 1998

Press E, Done AK: Solvent sniffing: physiologic effects and community control measures for intoxication from the intentional inhalation of organic solvents, I. Pediatrics 39:451–461, 1967

Price HL, Dripps RD: General anesthetics, in The Pharmacological Basis of Therapeutics, 5th Edition. Edited by Goodman LS, Gilman A. New York, Macmillan, 1975, pp 88–96

Pudiak CM, Bozarth MA: The effect of nitric oxide synthesis inhibition on intravenous cocaine self-administration. Prog Neuropsychopharmacol Biol Psychiatry 26:189–196, 2002

Rea TM, Nash JF, Zabik JE, et al: Effects of toluene inhalation on brain biogenic amines in the rat. Toxicology 31:143–1450, 1984

Reynolds JEF: Martindale: The Extra Pharmacopoeia, 28th Edition. London, Pharmaceutical Press, 1982, pp 745–746

Riegel AC, French ED: Acute toluene induces biphasic changes in rat spontaneous locomotor activity which are blocked by remoxipride. Pharmacol Biochem Behav 62:399–402, 1999

Riegel AC, Ali SF, French ED: Toluene-induced locomotor activity is blocked by 6-hydroxydopamine lesions of the nucleus accumbens and the mGluR2/3 agonist LY379268. Neuropsychopharmacology 28:1440–1447, 2003

Rupreht J, Dworacek B, Bonke B, et al: Tolerance to nitrous oxide in volunteers. Acta Anaesthesiol Scand 29:635–638, 1985

Saito K, Wada H: Behavioral approaches to toluene intoxication. Environ Res 62:53–62, 1993

Saracibar G, Hernandez ML, Echevarria E, et al: Toluene alters mu-opioid receptor expression in the rat brainstem. Ind Health 39:231–234, 2001

Schroeder HG: Acute and delayed chloroform poisoning. Br J Anaeseth 37:972–975, 1965

Schwartz AM: The cause, relief and prevention of headaches arising from contact with dynamite. N Engl J Med 235:541–544, 1946

Schwartz RH, Peary P: Abuse of isobutyl nitrite inhalation (rush) by adolescents. Clin Pediatr 25:308–310, 1986

Sellers EM, Naranjo CA, Harrison M, et al: Diazepam loading: simplified treatment of alcohol withdrawal. Clin Pharmacol Ther 34: 822–826, 1983

Sharp CW: Introduction to inhalant abuse, in Inhalant Abuse: A Volatile Research Agenda (NIDA Research Monograph 129). Edited by Sharp CW, Beuvais F, Spence R. Rockville, MD, National Institute on Drug Abuse, 1992, pp 1–10

Smelson DA, Losonczy MF, Davis CW, et al: Risperidone decreases craving and relapses in individuals with schizophrenia and cocaine dependence. Can J Psychiatry 47:671–675, 2002

Smith GB, Olsen RW: Functional domains of GABAA receptors. Trends Pharmacol Sci 16:162–168, 1995

Smith RA, Winter PM, Smith M, et al: Convulsions in mice after anesthesia. Anesthesiology 50:501–504, 1979

Stengard K, O'Connor WT: Acute toluene exposure decreases extracellular gamma-aminobutyric acid in the globus pallidus but not in striatum: a microdialysis study in awake, freely moving rats. Eur J Pharmacol 292:43–46, 1994

Stengard K, Hoglund G, Ungerstedt U: Extracellular dopamine levels within the striatum increase during inhalation exposure to toluene: a microdialysis study in awake, freely moving rats. Toxicol Lett 71:245–255, 1994

Stenqvist O: Nitrous oxide kinetics. Acta Anaesthesiol Scand 38:757–760, 1994

Substance Abuse and Mental Health Services Administration: Results from the 2010 National Survey on Drug Use and Health: Summary of National Findings, NSDUH Series H-41 (HHS Publ No SMA-11-4658). Rockville, MD, Substance Abuse and Mental Health Services Administration, 2011. Available at: http://www.samhsa.gov/data/nsduh/2k10nsduh/2k10results.htm. Accessed November 26, 2012.

Tobias JD: Tolerance, withdrawal, and physical dependency after long-term sedation and analgesia of children in the pediatric intensive care unit. Crit Care Med 28:2122–2132, 2000

Turle N, Saget A, Zouani B, et al: Neurochemical studies of narcosis: a comparison between the effects of nitrous oxide and hyperbaric nitrogen on the dopaminergic nigro-striatal pathway. Neurochem Res 23:997–1003, 1998

Vleeming W, Rambali B, Opperhuizen A: The role of nitric oxide in cigarette smoking and nicotine addiction. Nicotine Tob Res 4:341–348, 2002

von Euler G, Ogren SO, Li XM, et al: Persistent effects of subchronic toluene exposure on spatial learning and memory, dopamine-mediated locomotor activity and dopamine D2 agonist binding in the rat. Toxicology 77:223–232, 1993

Walker DJ, Zacny JP: Analysis of the reinforcing and subjective effects of different doses of nitrous oxide using a free-choice procedure. Drug Alcohol Depend 66:93–103, 2002

Wang T, French ED: NMDA, kainate, and AMPA depolarize nondopamine neurons in the rat ventral tegmentum. Brain Res Bull 36:39–43, 1995

Weiner JL, Gu C, Dunwiddie TV: Differential ethanol sensitivity of subpopulations of GABAA synapses onto rat hippocampal CA1 pyramidal neurons. J Neurophysiol 77:1306–1312, 1997

Whitwam JG, Morgan M, Hall GM, et al: Pain during continuous nitrous oxide administration. Br J Anaesth 48:425–429, 1976

Wiley JL, Bale AS, Balster RL: Evaluation of toluene dependence and cross-sensitization to diazepam. Life Sci 72:3023–3033, 2003

Wood RW, Grubman J, Weiss B: Nitrous oxide self-administration by the squirrel monkey. J Pharmacol Exp Ther 202:491–499, 1977

Wood RW, Coleman JB, Schuler R, et al: Anticonvulsant and antipunishment effects of toluene. J Pharmacol Exp Ther 230:407–412, 1984

Yamakura T, Harris RA: Effects of gaseous anesthetics nitrous oxide and xenon on ligand-gated ion channels: comparison with isoflurane and ethanol. Anesthesiology 93:1095–1101, 2000

Yanagita T, Takahashi S, Ishida K, et al: Voluntary inhalation of volatile anesthetics and organic solvents by monkeys. Jpn J Clin Pharmacol 1:13–16, 1970

Yavich L, Zvartau E: A comparison of the effects of individual organic solvents and their mixture on brain stimulation reward. Pharmacol Biochem Behav 48:661–664, 1994

You L, Muralidhara S, Dallas CE: Comparisons between operant response and 1,1,1-trichloroethane toxicokinetics in mouse blood and brain. Toxicology 93:151–163, 1994

Zimmet SV, Strous RD, Burgess ES, et al: Effects of clozapine on substance use in patients with schizophrenia and schizoaffective disorder: a retrospective survey. J Clin Psychopharmacol 20:94–98, 2000

9

Club Drugs and Synthetic Cannabinoid Agonists

Richard N. Rosenthal, M.D.

Ramon Solhkhah, M.D.

The use of "club drugs," which include γ-hydroxybutyrate (GHB), 3,4-methylenedioxymethamphetamine (MDMA; "Ecstasy"), and ketamine, particularly among adolescents and young adults, has raised concern (Chatlos 1996; Hill and Thomas 2011). Although these more recent studies of adolescents and adults have shown a slight decrease in drug use overall, adolescent substance abuse remains a public health concern, particularly as it relates to the use of designer drugs (Armentano 1995; Johnston et al. 2010). Moreover, given their popularity among a subgroup of the homosexual community, the club drugs also may represent a unique challenge in working with patients in this group.

Club drugs originally received their name from their use in nightclubs and "raves." Raves are all-night dance parties that feature "techno" music, which is intended to enhance drug effects. These parties tend to attract adolescents and young adults ages 15–25 years (Koesters et al. 2002). As part of the rave experience, partygoers are often looking for "euphoric transcendence," which is reached through the combination of frenetic dancing and club drug use (Weir 2000). Increasingly, however, clinicians must be concerned with nonclub uses of the club drugs, particularly among high school and college students (Pederson and Skrondal 1999). Although technically any drug used in a club could be considered a "club drug," general interest has focused on three agents: GHB, MDMA, and ketamine.

γ-Hydroxybutyrate and Related Compounds

GHB has been used both for legitimate clinical and clinical research purposes and for a range of illicit purposes. It was marketed legally in the United States until 1990, when the U.S. Food and Drug Administration (FDA) banned its sale to consumers. Except for the one indication described later in this section, GHB is a Schedule I controlled substance without other FDA-approved indications. The FDA also declared γ-butyrolactone (GBL) as a List I chemical and 1,4-butanediol (1,4-BD) as a Class I health hazard, practically designating these GHB precursors, which are also industrial solvents, as illicit and unapproved new drugs (Substance Abuse and Mental Health Services Administration 2013).

Epidemiology and Clinical Presentation

Emergency department (ED) episodes related to GHB as reported to the Drug Abuse Warning Network (DAWN) increased more than fivefold from 1994 to 2001, with weighted estimates of 3,340 GHB mentions in 2001, compared with 638 mentions in 1994 (Kissin and Ball 2002). More than 74% of GHB mentions in 2001 were concurrent mentions with other drugs, and 54% were concurrent mentions with alcohol. For the period of 2004–2011, DAWN-reported ED visits related to GHB had decreased but were relatively stable, moving from a low of 1,036 in 2005 to a high of 2,406 in 2011, but with no obvious trend (Substance Abuse and Mental Health Services Administration 2013). Fewer GHB mentions in 2011 also involved alcohol (35.8%) (Substance Abuse and Mental Health Services Administration 2013). In 2001, 58% of ED mentions of GHB were for patients ages 18–25 years, and GHB mentions typically involved patients who are white and male (Kissin and Ball 2002), a pattern that continued through 2011 (Substance Abuse and Mental Health Services Administration 2013). In 2011, 13% of GHB mentions were in patients ages 25–29 years, though a larger percentage (34%) were ages 35–44 years, suggesting an aging cohort of users. Although ED visits related to GHB are rare (<0.2% of drug/alcohol-related ED visits), the complaints that precipitate them may reflect the pattern of GHB sequelae in users in the community.

Miotto and colleagues (2001) surveyed 42 recreational users of GHB and found that 66% reported episodes of unpredictable loss of consciousness, and 26% had overdosed. Of daily users, 45% had experienced frequent amnesia during or after use of the drug, suggestive of blackouts typically attributed to severe alcohol abuse. The rate of adverse events was greater among those who used higher GHB doses and among those who used GHB together with other drugs of abuse.

Aside from the use of GHB and its analogs by bodybuilders for purported anabolic effects, the main abuse of this class of compounds is recreational use, which produces sedation, euphoria, and sexual disinhibition (Miotto et al. 2001). The sedative effects of GHB may be related to inhibition of dopamine release and a subsequent increase in the intraneuronal dopamine level (Itzhak and Ali 2002). In an attempt to sidestep the FDA ban on human use of GHB and its precursors, GBL and 1,4-BD, these drugs are frequently represented and sold on the Internet as cleaning fluids. Several "brands" sold over the Internet include GBL preparations such as Fire Water, Revivarant, Revivarant G, RenewTrient, GH Revitalizer, GH Release, Gamma-G, InvigorateX, Furomax, Insom-X, and Blue Nitro Vitality and 1,4-BD preparations such as Revitalize Plus, Serenity, Enliven, Zen, GHRE, SomatoPro, InnerG, NRG3, Weight Belt Cleaner, and Thunder Nectar (Centers for Disease Control and Prevention 1999; Hall and Maxwell 2000; Zvosec et al. 2001). Because GHB potentially causes coma and anterograde amnesia, especially in conjunction with alcohol, with which its effects are synergistic, it has reportedly been used as a drug to facilitate sexual assault. Reflecting street awareness of the side effects of loss of consciousness and decreased coordination, users usually avoid driving motor vehicles (Miotto at al. 2001).

Because GHB induces slow-wave sleep, a peak period of sleep for release of growth hormone (Gerra et al. 1994; Takahara et al. 1977), it has been marketed as a nonregulated anabolic health-food supplement to bodybuilders since the 1980s. However, Addolorato and colleagues (1999b) found no evidence of purported anabolic effects during long-term administration of GHB, and no other evidence from case reports or clinical trials exists for the efficacy of GHB in increasing muscle mass.

Acute Effects

When GHB is taken for recreational use as an intoxicant, typical acute effects described by misusers are euphoria, relaxation, and increased sexuality (Galloway et al. 1997; Miotto et al. 2001). On the street, GHB is taken in capfuls or teaspoons of a salty/sour liquid, which, because of variations in concentration, may range in dose from 0.5 to 5.0 g. Common side effects are nausea, headache, itching, and vomiting (Borgen et al. 2003). Doses of 10–20 mg/kg of GHB typically produce anxiolysis with hypotonia and amnesia, 20–30 mg/kg induces sleep, and 50–60 mg/kg induces anesthesia (Craig et al. 2000). In the context of rave-type parties, GHB or its precursors are often taken together with other club drugs (e.g., ketamine, MDMA) to offset the sedating properties of GHB and modulate the stimulants' adverse effects such as teeth grinding and jaw clenching, while increasing the subjective euphoria and disinhibition. GHB has also gained notoriety as a common drug of abuse at gay circuit parties. Similar to alcohol, GHB may cause impairment of judgment in addition to disinhibition when used to facilitate sexuality. In Liverpool, England, 61% of gay men identified in one study as infected with syphilis had used GHB as an aphrodisiac in the context of unprotected sex (Cook et al. 2001).

Chronic Effects

In a conditioned place preference paradigm, mice treated repeatedly for a week with 250 mg/kg of GHB showed place preference, suggesting that GHB cues are rewarding (Itzhak and Ali 2002). However, highly reinforcing drugs (e.g., cocaine, opioids) typically produce conditioned place preference after only two to three drug exposures, so GHB, which appears to require a greater number of exposures, may have less reinforcing effects (Nicholson and Balster 2001). Nonetheless, it appears that a small percentage of human users of GHB or its precursors become addicted. In addition to evidence of physiological dependence, including tolerance and withdrawal, evidence indicates that patients may quickly relapse to GHB or GBL use after complicated withdrawal (McDaniel and Miotto 2001), thus meeting the DSM-IV-TR criteria for substance dependence (American Psychiatric Association 2000). Part of the high relapse risk may be due to what McDaniel and Miotto (2001) have described as a protracted abstinence syndrome, characterized by dysphoria, anxiety, memory problems, and insomnia, which may last for 3–6 months after the acute withdrawal has stabilized.

Basic and Clinical Pharmacology

Biosynthetic and Metabolic Pathways

GHB is an endogenous, water-soluble, four-carbon fatty acid that is found in peripheral organs, including the heart, liver, kidney, and cardiac and skeletal muscle, as well as in the brain of mammals, where it is thought to play a role as a neurotransmitter (Maitre 1997; Nelson et al. 1981). This metabolite of γ-aminobutyric acid (GABA) appears to be synthesized in the central nervous system (CNS), and in rodents it has been shown to bind to high-affinity receptors in neurons of the hippocampus, cortex, striatum, olfactory bulb and tubercle, and dopaminergic nuclei (Maitre 1997). In the mitochondria, GABA is transaminated by GABA transaminase into succinic semialdehyde (SSA) (Figure 9–1). Most of the SSA is oxidized into succinate in the mitochondria for use in the Krebs cycle, but a small amount, 1%–2%, appears to be transported back into the cytosol, where it is reduced into GHB by SSA reductase, an enzyme found only in neurons (Maitre et al. 2000). In the brain, 1,4-BD is also converted into GHB (Snead et al. 1989), whereas peripheral lactonases appear to convert naturally occurring GBL into GHB, which then freely diffuses across the blood-brain barrier (Maitre 1997; Roth and Giarman 1968). In the liver, 1,4-BD is oxidized by alcohol dehydrogenase to γ-hydroxybutyraldehyde, which is oxidized to GHB by aldehyde dehydrogenase (Dyer et al. 2001). Inhibiting the enzyme GABA transaminase will block the formation of GHB from GABA; however, neither this effect nor the blocking of alcohol dehydrogenase affects the formation of GHB from 1,4-BD in the brain, demonstrating at least two different pathways for GHB synthesis in the CNS (Snead et al. 1989). GHB is ultimately metabolized to carbon dioxide (CO_2), which is eliminated through the lungs, although a small percentage is excreted in the urine (Galloway et al. 2000; Nicholson and Balster 2001).

GHB is rapidly absorbed from the gastrointestinal tract and is present in free form in the serum without protein binding (Li et al. 1998a), with peak

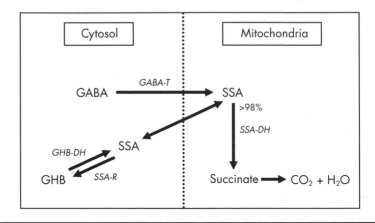

Figure 9–1.   γ-Hydroxybutyrate (GHB) synthesis in the neuron.

Succinic semialdehyde (SSA) is synthesized in the mitochondria through transamination of γ-aminobutyric acid (GABA) by GABA transaminase (GABA-T). Most of the SSA is oxidized by SSA dehydrogenase (SSA-DH) to form succinate, which is used for energy metabolism and results in the end products $CO_2 + H_2O$, which are expired. A small portion of SSA (<2%) is converted by SSA reductase (SSA-R) in the cytosol to GHB. GHB may also be oxidized back to SSA by GHB dehydrogenase (GHB-DH).

plasma concentrations usually appearing 40–60 minutes after ingestion, often more quickly (Borgen et al. 2003). However, absorption is capacity limited, and larger doses will increase the time to peak plasma concentration (Palatini et al. 1993). Food, especially that of high fat content, significantly reduces bioavailability of GHB, reducing peak plasma concentration and increasing median time to peak concentration (Borgen et al. 2003). Because the main enzyme for degradation of GHB is saturable and the elimination pharmacokinetics of GHB are nonlinear, plasma clearance of GHB decreases as the dose of GHB increases (Borgen et al. 2000). At low doses such as 12.5 mg/kg, the elimination half-life is as brief as 20 minutes, with clearance of 14 mL/min/kg, whereas at moderate doses such as 32 mg/kg, the mean clearance is reduced to 6.6 mL/min/kg and is further reduced by almost 40% with doses of approximately 60 mg/kg (Borgen et al. 2000; Roth and Giarman 1966; Scharf et al. 1998). Plasma levels of GHB are negligible 6 hours after a single 64-mg/kg (4.5-g) dose in healthy adults (Borgen et al. 2003). Because of the rapid elimination of the drug, the alteration in clearance with increased dose is not usually clinically relevant, except in the case of overdose, when coma may be extended with high doses, or when there is a pattern of high-dose administration at frequent intervals. The effect of the latter is discussed later in this chapter, in the subsection "Abstinence Syndrome."

Clinical Pharmacology

GHB has sedative, anxiolytic, and euphoric effects similar to those of ethanol, likely because of potentiation of cerebral GABAergic and dopaminergic activities. In general, GHB is thought to exert tonic inhibitory control over dopamine and GABA release through high-affinity GHB receptors (Howard and Feigenbaum 1997; Kemmel et al. 2003). Increases in neuronal pools of dopamine are mediated by induction of tyrosine hydroxylase (Gessa et al. 1966), the rate-limiting enzyme in the catecholaminergic synthetic pathway. There also may be a serotonergic effect of GHB that is mediated by increased transport of tryptophan into serotonergic cells (Gobaille et al. 2002). Although GHB does not interact directly with known sites of action of other drugs of abuse, including the $GABA_A$ receptor, in pharmacological doses it may be an agonist at $GABA_B$ sites (Nicholson and Balster 2001). It is likely that the rewarding properties of GHB mainly occur via disinhibition of ventral tegmental dopaminergic neurons rather than direct effects on the nucleus accumbens (Watson et al. 2010).

In addition, high-dose GHB causes epileptiform electroencephalogram (EEG) effects that are distinctly different from those of ethanol, and in preclinical studies it produced EEG changes that are more suggestive of petit mal absence seizures than of true sedation (Godschalk et al. 1977). However, the sedation caused by GHB is usually not thought to reflect absence seizures. Compared with the sedation induced by benzodiazepines and barbiturates, sedation induced by GHB at higher doses possesses distinct excitatory properties similar to those seen with dissociative anesthetics such as ketamine (Nicholson and Balster 2001; Winters and Kott 1979). This effect may contribute to its role as a club drug. GHB also differs from other sedative-hypnotics such as ethanol or benzodiazepines in that it consolidates rapid eye movement (REM) sleep.

GHB has been investigated as a potential treatment for several disorders including those related to sleep, such as narcolepsy (Scrima et al. 1990) and sleep apnea (Sériès et al. 1992), and those postulated to involve dopamine and

GABA systems, such as schizophrenia (Levy et al. 1983), alcohol withdrawal (Addolorato et al. 2000), and fibromyalgia (Staud 2011). GHB was developed under FDA orphan drug status as sodium oxybate (Xyrem), which was approved by the FDA in July 2002 as a Schedule III drug for the treatment of cataplexy in patients with narcolepsy. GHB reduces cataplexy and induces and consolidates the type of brain EEG changes seen in normal sleep, such as slow-wave sleep, without affecting REM sleep (Sériès et al. 1992). As such, it has shown efficacy in controlled clinical trials in patients with narcolepsy (Lammers et al. 1993; Scrima et al. 1990).

Another potential clinical use of GHB is in the treatment of alcohol withdrawal and alcohol dependence. In preclinical studies, GHB inhibited voluntary ethanol consumption in ethanol-preferring rats and suppressed the ethanol withdrawal syndrome in alcohol-dependent animals (Gessa et al. 2000). These results set the foundation for investigating the potential use of GHB in the clinical treatment of alcohol dependence. Although an alcohol treatment indication is not currently approved in the United States, in Europe several open studies and randomized clinical trials have suggested that GHB is efficacious in preventing or controlling symptoms of alcohol withdrawal (Addolorato et al. 1999a; Moncini et al. 2000; Nimmerrichter et al. 2002) and that GHB may have a role in reducing alcohol craving, increasing treatment retention (Moncini et al. 2000), and preventing relapse to drinking (Gallimberti et al. 1992, 2000) in detoxified alcoholic patients. In view of the addiction liability of GHB, it is not surprising that in some trials of GHB for alcohol dependence, more than 10% of the sample lost control over or became dependent on the study drug (Addolorato et al. 1996; Gallimberti et al. 2000). The potential role of GHB as a substitution pharmacotherapy for alcoholism is confounded by its short plasma half-life; the role of longer-acting GHB analogs remains to be explored (Galloway et al. 2000).

Toxicology

Overdose Effects

The most frequent presentation of GHB-related syndromes in EDs is that of overdose characterized by coma or stupor and respiratory depression and usually complicated by ingestion of other recreational drugs, but fatalities have been reported in the context of GHB and 1,4-BD use alone (Centers for Disease Control and Prevention 1997; Zvosec et al. 2001). Other common findings are bradycardia, respiratory acidosis, and vomiting (Chin et al. 1998). GHB is frequently taken together with other psychoactive substances, and alcohol acts synergistically with GHB to produce respiratory and CNS depression (Mamelak 1989). GHB overdose also presents certain unusual clinical characteristics: patients may rapidly shift from an unconscious, apneic state requiring respiratory support to a markedly agitated, combative state, and back again (Li et al. 1998a), as well as become combative on recovery of consciousness (Chin et al. 1998). These combative states are frequently triggered by the stimulus of intubation attempts, which indicate an exaggerated gag reflex (Li et al. 1998b; Ross 1995). Fortunately, since GHB became a Schedule I controlled substance in 2000, the prevalence of illicit GHB use, abuse, intoxication, and overdose has declined (Carter et al. 2009).

Abstinence Syndrome

The development of tolerance for GHB has been repeatedly described in clinical vignettes and confirmed in animal models. For example, with repeated GHB treatment in mice, tolerance develops to both the hypolocomotion and the cataleptic effects of the drug (Itzhak and Ali 2002). There is also preclinical evidence of cross-tolerance and cross-dependence of GHB with alcohol (Colombo et al. 1995; Fadda et al. 1989). As described in the earlier subsection on clinical pharmacology, GHB and its analogs have been used in humans in the treatment of alcohol withdrawal. Nicholson and Balster (2001) reviewed the evidence for cross-tolerance and cross-dependence of GHB with alcohol.

In clinical trials with GHB, discontinuation syndromes were rarely mentioned (Addolorato et al. 1999c). However, numerous reports now exist of withdrawal syndromes clearly related to GHB or its precursors GBL and 1,4-BD (Craig et al. 2000; Dyer et al. 2001; McDaniel and Miotto 2001; Mycyk et al. 2001; Sivilotti et al. 2001). Craig and colleagues (2000) identified several probable antecedent factors that contribute to GHB withdrawal, including a history of prolonged GHB abuse with gradual dose escalation, the experience of dysphoria, anxiety and tremor on stopping, and numerous attempts to cut down or stop GHB use.

It is important for the clinician to obtain a clear history of the pattern of use of GHB or its precursors once the patient recovers from acute overdose. In the case of frequent dosing, the patient may be at high risk for severe withdrawal. A case series of 38 published reports reported that among heavily dependent users of GHB or its precursors, characterized by their use of 30 g/day or more of GHB or by a dosing frequency of at least every 8 hours, more than half deteriorated rapidly into a delirium state after initiating abstinence (McDonough et al. 2004). This high risk for severe withdrawal exists because a dose causing intoxication severe enough to require clinical treatment for overdose would have to be large enough to overcome the tolerance associated with repeated dosing. Most reports suggest that the distinguishing characteristic of patients presenting with the most clinically severe GHB withdrawal is a pattern of dosing at 2- to 4-hour intervals around the clock (Dyer et al. 2001; Hernandez et al. 1998; McDaniel and Miotto 2001; Miotto et al. 2001). This pattern of use is necessary in GHB-dependent patients because of the drug's short half-life. Severe withdrawal syndromes, which typically include delirium in daily users of more than 25 g, have been described in numerous case studies and surveys (Chin 2001; Craig et al. 2000; Hernandez et al. 1998; Hodges and Everett 1998; Sivilotti et al. 2001; Zvosec et al. 2001). Such withdrawal syndromes share similarities in symptom patterns to withdrawal from both alcohol and benzodiazepines.

The onset of GHB withdrawal symptoms typically begins 1–5 hours after the last dose; initial symptoms include anxiety, tremor, tachycardia, nausea, and insomnia (Table 9–1). Untreated, the symptoms may progress within 24 hours to a more severe pattern that is similar to delirium tremens, with dysfunction of cognition and sensorium, bouts of severe agitation, and autonomic dysregulation lasting up to 2 weeks (Dyer et al. 2001). Concurrent abuse of other sedative-hypnotics, in particular alcohol, may exacerbate the GHB withdrawal syndrome. The more severe forms of withdrawal typically occur within 48 hours of the last use and are characterized by delirium with auditory or visual hallucinations and confusion, horizontal nystagmus, autonomic instability with hypertension and increased temperature, and episodic agitation. Autonomic dysregulation characterized by tachycardia, fever, hypertension, and diaphoresis is generally milder than that seen in delirium tremens, and although generalized seizures are not reported, myoclonus resembling tonic-clonic movements has been described (see Dyer et al. 2001; Miotto and Roth 2001).

Table 9–1.   γ-Hydroxybutyrate (GHB) withdrawal syndrome

Severity of withdrawal	Symptoms
Mild	Tremor, anxiety, insomnia, mood lability, abdominal cramping, nausea, vomiting, palpitations, diaphoresis, tachycardia, miosis
Severe	Delirium with auditory or visual hallucinations and confusion, delusional thinking, autonomic instability with hypertension, increased temperature, severe agitation, horizontal nystagmus

Source.   Dyer et al. 2001; Mycyk et al. 2001.

Treatment

Overdose

The general treatment of GHB overdose is supportive medical care with a focus on the respiratory system. Patients typically regain consciousness in 2–5 hours. Commonly used coma reversal agents such as intravenous naloxone, glucose (50% dextrose in water), and flumazenil have had little benefit in GHB overdose (Li et al. 1998a). In addition, physostigmine has been suggested as a treatment for GHB overdose, but the risks of bradycardia and asystole in the context of GHB's short duration of action outweigh any purported benefits (Boyer et al. 2001).

Abstinence Syndrome

Milder forms of withdrawal, typically seen with lower frequency of dosing or lower cumulative daily doses, may be successfully treated with benzodiazepines on an outpatient basis (Addolorato et al. 1999c; Galloway et al. 1997). Severe withdrawal states typically require medical support, high doses of intravenous benzodiazepines, and capacity for physical restraint to prevent the patient from harming self or others during bouts of psychotic agitation (Dyer et al. 2001; Miotto and Roth 2001; Mycyk et al. 2001). Reports of the failure of benzodiazepines to adequately control symptoms of GHB withdrawal (Friedman et al. 1996; Mullins and Fitzmaurice 2001) have raised the question of how best to treat the disorder. The probable explanation for the observed lack of response is underdosing of the benzodiazepines. Many case reports have found that patients in severe GHB withdrawal may require very high doses of intravenous benzodiazepines such as lorazepam, diazepam, or even midazolam to control agitation and autonomic dysregulation. The average intravenous dosage of lorazepam given over a 24-hour period in these cases has ranged from 8 to 10 mg/hour (Chin 2001; Craig et al. 2000). Craig and colleagues (2000) reported the case of a patient who needed 2,655 mg of diazepam equivalents (507 mg of lorazepam plus 120 mg of diazepam) over 90 hours to control agitation. For patients taking high doses of benzodiazepines, Miotto and Roth (2001) suggest the use of pulse oximetry to monitor for oxygen desaturation. After a diagnosis of GHB withdrawal is established, it is likely that early aggressive dosing with benzodiazepines under careful medical supervision will reduce the severity and chronicity of acute GHB withdrawal, but this approach remains to be validated.

Other sedative-hypnotic medications, such as barbiturates, may play a useful role in severe withdrawal from this group of drugs. For example, in a case series of GBL withdrawal, use of intravenous pentobarbital in the range of 1–2 mg/kg/hour lowered the total requirement for intravenous lorazepam (Sivilotti et al. 2001). Antipsychotic medications are often used to reduce psychotic agitation. However, because antipsychotic medications lower the seizure threshold and may contribute to loss of central control of temperature, leading to hyperthermia or neuroleptic malignant syndrome (NMS), they are not indicated as first-line medications for GHB withdrawal delirium (Dyer and Roth 2001; McDaniel and Miotto 2001; Sharma et al. 2001). Nonetheless, antipsychotic agents have been used most commonly as an adjunct to benzodiazepines in the management of GHB withdrawal (McDonough et al. 2004). In addition, Eiden and colleagues (2011) described a case of a patient tolerant to GBL who presented symptoms consistent with NMS, apparently precipitated by neuroleptics that were administered to control her symptoms of agitation and auditory and visual hallucinations. If antipsychotics are needed, second-generation agents are preferred because of their lower risk for dystonia, dyskinesia, and NMS (McDaniel and Miotto 2001; Olivera et al. 1990).

Freese et al. (2002) proposed that anticonvulsants such as gabapentin, which inhibit glutamate production, may reduce glutamate-induced excitotoxicity, thus reducing the severity of GHB withdrawal. However logical this may be, little evidence supports this intervention at present, except that the use of gabapentin, sodium valproate, or carbamazepine administered adjunctively with benzodiazepines has been described in a few published case reports (McDaniel and Miotto 2001).

Finally, some evidence indicates that GHB as a tapering dosage can be used to detoxify individuals from GHB. In a prospective case series, de Jong and colleagues (2012) successfully stabilized 23 GHB-dependent inpatients by titrating to 70% of the estimated self-administration dose with pharmaceutical GHB (150 mg/mL). The drug was first administered within 1.5–2 hours after the last patient self-administration dose and then every 3 hours over 1–2 days, followed by tapering the dosage by 0.3–0.45 g per dose each day. Objective and subjective withdrawal symptoms were used to monitor withdrawal, and although most experienced uncomfortable withdrawal symptoms during the GHB troughs in the first few days, none developed delirium or psychosis (de Jong et al. 2012).

GHB Dependence

Although the evidence base for this relatively rare disorder is not well developed, patients who are dependent on GHB appear to benefit from cognitive and motivational psychosocial therapies and from support of recovery in a manner similar to alcohol-dependent patients. However, because of the high likelihood of amnesia and cognitive dysfunction during the acute and subacute phases of GHB withdrawal, psychosocial interventions should, when possible, include significant others who can review and reinforce with the patient the negative consequences of GHB dependence.

3,4-Methylenedioxymethamphetamine ("Ecstasy")

MDMA is commonly known as Ecstasy. Other slang names include XTC, X, E, Adam, clarity, and lover's speed. MDMA is chemically similar to the stimulant amphetamine and the hallucinogen mescaline. Because MDMA has hallucinogenic effects, it is also discussed in Chapter 7, "Hallucinogens and Related Drugs." It was developed in the early 1900s as a chemical precursor in the synthesis of pharmaceutical agents and was patented by Merck in 1914. MDMA was initially thought to have appetite suppressant properties, but it was never marketed for that indication. The first reported "underground" synthesis of MDMA occurred in 1967. The United Kingdom placed MDMA on

Schedule I in 1977, and the United States did so in 1985. During the 1970s, MDMA was used by some psychotherapists to enhance the therapy process in the treatment of depression, trauma, and other psychiatric disorders (Moonzwe et al. 2011). Although this use was based on the drug's purported empathogenic or "relationship-enhancing" properties, until very recently it had not been shown in high quality studies to be effective in this role, and it remains an illegal substance with no accepted medical uses (Moonzwe et al. 2011). Recent small randomized trials (Mithoefer et al. 2011, 2013; Oehen et al. 2013) have demonstrated that at least two sessions of MDMA-assisted manualized psychotherapy appear safe and may be of both short- and longer-term benefit in patients with treatment-resistant posttraumatic stress disorder (PTSD). One study ($N=20$) demonstrated significant reductions in clinician-rated PTSD symptoms at 2 months (Mithoefer et al. 2011) and long-term follow-up (mean = 3.5 years) (Mithoefer et al. 2013), whereas the other, using an active control over three sessions, demonstrated significant reductions in self-rated but not clinician-rated PTSD symptoms at 1-year follow-up (Oehen et al. 2013). It is as yet unclear whether the mechanism of benefit is due to the direct psychopharmacological effects of MDMA, such as decreased fear responding, or due to general facilitation of targeted psychotherapeutic interventions delivered over extended (8-hour) sessions.

Epidemiology and Clinical Presentation

Before its designation as a Schedule I drug in the United States in 1985, MDMA had a low level of use (Green et al. 2012). Use of MDMA tapered off in the period immediately following its designation as a Schedule I drug (Koesters et al. 2002). However, the 1990s saw a resurgence in the use of MDMA, and its use continued to increase among adolescents in the early 2000s, becoming more commonly used than cocaine/crack. According to the Monitoring the Future Survey for 2009, 6.5% of twelfth-grade students had used MDMA at least once in their lifetime, and nearly 2% of twelfth-grade students had used MDMA in the month before being surveyed (Johnston et al. 2010). These numbers reached their peak in 2000–2002 and had been generally declining since then, although recently there may have been a rising trend (Johnston et al. 2010). High school students generally view MDMA as easily accessible and as having a low harm potential (Johnston et al. 2010).

MDMA is a white, tasteless powder in its pure form that may be ingested orally, smoked, injected, or inhaled (Karlsen et al. 2007). It is commonly taken orally, usually in a tablet or capsule. The onset of effect is typically sudden, within 30–60 minutes. These effects generally last 3–6 hours, but they may persist as long as 8 hours (Baylen and Rosenberg 2006; Gouzoulis-Mayfrank and Daumann 2006; Jerrard 1990). Intoxication with MDMA is usually described as occurring in three stages (Koesters et al. 2002; Parrott and Lasky 1998). The initial stage consists of disorientation. This leads to the second stage of "yielding to tingling and spasmodic jerking" (Koesters et al. 2002). The final ("target") stage of MDMA intoxication consists of the typical response of increased sociability, increased mental clarity, a feeling of emotional warmth and closeness to others, and a general sense of well-being (Cami et al. 2000; Koesters et al. 2002; Parrott and Lasky 1998). At higher doses, frank euphoria is experienced. A "hangover" is common the next day and can last for up to 48 hours. Side effects (including confusion, depression, insomnia, anxiety, and paranoia) have been reported to occur for weeks after ingestion (Curran and Travill 1997; Parrott and Lasky 1998).

The threshold dose of MDMA is 30 mg, but the average dose is 80–150 mg, with some users taking more than 200 mg. The lethal dose is estimated (from animal data) to be approximately 6,000 mg. On the street, concentrations of MDMA can vary greatly, and tablets may also contain other substances such as methylenedioxyamphetamine (MDA) and methylenedioxyethylamphetamine (MDE) (Sherlock et al. 1999). The presence of these other substances is often associated with emergency presentations because of their narrower "therapeutic" windows.

Basic and Clinical Pharmacology

Acutely, MDMA acts to increase serotonin, but with chronic use, decreases in serotonin are noted, suggesting loss of serotonergic neurons (Montoya et al. 2002; Sprague et al. 1998). Decreases in serotonin transporter (SERT) levels also have been reported (McCann et al. 1998; Schouw et al. 2012). MDMA's use is also correlated with secondary increases in dopamine in the basal ganglia (Sprague et al. 1998). MDMA acts primarily in the frontal cortex, leading to effects on cognition and memory. It also works on the limbic system, leading to MDMA's effects on mood, anxiety, and emotions. Metabolism occurs through the cytochrome P450 2D6 enzyme system, although 20% is excreted unchanged in the urine (Karlsen et al. 2007; Tucker et al. 1994).

Toxicology

In the emergency setting, MDMA intoxication is usually seen in conjunction with dehydration, hyperthermia, tachycardia, hypertension, liver failure, rhabdomyolysis, and/or renal failure, often mimicking NMS (Jonas and Graeme-Cook 2001; Karlsen et al. 2007; Lester et al. 2000; Montoya et al. 2002; Schwartz and Miller 1997). The physical symptoms may be accompanied by symptoms of anxiety, agitation, and even confusion (Montoya et al. 2002). Because these presentations are nonspecific, they lead to a wide differential diagnosis. Nevertheless, the clinician must have a high index of suspicion of a substance-induced basis for behavioral emergency presentations in most adolescents and young adults (Williams et al. 1998). The diagnosis is complicated by the fact that routine urine toxicology screens do not typically detect the presence of MDMA, although occasionally cross-reactivity with amphetamines may occur (Koesters et al. 2002; Shannon 2000). Although rare, death from MDMA overdose has been reported and is most commonly related to hyperthermia and hyponatremia (Rogers et al. 2009).

MDMA's toxicity may be related to its effects on serotonergic neurons and to oxidative stress and free radical formation (Bolla et al. 1998; Gouzoulis-Mayfrank and Daumann 2006; McCann et al. 2000; Montoya et al. 2002). In animal studies, these processes are associated with exaggerated pruning in those regions of the brain with high serotonergic activity, particularly the hippocampus and amygdala (Green et al. 2012; Ricaurte et al. 1988, 2000). These changes may be long lasting, persisting for as long as 7 years after MDMA exposure, although at least partial recovery may be possible with abstinence (Gouzoulis-Mayfrank and Daumann 2006; Hatzidimitriou et al. 1999).

The neurochemical changes caused by MDMA result in significant, observable functional impairment as well. These impairments occur in areas of the brain that have high concentrations of serotonergic neurons. Most notably affected are cognition and memory (Gouzoulis-Mayfrank and Daumann 2006; Montoya et al. 2002). Studies have shown decreases in word recall, as well as poorer functioning in general measures of memory (Montoya et al. 2002;

Morgan 1999; Rodgers 2000; Verkes et al. 2001). It remains unclear if this effect is dose related or independent of dose (Bolla et al. 1998). Moreover, these effects may be compounded when MDMA and marijuana are combined (Gouzoulis-Mayfrank et al. 2000; Taffe 2012).

Treatment

General principles of the treatment of MDMA intoxication are the same as those for intoxication with other stimulants, such as cocaine and methamphetamine. Overdoses of MDMA are generally treated with supportive care, because no specific pharmacological treatments have been identified (Shannon 2000; Solhkhah and Wilens 1998). This approach includes the use of routine laboratory tests to detect electrolyte abnormalities and to assess renal and hepatic functioning (Koesters et al. 2002). Adequate rehydration is crucial. Occasionally, the use of sedatives such as the benzodiazepines is indicated, particularly when extreme agitation is present. If pronounced hyperthermia, hypertension, or rhabdomyolysis is present, observation in an intensive care unit may be indicated. Observation may be combined with the use of dantrolene sodium (a skeletal muscle relaxant) at doses of 2–3 mg/kg intravenously three times a day.

MDMA has been associated with significant increases in heart rate and blood pressure, similar to the increases associated with amphetamine use (Lester et al. 2000). This effect may require acute treatment with antihypertensives such as calcium channel blockers or nitroprusside (Koesters et al. 2002). The use of MDMA during raves may lead to dehydration, hypertension, intracerebral hemorrhage, heart failure, liver failure, kidney damage, and malignant hyperthermia (Barrett and Taylor 1993; Baylen and Rosenberg 2006; Harries and De Silva 1992; Jonas and Graeme-Cook 2001). Its use is often associated with jaw clenching (trismus) and bruxism (Jerrard 1990; Karlsen et al. 2007; Shannon 2000). This effect explains the use of pacifiers or lollipops by teenagers on the dance floor.

As was previously mentioned, a hangover-like syndrome is common the next day after use of MDMA. MDMA withdrawal, which is thought to be caused by serotonin depletion, can last for weeks and includes symptoms of depression, anxiety, restlessness, and insomnia (Allen et al. 1993; McGuire et al. 1994). No specific treatments are currently indicated for this withdrawal syndrome, although the antidepressant bupropion may be helpful (Solhkhah and Wilens 1998; Solhkhah et al. 2001). Teenage lore has it that use of selective serotonin reuptake inhibitors (SSRIs) may alleviate those symptoms acutely, but some preliminary data may in fact support the opposite effect. In addition, MDMA use may be associated with sexual dysfunction (Baylen and Rosenberg 2006; Buffum and Moser 1986). This effect has led to use of a combination of MDMA and sildenafil (Viagra; "sexctasy").

Ketamine

Ketamine [2(2-chlorophenyl)-2-(methylamino)-cyclohexanone] is a Schedule III cyclohexane injectable anesthetic approved for human and veterinary use. It is known by the slang names K, Special K, Vitamin K, and Cat Valium (Bobo and Miller 2002; Canet and Castillo 2012; Covvey et al. 2012). Because it has hallucinogenic effects, it is also discussed in Chapter 7, "Hallucinogens and Related Drugs." Ketamine is produced in a liquid form or as a white powder and is usually ingested orally or intranasally but is occasionally administered intramuscularly. It is a phencyclidine (PCP) analog that was first developed in 1962. It has amnestic, analgesic, and anesthetic properties (Canet and Castillo 2012; Covvey et al. 2012) and has recently gained interest as a possible antidepressant (at a dose of 0.5 mg/kg), particularly for patients with treatment-resistant major depressive disorder or bipolar depression (Covvey et al. 2012; Diazgranados et al. 2010). The antidepressant effects of ketamine seem to be rapid and consistent and can be evident after a single dose (Covvey et al. 2012; Murrough 2012).

Epidemiology and Clinical Presentation

As with the other club drugs, the use of ketamine has increased over the past decade. Although ketamine use remains much less common than use of MDMA, it is still an important cause of emergency presentations (Koesters et al. 2002). Estimates of lifetime use vary between 0.1% and 4% of the population (Kalsi et al. 2011). The use of ketamine leads to dose-dependent dissociative episodes (Bowdle et al. 1988). Emergence from ketamine-induced anesthetic effects leads to a variety of symptoms that are generally described as psychedelic by users, including "intense alterations in mood, perception, thinking, body awareness, and self-control" (Bowdle et al. 1988).

Basic and Clinical Pharmacology

Ketamine is a noncompetitive *N*-methyl-D-aspartate receptor antagonist and is generally considered a psychotomimetic or schizophrenomimetic. Ketamine also appears to have cholinergic, opioidergic, and glutamatergic effects (Covvey et al. 2012; Koesters et al. 2002; Stone et al. 2012). The drug has been shown to increase plasma cortisol and prolactin levels, although the physiological significance of these effects is unclear (Krystal et al. 1994). Large doses of ketamine produce reactions similar to those produced by PCP, which include dreamlike states, dissociation, and hallucinations (Koesters et al. 2002; Krystal et al. 1994; Murrough 2012). Important differences between ketamine and PCP include ketamine's lower potency, shorter duration of action, and tendency to cause less agitation. In general, the psychotic symptoms associated with ketamine include both positive and negative symptoms and may include catatonia (informally described as a "K-hole") (Koesters et al. 2002; Krystal et al. 1994). Functionally, ketamine leads to increased glutamatergic neurotransmission, predominantly in the anterior cingulate cortex (Stone et al. 2012). Ketamine is metabolized via the cytochrome P450 system and has two major metabolites: dehydronorketamine and norketamine (Kalsi et al. 2011). Excretion is entirely via the urine.

For recreational use, ketamine is often snorted, is sometimes smoked with marijuana or tobacco products, and also may be injected intramuscularly (Weiner et al. 2000). The typical street dose of ketamine ranges from 30 to 300 mg. These amounts are in contrast to the clinical doses used for anesthesia, which range from 2 to 10 mg/kg. Ketamine has a half-life of less than 2 hours (Koesters et al. 2002; Reich and Silvay 1989).

At low doses, ketamine may result in impairment of attention, learning ability, and memory; at high doses, it has been associated with delirium, amnesia, impaired motor function, hypertension, depression, and respiratory depression (Krystal et al. 1994). Another mechanism of action appears to be a blocking of the reuptake of catecholamines. This effect leads to an increase in heart rate and blood pressure (Reich and Silvay 1989).

Toxicology

In overdose, ketamine may lead to hyperthermia, seizures, hypertensive crisis, coma, and even death. Ketamine also may produce nonspecific abdominal pain ("K-cramps") (Kalsi et al. 2011). These symptoms are generally thought to result from ketamine's catecholaminergic effects (Reich and Silvay 1989). Ketamine is physically addicting, with a short-term (~48-hour) withdrawal syndrome (Critchlow 2006; Jansen and Darracot-Cankovic 2001; Winstock and Mitcheson 2012). Recent animal studies indicate that chronic ketamine use may lead to cognitive impairments (Kalsi et al. 2011; Venancio et al. 2011).

In the ED setting, the diagnosis of ketamine intoxication is a clinical one. Ketamine is not routinely detected by urine toxicology tests, although it can be detected with high-performance liquid chromatography (Koesters et al. 2002). As with MDMA, the initial assessment for ketamine intoxication includes the use of routine laboratory tests to detect electrolyte abnormalities and to evaluate renal and hepatic functioning (Koesters et al. 2002). It is worth noting that although ketamine's median lethal dose in animals is 100-fold the typical intravenous therapeutic dose, deaths due to ketamine overdose have been reported (Kalsi et al. 2011).

Treatment

No specific treatments for ketamine intoxication are currently indicated (Solhkhah and Wilens 1998). General supportive care, including providing the patient with a quiet, low-stimulus environment, can be helpful (Koesters et al. 2002; White et al. 1982). Benzodiazepines may be useful, particularly if agitation is present, although clinicians must be mindful of a possible interaction leading to a prolonged half-life for ketamine (Lahti et al. 1995; Lo and Cumming 1975). In general, because of the short half-life of ketamine, patients usually require observation only for several hours and then can be released home (Koesters et al. 2002).

As with many other hallucinogens, ketamine use may be associated with flashbacks. These flashbacks are generally milder and less frequent than those associated with PCP use (Fine and Finestone 1973). Generally, treatment with an antipsychotic is not required and can occasionally make symptoms worse (Solhkhah et al. 2000).

Synthetic Cannabinoids

Spice, Spice Gold, Spice Diamond, K2, Kush, Blaze, Aroma, Magma, Sence, King Krypto, Colorado Chronic, and Red X Dawn are the names most commonly applied to herbal products containing a class of synthetic cannabinoid drugs that activate cannabinoid-1 (CB_1) receptors. Although these drugs have agonist properties at G protein–coupled CB_1 receptors, most have a chemical structure that is not derived from delta-9-tetrahydrocannabinol (Δ^9-THC) and, until recently, were sold legally on Internet sites and through other retail channels such as "head shops" (Seely et al. 2011). In addition, because of their chemical structure, they were not detectible in standard assays for drugs of abuse (Auwärter et al. 2009). Spice and related products marketed as incense or as plant food (e.g., Bonsai-18) and labeled "not for human consumption" are smoked or consumed orally as an infusion of a mixture of herbs such as mugwort and skullcap that has been processed with the synthetic cannabinoids (Vardakou et al. 2010). Other common herbs that have been used in Spice-type preparations include aromatic herbs, marshmallow, red clover, rose, and vanilla, as well as others purported to have mild psychoactive effects such as Bay Bean (*Canavalia maritima*), Blue Lotus (*Nymphaea caerulea*), dwarf skullcap (*Scutellaria nana*), Indian warrior (*Pedicularis densiflora*), Lion's Tail (*Leonotis leonurus*), Lousewort (*Pedicularis sp.*), Maconha Brava (*Zornia latifolia*), and Siberian motherwort (*Leonurus sibiricus*) (Seely et al. 2011). Because of a prior lack of regulation, there has been inconsistent appraisal and monitoring of the manufacture and distribution of these products, leading to a variety of contents and potency since the first products became available for purchase in the early 2000s and over the Internet in 2004 (Auwärter et al. 2009; Seely et al. 2011).

With the increasing popularity of Spice, there have been concomitant reports from EDs of Spice-related adverse effects, such as convulsions, anxiety attacks, dangerously elevated heart rates, increased blood pressure, vomiting, and disorientation. In response to these adverse effects and the rise in Spice's popularity, in March 2011, the U.S. Drug Enforcement Administration (DEA) used its emergency scheduling authority to temporarily place five of the extant synthetic cannabinoids (JWH-018, JWH-073, JWH-200, CP-47,497, and cannabicyclohexanol, the CP-47,497 dimethyloctyl homologue) commonly found in Spice and other products under Schedule I of the Controlled Substances Act for a 1-year observation period. Eighteen states in the United States had already controlled one or more of the five synthetic cannabinoids as of January 2011 (U.S. Department of Justice 2011). The public safety concerns about Spice are also present in many other countries, and beginning in

2009, synthetic cannabinoid receptor agonists have been controlled in several European countries, including Austria, Denmark, Estonia, France, Germany, Hungary, Ireland, Italy, Latvia, Lithuania, Luxembourg, the Netherlands, Poland, Romania, Russia, Sweden, Switzerland, and the United Kingdom, as well as in Canada (Dargan et al. 2011; Vardakou et al. 2010).

Epidemiology and Clinical Presentation

Acute Effects

Δ^9-THC causes physical relaxation, perceptual changes, mild euphoria, reduced motor coordination, increased appetite, and decreased information processing in humans (Seely et al. 2011). The typical acute effects of synthetic cannabinoids are similar in to those of Δ^9-THC: reddened conjunctivae, xerostomia, increased appetite, impaired time sense, and mood changes ranging from euphoria to dysphoria, with alterations in perception. However, synthetic cannabinoids also produce frequent anxiety, light-headedness, increased heart rate, and palpitations, with hallucinations reported by a quarter of respondents in one survey of users (Vandrey et al. 2012; Vardakou et al. 2010). The duration of effects depends on the admixture of the various synthetic cannabinoids in the herbal product. For example, compared with Δ^9-THC, the effects of CP-47,497-C8 are longer lasting (i.e., 5–6 hours), whereas JWH-018 effects typically last about 1–2 hours (Vardakou et al. 2010).

Cannabidiol, another compound found in cannabis, may have antipsychotic and other ameliorating effects and thus may be relatively protective in natural cannabis use (Bhattacharyya et al. 2010). Because its components are CB_1 and CB_2 agonists, Spice is lacking in cannabidiol; thus, its active CB_1 agonist effects, which produce sedation and dysphoria and are probably psychotogenic, are not counterbalanced by it (Alverio et al. 2011; Russo and Guy 2006). In one case study, a man who had repeated psychotic episodes in the context of cannabis abuse and had been stable for 2 years on antipsychotic medication had an immediate exacerbation of his schizophrenia symptoms in the context of Spice use, as well as the onset of new command auditory and persecutory hallucinations (Müller et al. 2010). Because of the increased prevalence of synthetic cannabis use in New Orleans, Louisiana, three cases of acute psychosis caused by smoking Spice occurred in one 12-hour period (Rodgman et al. 2011). These findings were replicated in a small set ($N=15$)

of male inpatients with histories of psychotic illness, among whom 13 (87%) had used synthetic cannabinoids in the form of the product Aroma (containing JWH-018) over the preceding 12 months; of those who had used Aroma, 69% had psychotic symptoms following use, with 38% having a full relapse of psychosis within 24 hours (Every-Palmer 2011). The capacity of synthetic cannabinoids to induce a recurrent psychosis independent of a family history of psychosis or an underlying diathesis for it is currently unclear. However, Spice can induce acute psychosis (visual hallucinations, disorganized and bizarre behavior) in individuals without histories of psychotic symptoms (Peglow et al. 2012).

Chronic Effects
Case reports have described apathy and cognitive impairment resulting from the chronic use of synthetic cannabinoids (Zimmermann et al. 2009).

Basic and Clinical Pharmacology

Spice or K2 products typically contain synthetic compounds including nonclassic cannabinoids (e.g., CP-47,497) and synthetic aminoalkylindole derivatives such as JWH-018, as well as the classic cannabinoid HU-210, a dibenzopyran derivative that is a Schedule I controlled substance in the United States (Seely et al. 2011). Although most classic cannabinoids are CB_1 and CB_2 partial agonists, CP-47,497, JWH-018, and HU-210 also bind and activate CB_1 receptors, but as full agonists with a higher affinity (CP-47,497, 20-fold; JWH-018, fourfold) and a stronger potency than Δ^9-THC (Mackie 2008; Vardakou et al. 2010). Although the safety of these moieties has not been tested, scores of other cannabinomimetic compounds have been synthesized in recent years (Huffman and Padgett 2005).

Toxicology

Overdose Effects
Spice or K2 use is associated with many effects similar to those produced by cannabis, as well as effects that are not typically seen after cannabis use (Seely et al. 2011). Although Spice and K2 have not been formally tested in laboratory and Phase I safety trials to determine what constitutes actual overdoses, agitation, lethargy, anxiety, irritability, nausea, vomiting, tachycardia, elevated

blood pressure, chest pain, tremors, numbness, tingling, seizures, hallucinations, paranoia, and nonresponsiveness after synthetic cannabinoid use have been reported by the DEA and by poison control and ED physicians (Faircloth et al. 2012; Seely et al. 2011).

Abstinence Syndrome

Chronically administered Δ^9-THC causes receptor downregulation (Rodriguez et al. 2001) and desensitization (Sim et al. 1996), leading to tolerance to its acute effects. Similarly, observations from case reports suggest that tolerance to the effects of various synthetic cannabinoids with dose escalation can develop relatively quickly, which may not be surprising given their potent effects at CB_1 and CB_2 receptors as compared with Δ^9-THC (Zimmermann et al. 2009). Zimmermann et al. (2009) reported a case of withdrawal symptoms developing 4–7 days after cessation of daily high-dose (3 g) Spice smoking, with symptoms including profuse sweating, nausea, tremor, headache, increased blood pressure, tachycardia, drug craving, dissociative phenomena, nightmares, and restlessness. An international Internet survey of Spice use conducted by Vandrey and colleagues (2012) found that 38% of 168 appropriate study completers had previously experienced symptoms of tolerance and that withdrawal symptoms were present among the frequent users, with symptoms including headaches, anxiety/nervousness, coughing, sleep disturbance, anger/irritability, impatience, difficulty concentrating, restlessness, nausea, and depressed mood.

Treatment

As with cannabis-induced psychosis, the treatment of synthetic cannabinoid overdose is supportive care and reassurance (Rodgman et al. 2011). Severe anxiety can be treated symptomatically with benzodiazepines, and tachycardia, if severe, can be treated with β-blockers (Rodgman et al. 2011). In the survey by Vandrey et al. (2012), almost half of the 168 respondents had symptoms that met DSM-IV-TR criteria for abuse or dependence, yet none had sought or received treatment. Because no studies of the treatment of synthetic cannabinoid dependence have been published, it behooves the clinician to rely on general knowledge of substance dependence treatment and a working knowledge of the pharmacology of these drugs. Clearly, familiarity with the pharmacology, acute effects, withdrawal symptoms, and characteristics of cannabis and treatment of the dependence syndrome should inform the general approach to the treatment of on synthetic cannabis analog dependence.

Conclusion

There is an epidemic of club drug use, which is of greatest concern among adolescents. Use of club drugs is particularly problematic among individuals with psychiatric illness, including mood disorders, anxiety disorders, and attention-deficit/hyperactivity disorder (American Academy of Child and Adolescent Psychiatry 1998; Armentano 1995). Clinicians need to be aware of the ever-changing patterns of drug abuse. The club drugs as a group are not benign, although youths often perceive them as such (Johnston et al. 2010). Use of these drugs often has serious and occasionally fatal consequences.

References

Addolorato G, Castelli E, Stefanini GF, et al: An open multicentric study evaluating 4-hydroxybutyric acid sodium salt in the medium-term treatment of 179 alcohol dependent subjects. Alcohol Alcohol 31:341–345, 1996

Addolorato G, Balducci G, Capristo E, et al: Gamma-hydroxybutyric acid (GHB) in the treatment of alcohol withdrawal syndrome: a randomized comparative study versus benzodiazepine. Alcohol Clin Exp Res 23:1596–604, 1999a

Addolorato G, Capristo E, Gessa GL, et al: Long-term administration of GHB does not affect muscular mass in alcoholics. Life Sci 65:PL191–PL196, 1999b

Addolorato G, Caputo F, Capristo E, et al: A case of gamma-hydroxybutyric acid withdrawal syndrome during alcohol addiction treatment: utility of diazepam administration. Clin Neuropharmacol 22:60–62, 1999c

Addolorato G, Caputo F, Capristo E, et al: Gamma-hydroxybutyric acid: efficacy, potential abuse, and dependence in the treatment of alcohol addiction. Alcohol 20:217–222, 2000

Allen RP, McCann UD, Ricaurte GA: Persistent effects of +/- 3,4-methylenedioxy-methamphetamine (MDMA, "ecstasy") on human sleep. Sleep 16:560–564, 1993

Alverio C, Reddy A, Hernandez E, et al: Synthetic cannabis "Spice," more potent than natural cannabis and may have increased risk for psychosis. Presented at the American Academy of Addiction Psychiatry Annual Meeting, Scottsdale, AZ, December 2011

American Academy of Child and Adolescent Psychiatry: Practice parameters for the assessment and treatment of children and adolescents with substance abuse disorders. J Am Acad Child Adolesc Psychiatry 37:122–126, 1998

American Psychiatric Association: Diagnostic and Statistical Manual of Mental Disorders, 4th Edition, Text Revision. Washington, DC, American Psychiatric Association, 2000

Armentano M: Assessment, diagnosis, and treatment of the dually diagnosed adolescent. Pediatr Clin North Am 42:479–490, 1995

Auwärter V, Dresen S, Weinmann W, et al: "Spice" and other herbal blends: harmless incense or cannabinoid designer drugs? J Mass Spectrom 44:832–837, 2009

Barrett PJ, Taylor GT: "Ecstasy" ingestion: a case report of severe complications. J R Soc Med 86:233–234, 1993

Baylen CA, Rosenberg H: A review of the acute subjective effects of MDMA/ecstasy. Addiction 101:933–947, 2006

Bhattacharyya S, Morrison PD, Fusar-Poli P, et al: Opposite effects of delta-9-tetrahydrocannabinol and cannabidiol on human brain function and psychopathology. Neuropsychopharmacology 35:764–774, 2010

Bobo WV, Miller SC: Ketamine as a preferred substance of abuse. Am J Addict 11:332–334, 2002

Bolla KI, McCann UD, Ricaurte GA: Memory impairment in abstinent MDMA ("ecstasy") users. Neurology 51:1532–1537, 1998

Borgen L, Lane E, Lai A: Xyrem (sodium oxybate): a study of dose proportionality in healthy human subjects. J Clin Pharmacol 40:1053, 2000

Borgen LA, Okerholm R, Morrison D, et al: The influence of gender and food on the pharmacokinetics of sodium oxybate oral solution in healthy subjects. J Clin Pharmacol 43:59–65, 2003

Bowdle TA, Radant AD, Crowley DS, et al: Psychedelic effects of ketamine in healthy volunteers: relationship to steady-state plasma concentrations. Anesthesiology 88:82–88, 1988

Boyer EW, Quang L, Woolf A, et al: Use of physostigmine in the management of gamma-hydroxybutyrate overdose (letter). Ann Emerg Med 38:346, 2001

Buffum J, Moser C: MDMA and human sexual dysfunction. J Psychoactive Drugs 18:355–359, 1986

Cami J, Farre M, Mas M, et al. Human pharmacology of 3,4-methylenedioxymethamphetamine ("ecstasy"): psychomotor performance and subjective effects. J Clin Psychopharmacol 20:455–466, 2000

Canet J, Castillo J: Ketamine: a familiar drug we trust. Anesthesiology 116:35–46, 2012

Carter LP, Pardi D, Gorsline J, et al: Illicit gamma-hydroxybutyrate (GHB) and pharmaceutical sodium oxybate (Xyrem): differences in characteristics and misuse. Drug Alcohol Depend 104:1–10, 2009

Centers for Disease Control and Prevention: Gamma hydroxy butyrate use—New York and Texas, 1995–96. JAMA 277:1511, 1997

Centers for Disease Control and Prevention: Adverse events associated with ingestion of gamma-butyrolactone—Minnesota, New Mexico, and Texas, 1998–1999. MMRW Morb Mortal Wkly Rep 48:137–140, 1999

Chatlos JC: Recent trends and a developmental approach to substance abuse in adolescents. Child Adolesc Psychiatr Clin N Am 5:1–27, 1996

Chin RL: A case of severe withdrawal from gamma-hydroxybutyrate. Ann Emerg Med 37:551–552, 2001

Chin RL, Sporer KA, Cullison B, et al: Clinical course of gamma-hydroxybutyrate overdose. Ann Emerg Med 31:716–722, 1998

Colombo G, Agabio R, Lobina C, et al: Cross-tolerance to ethanol and gamma-hydroxybutyric acid. Eur J Pharmacol 273:235–238, 1995

Cook PA, Clark P, Bellis MA, et al: Re-emerging syphilis in the UK: a behavioral analysis of infected individuals. Commun Dis Public Health 4:253–258, 2001

Covvey JR, Crawford AN, Lowe DK: Intravenous ketamine for treatment-resistant major depressive disorder. Ann Pharmacother 46:117–123, 2012

Craig K, Gomez HF, McManus JL, et al: Severe gamma-hydroxybutyrate withdrawal: a case report and literature review. J Emerg Med 18:65–70, 2000

Critchlow DG: A case of ketamine dependence with discontinuation symptoms. Addiction 101:1212–1213, 2006

Curran HV, Travill RA: Mood and cognitive effects of +/-3,4 methylenedioxymethamphetamine (MDMA, "ecstasy"): week-end "high" followed by a mid-week low. Addiction 92:821–831, 1997

Dargan PI, Hudson S, Ramsey J, et al: The impact of changes in UK classification of the synthetic cannabinoid receptor agonists in "spice." Int J Drug Policy 22:274–277, 2011

de Jong CA, Kamal R, Dijkstra BA, et al: Gamma-hydroxybutyrate detoxification by titration and tapering. Eur Addict Res 18:40–45, 2012

Diazgranados N, Ibrahim L, Brutsche NE, et al: A randomized add-on trial of N-methyl-o-aspartate antagonist in treatment-resistant bipolar depression. Arch Gen Psychiatry 67:793–802, 2010

Dyer JE, Roth B: In reply (letter). Ann Emerg Med 38:606, 2001

Dyer JE, Roth B, Hyma BA: Gamma-hydroxybutyrate withdrawal syndrome. Ann Emerg Med 37:147–153, 2001

Eiden C, Capdevielle D, Deddouche C, et al: Neuroleptic malignant syndrome-like reaction precipitated by antipsychotics in a patient with gamma-butyrolactone withdrawal. J Addict Med 5:302–303, 2011

Every-Palmer S: Synthetic cannabinoid JWH-018 and psychosis: an explorative study. Drug Alcohol Depend 117:152–157, 2011

Fadda F, Columbo G, Mosca E, et al: Suppression by gamma-hydroxybutyric acid of ethanol withdrawal syndrome in rats. Alcohol Alcohol 24:447–451, 1989

Faircloth J, Khandheria B, Shum S: Case report: adverse reaction to synthetic marijuana. Am J Addict 21:289–290, 2012

Fine J, Finestone SC: Sensory disturbances following ketamine anesthesia: recurrent hallucinations. Anesth Analg 52:428–430, 1973

Freese TE, Miotto K, Reback CJ: The effects and consequences of selected club drugs. J Subst Abuse Treat 23:151–156, 2002

Friedman J, Westlake R, Furman M: "Grievous bodily harm": gamma hydroxybutyrate abuse leading to Wernicke-Korsakoff syndrome. Neurology 46:469–471, 1996

Gallimberti L, Ferri M, Ferrara SD, et al: Gamma-hydroxybutyric acid in the treatment of alcohol dependence: a double-blind study. Alcohol Clin Exp Res 16:673–676, 1992

Gallimberti L, Spella MR, Soncini CA, et al: Gamma-hydroxybutyric acid in the treatment of alcohol and heroin dependence. Alcohol 20:257–262, 2000

Galloway GP, Frederick SL, Staggers FE Jr, et al: Gamma-hydroxybutyrate: an emerging drug of abuse that causes physical dependence. Addiction 92:89–96, 1997

Galloway GP, Frederick-Osborne SL, Seymour R, et al: Abuse and therapeutic potential of gamma-hydroxybutyric acid. Alcohol 20:263–269, 2000

Gerra G, Caccavari R, Fontanesi B, et al: Flumazenil effects on growth hormone response to gamma-hydroxybutyric acid. Int Clin Psychopharmacol 9:211–215, 1994

Gessa G, Vargiu L, Crabai F, et al: Selective increase of brain dopamine induced by gamma-hydroxybutyrate. Life Sci 5:1921–1930, 1966

Gessa GL, Agabio R, Lobina C, et al: Mechanism of the antialcohol effect of gamma-hydroxybutyric acid. Alcohol 20:271–276, 2000

Gobaille S, Schleef C, Hechler V, et al: Gamma-hydroxybutyrate increases tryptophan availability and potentiates serotonin turnover in rat brain. Life Sci 70:2101–2112, 2002

Godschalk M, Dzoljic M, Bonta I: Slow wave sleep and a state resembling absence epilepsy induced in the rat by gamma-hydroxybutyrate. Eur J Pharmacol 44:105–111, 1977

Gouzoulis-Mayfrank E, Daumann J: Neurotoxicity of methylenedioxyamphetamines (MDMA; ecstasy) in humans: how strong is the evidence for persistent brain damage? Addiction 101:348–361, 2006

Gouzoulis-Mayfrank E, Daumann J, Tuchtenhagen F, et al: Impaired cognitive performance in drug free users of recreational ecstasy (MDMA). J Neurol Neurosurg Psychiatry 68:719–725, 2000

Green AR, King MV, Shortall SE, et al: Lost in translation: preclinical studies on MDMA provide mechanisms of action, but do not allow accurate prediction of adverse events in humans. Br J Pharmacol 166:1521–1522, 2012

Hall J, Maxwell J: Patterns and Trends of GHB, GBL, and 1,4BD Abuse. Austin, Texas Commission on Drug and Alcohol Abuse, 2000. Available at: http://www.tcada.state.tx.us/research/presentation/Patterns_trends_GHB/sld001.htm. Accessed November 27, 2012.

Harries DP, De Silva R: "Ecstasy" and intracerebral haemorrhage. Scott Med J 37:150–152, 1992

Hatzidimitriou G, McCann UD, Ricaurte GA: Altered serotonin innervation patterns in the forebrain of monkeys treated with (+/-)3,4-methylenedioxymethamphetamine seven years previously: factors influencing abnormal recovery. J Neurosci 19:169–172, 1999

Hernandez M, McDaniel CH, Costanza CD, et al: GHB-induced delirium: a case report and review of the literature of gamma hydroxybutyric acid. Am J Drug Alcohol Abuse 24:179–183, 1998

Hill SL, Thomas SH: Clinical toxicology of newer recreational drugs. Clin Toxicol (Phila) 49:705–719, 2011

Hodges B, Everett J: Acute toxicity from home-brewed gamma hydroxybutyrate. J Am Board Fam Pract 11:154–157, 1998

Howard SG, Feigenbaum JJ: Effect of gamma-hydroxybutyrate on central dopamine release in vivo: a microdialysis study in awake and anesthetized animals. Biochem Pharmacol 53:103–110, 1997

Huffman JW, Padgett LW: Recent developments in the medicinal chemistry of cannabinomimetic indoles, pyrroles and indenes. Curr Med Chem 12:1395–1411, 2005

Itzhak Y, Ali SF: Repeated administration of gamma-hydroxybutyric acid (GHB) to mice: assessment of the sedative and rewarding effects of GHB. Ann N Y Acad Sci 965:451–460, 2002

Jansen KL, Darracot-Cankovic R: The nonmedical use of ketamine, part two: A review of problem use and dependence. J Psychoactive Drugs 33:151–158, 2001

Jerrard DA: "Designer drugs": a current perspective. J Emerg Med 8:733–741, 1990

Johnston LD, O'Malley PM, Bachman JG, et al: Monitoring the Future National Results on Adolescent Drug Use: Overview of Key Findings, 2009 (NIH Publ No 10-7583). Bethesda, MD, National Institute on Drug Abuse, 2010

Jonas MM, Graeme-Cook FM: Case 6-2001: a 17-year-old girl with marked jaundice and weight loss. N Engl J Med 344:591–599, 2001

Kalsi SS, Wood DM, Dargan PI: The epidemiology and patterns of acute and chronic toxicity associated with recreational ketamine use. Emerging Health Threats Journal 4:7107, 2011

Karlsen SN, Spigset O, Slordal L: The dark side of ecstasy: neuropsychiatric symptoms after exposure to 3,4-methylenedioxymethamphetamine. Basic Clin Pharmacol Toxicol 102:15–24, 2007

Kemmel V, Taleb O, Andriamampandry C, et al: Gamma-hydroxybutyrate receptor function determined stimulation of rubidium and calcium movements from NCB-20 neurons. Neuroscience 116:1021–1031, 2003

Kissin W, Ball J: The DAWN Report: Club Drugs, 2001 Update. Rockville, MD, Substance Abuse and Mental Health Services Administration, October 2002. Available at: http://www.oas.samhsa.gov/2k2/DAWN/clubdrugs2k1.pdf. Accessed November 27, 2012.

Koesters SC, Rogers PD, Rajasingham CR: MDMA ("ecstasy") and other "club drugs": the new epidemic. Pediatr Clin North Am 49:415–433, 2002

Krystal JH, Karper LP, Siebyl JP, et al: Subanesthetic effects of the noncompetitive NMDA antagonist, ketamine, in humans: psychotomimetic, perceptual, cognitive, and neuroendocrine responses. Arch Gen Psychiatry 51:199–214, 1994

Lahti AC, Koffel B, LaPorte D, et al: Subanesthetic doses of ketamine stimulate psychosis in schizophrenia. Neuropsychopharmacology 13:9–19, 1995

Lammers GJ, Arends J, Declerck AC, et al: Gammahydroxybutyrate and narcolepsy: a double-blind placebo-controlled study. Sleep 16:216–220, 1993

Lester SJ, Baggott M, Welm S, et al: Cardiovascular effects of 3,4-methylenedioxymethamphetamine: a double-blind, placebo-controlled trial. Ann Intern Med 113:969–973, 2000

Levy MI, Davis BM, Mohs RC, et al: Gamma-hydroxybutyrate in the treatment of schizophrenia. Psychiatry Res 9:1–8, 1983

Li J, Stokes SA, Woeckener A: A tale of novel intoxication: seven cases of gamma-hydroxybutyric acid overdose. Ann Emerg Med 31:723–728, 1998a

Li J, Stokes SA, Woeckener A: A tale of novel intoxication: a review of the effects of gamma-hydroxybutyric acid with recommendations for management. Ann Emerg Med 31:729–736, 1998b

Lo JN, Cumming JF: Interaction between sedative premedicants and ketamine in man in isolated perfused rat livers. Anesthesiology 43:307–312, 1975

Mackie K: Cannabinoid receptors: where they are and what they do. J Neuroendocrinol 20 (suppl 1):10–14, 2008

Maitre M: The gamma-hydroxybutyrate signaling system in brain: organization and functional implications. Prog Neurobiol 51:337–361, 1997

Maitre M, Andriamampandry C, Kemmel V, et al: Gamma-hydroxybutyric acid as a signaling molecule in brain. Alcohol 20:277–283, 2000

Mamelak M: Gamma-hydroxybutyrate: an endogenous regulator of energy metabolism. Neurosci Biobehav Rev 13:187–198, 1989

McCann UD, Szabo Z, Scheffel U, et al: Positron emission tomographic evidence of toxic effect of MDMA ("ecstasy") on brain serotonin neurons in human beings. Lancet 352:1433–1437, 1998

McCann UD, Eligulashvili V, Ricaurte GA: +/- 3,4-Methylenedioxymethamphetamine ("ecstasy")–induced serotonin neurotoxicity: clinical studies. Neuropsychobiology 42:11–16, 2000

McDaniel CH, Miotto KA: Gamma hydroxybutyrate (GHB) and gamma butyrolactone (GBL) withdrawal: five case studies. J Psychoactive Drugs 33:143–149, 2001

McDonough M, Kennedy N, Glasper A, et al: Clinical features and management of gamma-hydroxybutyrate (GHB) withdrawal: a review. Drug Alcohol Depend 75:3–9, 2004

McGuire PK, Cope H, Fahy TA: Diversity of psychopathology associated with use of 3,4-methylenedioxymethamphetamine ("ecstasy"). Br J Psychiatry 165:391–395, 1994

Miotto K, Roth B: GHB Withdrawal. Austin, Texas Commission on Alcohol and Drug Abuse, 2001. Available at: http://www.tcada.state.tx.us/research/populations/GHB_Withdrawal.pdf. Accessed November 27, 2012.

Miotto K, Darakjian J, Basch J, et al: Gamma-hydroxybutyric acid: patterns of use, effects and withdrawal. Am J Addict 10:232–241, 2001

Mithoefer MC, Wagner MT, Mithoefer AT, et al: The safety and efficacy of {+/-}3,4-methylenedioxymethamphetamine-assisted psychotherapy in subjects with chronic, treatment-resistant posttraumatic stress disorder: the first randomized controlled pilot study. J Psychopharmacol 25:439–452, 2011

Mithoefer MC, Wagner MT, Mithoefer AT, et al: Durability of improvement in posttraumatic stress disorder symptoms and absence of harmful effects or drug dependency after 3,4-methylenedioxymethamphetamine-assisted psychotherapy: a prospective long-term follow-up study. J Psychopharmacol 27:28–39, 2013

Moncini M, Masini E, Gambassi F, et al: Gamma-hydroxybutyric acid and alcohol-related syndromes. Alcohol 20:285–291, 2000

Montoya AG, Sorrentino R, Lukas SE, et al: Long-term neuropsychiatric consequences of "ecstasy" (MDMA): a review. Harv Rev Psychiatry 10:212–220, 2002

Moonzwe LS, Schensul JJ, Kostick KM: The role of MDMA (ecstasy) in coping with negative life situations among urban young adults. J Psychoactive Drugs 43:199–210, 2011

Morgan MJ: Memory deficits associated with recreational use of "ecstasy" (MDMA). Psychopharmacology (Berl) 141:30–36, 1999

Müller H, Sperling W, Kohrmann M, et al: The synthetic cannabinoid spice as a trigger for an acute exacerbation of cannabis induced recurrent psychotic episodes. Schizophr Res 118:309–310, 2010

Mullins ME, Fitzmaurice SC: Lack of efficacy of benzodiazepines in treating gamma hydroxybutyrate withdrawal. J Emerg Med 20:418–420, 2001

Murrough JW: Ketamine as a novel antidepressant: from synapse to behavior. Clin Pharmacol Ther 91:303–309, 2012

Mycyk MB, Wilemon C, Aks SE: Two cases of withdrawal from 1,4-butanediol use. Ann Emerg Med 38:345–346, 2001

Nelson T, Kaufman E, Kline J, et al: The extraneuronal distribution of gamma-hydroxybutyrate. J Neurochem 37:1345–1348, 1981

Nicholson KL, Balster RL: GH: a new and novel drug of abuse. Drug Alcohol Depend 63:1–22, 2001

Nimmerrichter AA, Walter H, Gutierrez-Lobos KE, et al: Double-blind controlled trial of gamma-hydroxybutyrate and clomethiazole in the treatment of alcohol withdrawal. Alcohol 37:67–73, 2002

Oehen P, Traber R, Widmer V, et al: A randomized, controlled pilot study of MDMA (± 3,4-Methylenedioxymethamphetamine)-assisted psychotherapy for treatment of resistant, chronic Post-Traumatic Stress Disorder (PTSD). J Psychopharmacol 27:40–52, 2013

Olivera AA, Kiefer MW, Manley NK: Tardive dyskinesia in psychiatric patients with substance abuse disorders. Am J Drug Alcohol Abuse 16:57–66, 1990

Palatini P, Tedeschi L, Frison G, et al: Dose-dependent absorption and elimination of gamma-hydroxybutyric acid in healthy volunteers. Eur J Clin Pharmacol 45:353–356, 1993

Parrott AC, Lasky J: Ecstasy (MDMA) effects upon mood and cognition: before, during and after a Saturday night dance. Psychopharmacology (Berl) 139:261–268, 1998

Pederson W, Skrondal A: Ecstasy and new patterns of drug use: a normal population study. Addiction 94:1695–1706, 1999

Peglow S, Buchner J, Briscoe G: Synthetic cannabinoid induced psychosis in a previously nonpsychotic patient. Am J Addict 21:287–288, 2012

Reich DL, Silvay G: Ketamine: an update on the first twenty-five years of clinical experience. Can J Anaesth 36:186–197, 1989

Ricaurte GA, Forno LS, Wilson MA, et al: (+/-)3,4-Methylenedioxymethamphetamine selectively damages central serotonergic neurons in nonhuman primates. JAMA 260:51–55, 1988

Ricaurte GA, Yuan J, McCann UD: +/- 3,4-Methylenedioxymethamphetamine ("ecstasy")-induced serotonin neurotoxicity: studies in animals. Neuropsychobiology 42:5–10, 2000

Rodgers J: Cognitive performance amongst recreational users of "ecstasy." Psychopharmacology (Berl) 151:19–24, 2000

Rodgman C, Kinzie E, Leimbach E: Bad Mojo: use of the new marijuana substitute leads to more and more ED visits for acute psychosis. Am J Emerg Med 29:232, 2011

Rodriguez JJ, Mackie K, Pickel VM: Ultrastructural localization of the CB1 cannabinoid receptor in mu-opioid receptor patches of the rat caudate putamen nucleus. J Neurosci 21:823–833, 2001

Rogers G, Elston J, Garside R, et al: The harmful health effects of recreational ecstasy: a systematic review of observational evidence. Health Technol Assess 13:iii–iv, ix–xii, 2009

Ross T: Gamma hydroxybutyrate overdose: two cases illustrate the unique aspects of this dangerous recreational drug. J Emerg Nurs 21:374–376, 1995

Roth RH, Giarman NJ: Gamma-butyrolactone and gamma-hydroxybutyric acid, I: distribution and metabolism. Biochem Pharmacol 15:1333–1348, 1966

Roth RH, Giarman NJ: Evidence that central nervous system depression by 1,4-butanediol is mediated through a metabolite, gamma-hydroxybutyrate. Biochem Pharmacol 17:735–739, 1968

Russo E, Guy GW: A tale of two cannabinoids: the therapeutic rationale for combining tetrahydrocannabinol and cannabidiol. Med Hypotheses 66:234–246, 2006

Scharf MB, Lai AA, Branigan B, et al: Pharmacokinetics of gammahydroxybutyrate (GHB) in narcoleptic patients. Sleep 21:507–514, 1998

Schouw ML, Gevers S, Caan MW, et al: Mapping serotonergic dysfunction in MDMA (ecstasy) users using pharmacological MRI. Eur Neuropsychopharmacol 22:537–545, 2012

Schwartz RH, Miller NS: MDMA (ecstasy) and the rave: a review. Pediatrics 100:705–708, 1997

Scrima L, Hartman PG, Johnson FH, et al: The effects of gamma-hydroxybutyrate on the sleep of narcolepsy patients: a double blind study. Sleep 13:479–490, 1990

Seely KA, Prather PL, James LP, et al: Marijuana-based drugs: innovative therapeutics or designer drugs of abuse? Mol Interv 11:36–51, 2011

Sériès F, Sériès I, Cormier Y: Effects of enhancing slow-wave sleep by gamma-hydroxybutyrate on obstructive sleep apnea. Am Rev Respir Dis 145:1378–1383, 1992

Shannon M: Methylenedioxymethamphetamine (MDMA, "ecstasy"). Pediatr Emerg Care 16:377–380, 2000

Sharma AN, Lombardi MH, Illuzzi FA, et al: Management of gamma-hydroxybutyrate withdrawal. Ann Emerg Med 38:605–607, 2001

Sherlock K, Wolff K, Hay AW, et al: Analysis of illicit ecstasy tablets: implications for clinical management in the accident and emergency department. Emerg Med J 16:194–197, 1999

Sim LJ, Hampson RE, Deadwyler SA, et al: Effects of chronic treatment with delta9-tetrahydrocannabinol on cannabinoid stimulated [35S]GTPgammaS autoradiography in rat brain. J Neurosci 16:8057–8066, 1996

Sivilotti ML, Burns MJ, Aaron CK, et al: Pentobarbital for severe gamma-butyrolactone withdrawal. Ann Emerg Med 38:660–665, 2001

Snead OC 3rd, Furner R, Liu CC: In vivo conversion of gamma-aminobutyric acid and 1,4-butanediol to gamma-hydroxybutyric acid in rat brain: studies using stable isotopes. Biochem Pharmacol 38:4375–4380, 1989

Solhkhah R, Wilens TE: Pharmacotherapy of adolescent alcohol and other drug use. Alcohol Health Res World 22:122–125, 1998

Solhkhah R, Finkel J, Hird S: Possible risperidone-induced visual hallucinations. J Am Acad Child Adolesc Psychiatry 39:1074–1075, 2000

Solhkhah R, Wilens TE, Prince JB, et al: Bupropion sustained release for substance abuse, ADHD, and mood disorders in adolescents (NR31), in New Research Abstracts, Annual Meeting of the American Psychiatric Association. Washington, DC, American Psychiatric Association, 2001

Sprague JE, Everman SL, Nichols DE: An integrated hypothesis for the serotonergic axonal loss induced by 3,4-methylenedioxymethamphetamine. Neurotoxicology 19:427–441, 1998

Staud R: Sodium oxybate for the treatment of fibromyalgia. Expert Opin Pharmacother 12:1789–1798, 2011

Stone JM, Dietrich C, Edden R, et al: Ketamine effects on brain GABA and glutamate levels with 1H-MRS: relationship to ketamine-induced psychopathology. Mol Psychiatry 17:664–665, 2012

Substance Abuse and Mental Health Services Administration: Drug Abuse Warning Network, 2011: National Estimates of Drug-Related Emergency Department Visits. HHS Publ No SMA 13-4760, DAWN Series D-39. Rockville, MD, Substance Abuse and Mental Health Services Administration, 2013

Taffe MA: Δ9-Tetrahydrocannabinol attenuates MDMA-induced hyperthermia in Rhesus monkeys. Neuroscience 201:125–133, 2012

Takahara J, Yunoki S, Yakushiji W, et al: Stimulatory effects of gamma-hydroxybutyric acid on growth hormone and prolactin release in humans. J Clin Endocrinol Metab 44:1014–1017, 1977

Tucker GT, Lennard MS, Ellis SW, et al: The demethylation of methylenedioxymethamphetamine ("ecstasy") by debrisoquine hydroxylase (CYP2D6). Biochem Pharmacol 47:1151–1156, 1994

U.S. Department of Justice: Schedules of Controlled Substances: Temporary Placement of Five Synthetic Cannabinoids Into Schedule I Federal Register 76, Number 40:11075–11078 (Tuesday, March 1, 2011)] [FR Doc No: 2011–4428]

U.S. Drug Enforcement Administration: Chemicals Used in "Spice" and "K2" Type Products Now Under Federal Control and Regulation. March 1, 2011. Available at: http://www.justice.gov/dea/pubs/pressrel/pr030111.html. Accessed November 27, 2012.

Vandrey R, Dunn KE, Fry JA, et al: A survey study to characterize use of Spice products (synthetic cannabinoids). Drug Alcohol Depend 120:238–241, 2012

Vardakou I, Pistos C, Spiliopoulou CH: Spice drugs as a new trend: mode of action, identification and legislation. Toxicol Lett 197:157–162, 2010

Venancio C, Magalhaes A, Antunes L, et al: Impaired spatial memory after ketamine administration in chronic low doses. Curr Neuropharmacol 9:251–255, 2011

Verkes RJ, Gilsman HJ, Pieters MS, et al: Cognitive performance and serotonergic function in users of ecstasy. Psychopharmacology (Berl) 153:196–202, 2001

Watson J, Guzzetti S, Franchi C, et al: Gamma-hydroxybutyrate does not maintain self-administration but induces conditioned place preference when injected in the ventral tegmental area. Int J Neuropsychopharmacol 13:143–153, 2010

Weiner AL, Vieira L, McKay CA, et al: Ketamine abusers presenting to the emergency department: a case series. J Emerg Med 18:447–451, 2000

Weir E: Raves: a review of the culture, the drugs and the prevention of harm. CMAJ 162:1843–1848, 2000

White PF, Way WL, Trevor AJ: Ketamine: its pharmacology and therapeutic uses. Anesthesiology 56:119–136, 1982

Williams H, Dratcu L, Taylor R, et al: "Saturday night fever:" ecstasy related problems in a London accident and emergency department. Emerg Med J 15:322–326, 1998

Winstock AR, Mitcheson L: New recreational drugs and the primary care approach to patients who use them. BMJ 344:E288, 2012

Winters WD, Kott KS: Continuum of sedation, activation and hypnosis or hallucinosis: a comparison of low dose effects of pentobarbital, diazepam or gamma-hydroxybutyrate in the cat. Neuropharmacology 18:877–884, 1979

Zimmermann US, Winkelmann PR, Pilhatsch M, et al: Withdrawal phenomena and dependence syndrome after the consumption of "spice gold." Deutsches Arzteblatt Int 106:464–467, 2009

Zvosec DL, Smith SW, McCutcheon JR, et al: Adverse events, including death, associated with use of 1,4-butanediol. N Engl J Med 344:87–94, 2001

10

Treatment of
Substance Use Disorders

Nancy M. Petry, Ph.D.

David M. Ledgerwood, Ph.D.

James R. McKay, Ph.D.

Psychotherapy and pharmacotherapy are frequently combined in treating substance use disorders. Medication is often used to reduce cravings for or use of a substance. The focus of psychotherapy, on the contrary, may be to encourage abstinence, teach the patient new coping skills, or improve motivation to address drug or alcohol problems.

Several psychosocial treatments for alcohol and other substance use disorders are widely used in research and clinical settings. In this chapter, we discuss

We thank Mary E. McCaul, Ph.D., for her contributions to the original version of this chapter.

six of these psychotherapies as they are applied to alcohol, cocaine, and opioid dependence: brief interventions; motivational interviewing/motivational enhancement therapy; cognitive-behavioral therapies; behavioral treatments, including community reinforcement approach and contingency management; behavioral couples therapy; and 12-step facilitation. We also describe studies that examined the efficacy of a medication in combination with one or more of the six psychotherapies. In the second section of the chapter, we highlight research that directly studied the interaction between psychosocial and pharmacological treatments.

Psychotherapies for Substance Use Disorders

Brief Interventions

Brief interventions focus on changing behavior in just a few sessions. This type of counseling strategy can range in duration from 5 minutes up to four 60-minute sessions. Fleming and Manwell (1999) described five steps common in many brief interventions: 1) provide assessment and feedback; 2) negotiate a goal with respect to abstinence or minimal use; 3) use behavior modification techniques, such as identifying high-risk situations; 4) provide bibliotherapy by making available informational materials on substance use and its consequences; and 5) ensure follow-up to check on progress.

Numerous meta-analyses have been published after examining the effects of brief interventions in a variety of patient populations, and they generally concur that brief interventions are efficacious in reducing alcohol use (e.g., Kaner et al. 2007; Moyer et al. 2002; Sullivan et al. 2011). The beneficial effects can extend for up to 1 year. Longer interventions tend not to improve outcomes relative to shorter interventions, and brief treatments can be effectively delivered by nonphysicians. However, subgroup analyses find that the effect is stronger in men than in women. More research is needed to evaluate the potential benefits of brief interventions in women and to examine long-term effects of brief interventions.

Brief interventions also have been extended to individuals with illicit drug use disorders. Emerging evidence suggests that brief treatments also may be effective in reducing cocaine and opioid use (Bernstein et al. 2005; Humeniuk et al. 2012; Madras et al. 2009), although the long-term effects require further evaluation.

Brief interventions have been applied in pharmacotherapy trials, primarily with alcohol-dependent individuals. For example, Kranzler and colleagues (2003) reported on brief (four-session) coping skills training for heavy drinkers. Patients were randomly assigned to one of four conditions: daily administration of placebo, daily administration of naltrexone, targeted administration of placebo, or targeted administration of naltrexone. Patients in the targeted conditions were taught to consume their medication during high-risk situations. Patients in both the targeted naltrexone and the placebo conditions reduced their drinking as long as medication was available at least 3 days per week. Among patients randomly assigned to daily medication administration, drinking was reduced among those patients receiving active naltrexone but not among those receiving placebo. Thus, brief interventions may be useful when provided in conjunction with medications that reduce alcohol use among heavy drinkers.

Motivational Interviewing/ Motivational Enhancement Therapy

Motivational interviewing was developed by Miller and Rollnick (2002) and is based partially on the transtheoretical stages of change model (Prochaska and DiClemente 1986). The emphasis of motivational interviewing is on increasing patients' motivation to reduce or abstain from substances by encouraging commitment to behavior change and helping patients use their own coping and interpersonal resources. Motivational interviewing techniques include expression of empathy and a nonconfrontational style. The patient's ambivalence about substance use is addressed, and the therapist provides feedback about the patient's strengths and difficulties, gives direct advice, and supports the patient's self-efficacy (Miller and Rollnick 2002). Motivational interviewing may be particularly appealing because it is a brief therapy that can easily be used in numerous settings where patients receive pharmacotherapy for substance use disorders.

The efficacy of motivational interviewing has been addressed in alcohol and drug abuse treatment. The National Institute on Alcohol Abuse and Alcoholism (NIAAA) Project MATCH used a brief, four-session, manual-based version of motivational interviewing they termed *motivational enhancement therapy* (MET) and compared it with 12-session interventions consisting of either cognitive-behavioral therapy (CBT) or 12-step facilitation. The brief

MET was as efficacious as the two longer treatments in improving drinking-related outcomes, and MET showed greater efficacy with angry patients (Project MATCH Research Group 1997). Subsequent studies have confirmed benefits of motivational interviewing and MET approaches for reducing alcohol use in several populations (Adamson and Sellman 2008; LaBrie et al. 2008), but this approach has not universally been found to be superior to other active treatments (Nyamathi et al. 2010).

A few pharmacotherapy trials for alcohol have used motivational interviewing or MET. For example, Anton et al. (2004) conducted a double-blind study examining the efficacy of nalmefene for preventing relapse in recently abstinent alcohol-dependent patients ($N=270$). MET was also applied in attempt to further reduce alcohol use and encourage medication adherence. More than 90% of prescribed medication doses were taken, and 90% of patients attended their first two MET sessions. Patients in all groups experienced fewer heavy drinking days, more abstinent days, and decreased cravings for alcohol with treatment, but medication effects were not noted on any alcohol-related variable. Other clinical trials have similarly used MET or motivational interviewing as a base psychosocial intervention and found relatively high rates of medication adherence, alcohol abstinence, and therapy attendance (Heffner et al. 2010; Kranzler et al. 2004). Although MET may have contributed to greater abstinence and treatment adherence in these studies, efficacy trials of MET within the context of pharmacotherapy trials for alcohol are needed.

Fewer published reports have examined the use of motivational interviewing or MET with cocaine- and opioid-dependent patients. One pilot study reported that a single session of motivational interviewing was associated with reductions in drug use and sex work among 25 street sex workers who were using illicit drugs, primarily heroin and cocaine (Yahne et al. 2002). In another study (Stotts et al. 2001), 105 cocaine-dependent patients were randomly assigned to receive either 1) standard cocaine detoxification and standard treatment, consisting of assessment and psychoeducation, or 2) standard treatment plus MET. The MET patients provided more cocaine-free urine samples and were more likely to use behavioral coping skills than were the patients who received standard treatment. Some studies have found that MET is particularly beneficial to cocaine- and opioid-dependent patients who present to treatment with low motivation for change (Rohsenow et al. 2004). Additional studies have found that adding MET sessions to CBT for cocaine dependence can result in improved treatment attendance and greater desire for abstinence but not necessarily enhanced drug abstinence (McKee et al. 2007).

Other studies have found mixed results for motivational interviewing or MET compared with other psychotherapeutic approaches. In one randomized clinical trial (N=198) that compared cocaine-dependent individuals receiving motivational interviewing with those receiving assessment control condition, no significant differences were found in number of cocaine use days in the overall sample (Stein et al. 2009). However, when only those who used cocaine for 15 days or more per month were examined, motivational interviewing resulted in superior outcomes. Another study comparing (N=44) individuals with co-occurring psychotic and substance use disorders found that primary cocaine–using individuals responded better to a two-session motivational interviewing treatment, whereas primary cannabis–abusing participants responded better to a standard psychiatric interview (Martino et al. 2006). Thus, more studies are needed to establish the circumstances in which motivational interviewing or MET work best.

Very few studies have used motivational interviewing or MET in medication trials, but those that did used motivational interviewing or MET primarily to enhance compliance with medications. For example, motivational interviewing was as effective as an information-based video in enhancing medication compliance among individuals with co-occurring cocaine dependence and HIV (Ingersoll et al. 2011). Results from studies that examined the interaction between motivational interviewing and medications are presented in the final section of this chapter ("Interactions of Psychotherapy and Pharmacological Treatments").

Cognitive-Behavioral Therapies

CBT is based on the theoretical assumption that alcohol and other substance use problems are related to maladaptive social learning and adverse life situations. CBT interventions are designed to improve interpersonal and coping skills, reduce the risk of relapse, and increase self-efficacy. The patient and therapist discuss triggers that may be cues for substance use. Patients are made aware that triggers may be internal (such as feelings, thoughts, or cravings) or external (such as interactions with drug-using friends, proximity to a liquor shop, or an argument with a spouse). To cope with urges to use drugs or drink in the presence of triggers, patients are taught problem-solving and coping techniques.

Several randomized clinical trials have established the efficacy of CBT for treating substance use disorders compared with no-treatment control conditions, and recent meta-analyses have found CBT to have low to moderate effect sizes (Dutra et al. 2008; Magill and Ray 2009). Although some studies have found CBT to be more effective than other treatments, other studies have found this method to yield similar results to comparator treatment approaches (Carroll 1996). In Project MATCH, for instance, CBT, MET, and 12-step facilitation produced similar outcomes, with each therapy leading to substantial improvement in alcohol-related symptoms during the 12-week treatment period (Project MATCH Research Group 1997).

One benefit of CBT may be that it contributes to longer-term recovery once treatment has ended (Carroll et al. 1994b; O'Malley et al. 1996; Rawson et al. 2006). This continued reduction in symptoms is not generally seen with other therapies, in which a gradual return to baseline levels of use and associated problems is more typical. According to the theory underlying CBT, this continued improvement may result from the enhanced coping and relapse prevention skills that are acquired by the patient during treatment.

Several pharmacotherapy trials for alcohol-dependent patients have used CBT as the platform psychotherapy (Brown et al. 2009; Davidson et al. 2007; Johnson et al. 1996, 2000; Kranzler et al. 1995; Mason et al. 1999). For example, alcohol-dependent patients in a placebo-controlled clinical trial of naltrexone received 12 sessions of manual-based CBT (Anton et al. 1999). Patients taking naltrexone reported reduced drinking and longer time to relapse, compared with the placebo group, during the treatment period. However, both groups had substantial engagement in the psychotherapy, as evidenced by high rates of treatment completion and attendance at sessions. A more recent study tested an enhanced CBT (called *broad-spectrum treatment*) against MET in 149 alcohol-dependent patients also receiving naltrexone (Davidson et al. 2007). Patients receiving enhanced CBT experienced a significantly higher percentage of abstinent days, and benefits for CBT were particularly evident in patients who reported high support for drinking in their social environments. Anton et al. (2001) suggested that combining naltrexone treatment with CBT offers the patient an opportunity to hone relapse prevention skills during high-risk situations that are better managed with the anticraving and reward reduction properties of naltrexone. This conclusion is consistent with findings that patients who receive CBT experience longer-term improvement in substance use (Carroll et al. 1994b; O'Malley et al. 1996; Rawson et al. 2006).

CBT also has been studied in cocaine and opioid users who are receiving pharmacological treatment. CBT has been used as the base psychosocial treatment in studies examining the efficacy of medication for cocaine dependence (Oliveto et al. 2011). Additional studies have examined the effectiveness of CBT compared with no treatment or other active treatments in patients who are maintained on medication treatments (Nunes et al. 2006; Rosenblum et al. 1999). Nunes et al. (2006), for example, compared an enhanced CBT intervention (which included motivational interviewing and behavioral incentive components) with standard treatment in opioid-dependent outpatients ($N=69$) receiving naltrexone. Although 6-month retention was low in both groups, it was higher for the enhanced CBT (22%) than for the standard care condition (9%).

CBT also has been used to encourage engagement in methadone treatment and to reduce risky behaviors. Goldstein et al. (2002) randomly assigned patients to an outreach intervention that involved street-level outreach, individual counseling, and CBT groups or to a no-intervention condition in a study designed to encourage reengagement of patients who dropped out of methadone treatment. Intervention subjects who participated in at least two CBT groups (72%) were significantly more likely to return to methadone treatment than were intervention subjects who participated in no or one CBT group (53%) or comparison subjects (50%). It is important to note that there were no differences in treatment reentry as a function of level of exposure to outreach or individual counseling services. In another study, O'Neill et al. (1996) randomly assigned methadone-maintained pregnant injecting drug users to either standard methadone treatment or standard treatment plus six sessions of CBT directed at reducing HIV risk behaviors. Patients receiving CBT reported safer injecting practices (i.e., reduced frequency of sharing needles) at follow-up, compared with intake. The risk behaviors of the patients in standard treatment remained the same or increased.

Thus, although CBT may not be superior to other types of interventions in increasing abstinence during treatment, studies suggest that CBT may have other beneficial effects. CBT may have a longer-term effect on abstinence than that seen with other treatments. Furthermore, this treatment also may be used to encourage other behaviors, such as safe needle practices or engagement in pharmacotherapy.

Behavioral Treatments

Behavioral treatments, including community reinforcement approach (CRA) and contingency management (CM), are based on the principle that drugs of abuse induce positive effects and that these effects reinforce continued substance use. In CRA and CM treatments, the therapist rearranges the patient's environment so that drug use is less reinforcing than abstinence.

In CRA with alcohol-dependent patients, reinforcement of disulfiram compliance is one of the primary components of treatment, such that use of alcohol loses its reinforcing aspects and, in fact, becomes aversive. Furthermore, reinforcement from other sources is increased. Positive reinforcement for not drinking comes in the form of scheduling other recreational activities and reorganizing daily life by breaking down practical barriers. For example, the therapist may assist the patient in obtaining a telephone, a place to live, or transportation to treatment.

Strong evidence exists for the efficacy of CRA in treatment of alcohol use disorders (Miller et al. 1995). In controlled studies conducted on both an inpatient (Azrin 1976) and an outpatient basis (Azrin et al. 1982; Smith et al. 1998), patients receiving CRA demonstrated substantial enhancements in abstinence rates and psychosocial functioning, compared with patients receiving other treatments. However, fewer studies of CRA have been undertaken of late, potentially because of concern that coordinating community resources is overly burdensome (Kadden 2001).

CM treatments are based on principles similar to those underlying CRA, but CM extends positive reinforcement for not using substances to include tangible rewards. For example, every time the patient provides a substance-negative urine specimen or ingests medication, he or she earns a reward, such as a voucher exchangeable for retail goods and services (Higgins et al. 1994) or a chance to win $1–$100 prizes (Petry et al. 2000). An extensive literature exists on the use of CM for treatment of substance use disorders, and a meta-analysis (Dutra et al. 2008) of psychosocial treatments for substance use disorders found CM to have the largest effect size of all interventions. CM is effective in a range of populations, including patients dependent on alcohol (Petry et al. 2000), cocaine (Higgins et al. 2007; Petry et al. 2005a), marijuana (Budney et al. 2006), and multiple substances (Peirce et al. 2006; Petry et al. 2005b, 2011).

Studies have shown that CM can be used to reinforce adherence to medications as well. Petry et al. 2012) conducted a meta-analysis of studies that used CM procedures to promote medication adherence. Reinforcers have been successfully applied in more than 20 studies to increase adherence to medications for a variety of conditions including tuberculosis, substance use (e.g., naltrexone), hepatitis, HIV, and psychotic disorders. The overall effect size was large, indicating that CM procedures can have pronounced benefits for improving medication adherence. These studies suggest that behavioral treatments can be effective inventions for reducing substance use, and they also can be applied as adjuncts to pharmacotherapy.

Behavioral Couples Therapy

Behavioral couples therapy (BCT) is based on the principle that individuals with substance use disorders have high levels of relationship distress, and this distress is often associated with poor treatment outcomes and elevated relapse rates (Epstein and McCrady 1998; Powers et al. 2008). BCT has its basis in social learning theory and family systems models, and it assumes a reciprocal connection between substance use and relationship functioning such that substance use affects the quality and nature of a couple's relationship. In turn, aspects of the relationship can also influence substance use. Thus, BCT focuses on improving how the couple interacts by working on communication and problem-solving skills and enhancing social support (Ruff et al. 2010).

BCT has received relatively strong support in randomized clinical trials. Indeed, meta-analyses examining the efficacy of BCT for alcohol and drug use disorders reported superior outcomes of BCT on frequency of substance use, consequences of substance use, and relationship satisfaction variables when compared with other active treatments (Powers et al. 2008). Several studies with alcohol-dependent patients showed that BCT improves relationship adjustment and reduces drinking (McCrady et al. 1991; O'Farrell et al. 1992). Trials for illicit substances are less frequent, but the few studies that have examined BCT for drug use have found similarly promising results (e.g., Winters et al. 2002). Furthermore, the benefits of BCT often extend to behavior problems among children of substance users (Kelley and Fals-Stewart 2007), and BCT also has shown efficacy with various subject groups, including gay and lesbian couples (Fals-Stewart et al. 2009) and couples who are coping with co-occurring psychiatric conditions (Rotunda et al. 2008).

A recent critical review found that BCT has, on average, medium to large effect sizes for improving marital adjustment but that these effect sizes tend to diminish at 1- or 2-year follow-up (Ruff et al. 2010). Others, however, have found that the longer-term effectiveness of BCT can be improved by including concurrent individual relapse prevention (O'Farrell et al. 1998).

The inclusion of BCT in investigations to support pharmacotherapy is rare. Some studies have involved a spouse or significant other in observing medication ingestion. In a 6-month study, patients who consumed disulfiram (200 mg/day) under observation of a significant other significantly increased the number of abstinent days and decreased the total number of drinks, relative to patients who received placebo under observation (Chick et al. 1992).

BCT also can reduce drug use and improve psychosocial problems when combined with standard methadone treatment. Fals-Stewart et al. (2001) randomly assigned 36 men initiating methadone treatment to standard care (methadone plus twice-weekly individual drug abuse counseling) or to methadone plus weekly couples therapy with their partner and once-weekly individual drug abuse counseling. Patients in the couples therapy condition had reduced opioid and cocaine use during treatment and higher levels of relationship satisfaction posttreatment, compared with subjects in standard care. In a second study, Fals-Stewart and O'Farrell (2003) randomly assigned 124 opioid-dependent men receiving naltrexone treatment to either individual counseling or BCT. Patients in BCT were less likely to use opioids, cocaine, alcohol, or other drugs during treatment, compared with patients in individual treatment. BCT patients reported greater abstinence at 1-year follow-up and had more consecutive days abstinent, compared with the patients who received individual therapy.

Other studies that have included family counseling as the psychotherapeutic intervention in medication trials highlight challenges of this approach. One study evaluated family counseling in conjunction with naltrexone treatment (Carroll et al. 2001). Opioid-dependent patients ($N=127$) were randomly assigned to receive standard naltrexone treatment, naltrexone treatment with CM for consuming naltrexone, or naltrexone treatment with CM plus family counseling. Of the patients assigned to the family counseling condition, 48% never attended even one of their family sessions, suggesting considerable difficulty engaging families of opioid-dependent patients in treatment. Among those who attended one or more sessions, family counseling appeared to increase retention and opioid abstinence rates, compared with the other two treatment conditions. Compared with patients in the non–family therapy conditions, patients who attended the family therapy sessions showed decreases in family problems during the trial, suggesting treatment-specific effects.

These findings suggest that BCT may improve outcomes on several levels when provided along with methadone or naltrexone treatment in polydrug-using patients. However, the Carroll et al. (2001) study also found that engaging family members in treatment may be no easy task. Thus, additional strategies to encourage family involvement may increase the effectiveness of this approach.

12-Step Facilitation

Alcoholics Anonymous (AA), a self-help organization, is the most widely accessed resource for individuals with alcohol problems (McCrady and Miller 1993). The philosophy is based on the concept of alcoholism as a chronic disease that cannot be cured but that can be halted by means of complete abstinence. AA has described 12 principles or steps to guide those in recovery. Narcotics Anonymous and Cocaine Anonymous fellowships also exist, with similar principles.

Although individuals with substance use disorders are commonly encouraged to attend 12-step meetings, few data exist regarding the efficacy of these interventions. Observational data indicate that 12-step involvement can be associated with improved substance use outcomes in alcohol- (e.g., Gossop et al. 2003, 2008) and cocaine-dependent patients (McKay et al. 1994), but patients who attend 12-step meetings may differ in important ways from those who do not (Ye and Kaskutas 2009).

Although randomized studies of AA do not exist, 12-step facilitation, a manual-based psychotherapy to promote AA participation, was equally efficacious to CBT and MET in a large randomized study of treatments for alcohol dependence (Project MATCH Research Group 1997). Other randomized studies found that active and directive 12-step facilitation interventions (Timko and DeBenedetti 2007; Walitzer et al. 2009) were more efficacious than usual care treatments in promoting engagement in 12-step meetings and outcomes.

A common belief is that AA discourages use of treatment medications, which are considered "crutches." However, in a survey of a large sample of AA members, more than one-half of the respondents reported that the use of re-lapse-preventing medication either was or might be a good idea; only 12% reported that they would tell another member to stop taking it (Rychtarik et al. 2000). Given the positive outcomes associated with 12-step attendance and the apparent tolerance of medication use among most AA members, use of this treatment approach in combination with pharmacotherapy seems appropriate.

The Veterans Affairs Cooperative Studies Group completed a multisite, placebo-controlled study of naltrexone for treatment of alcohol dependence (Krystal et al. 2001). For 13 months, participants received 12-step facilitation counseling and were encouraged to attend AA meetings. The 12-step facilitation approach was adapted to promote use of pharmacotherapy, introduce basic relapse prevention principles, and reinforce abstinence and continued treatment. Although no differences in outcomes were noted between those receiving naltrexone and those receiving placebo, moderate to high rates of medication and counseling compliance were noted in the first 3 months, along with high rates of alcohol abstinence and a relatively low proportion of drinking days in both groups. A trial of sertraline for the treatment of alcohol dependence (Pettinati et al. 2001) also incorporated 12-step facilitation and support group attendance, in conjunction with brief physician visits. This research suggested that 12-step-oriented interventions can be combined successfully with pharmacotherapy to engage and retain alcohol-dependent patients in treatment.

Interactions of Psychotherapy and Pharmacological Treatments

Pharmacotherapy studies typically use one of the psychotherapies reviewed earlier as a platform for evaluation of one or more pharmacotherapies. Relatively few studies have simultaneously manipulated the type or dose of both medication and psychotherapy as a specific test of treatment interactions. Such interaction studies can provide information on the relative efficacy of psychotherapy and medication approaches, and they can explore how combining medication and psychotherapy may differentially affect substance use, compared with either treatment method alone.

O'Malley et al. (1992) conducted a double-blind study combining naltrexone and CBT for alcoholism. Patients were randomly assigned to participate in cognitive-behavioral coping skills treatment or supportive therapy and to receive 50 mg/day of naltrexone or placebo. Naltrexone-treated patients who received supportive therapy had more continuous abstinence than did the other treatment groups. However, naltrexone-treated patients who received CBT had a lower level of craving and lower risk of relapse than did the other three groups. This interaction would not have been observed in a study that manipulated only psychosocial treatment or only medication.

Anton et al. (2005) conducted a 2×2 study in which alcohol-dependent patients were randomly assigned to receive naltrexone or placebo and CBT or MET. CBT was provided in 12 weekly sessions, whereas MET was delivered in 4 sessions. Although there was a main effect for naltrexone on increased time to first relapse, the combination of CBT and naltrexone had the best outcomes on several other measures, including a lower relapse rate, fewer participants with multiple relapses, increased time between multiple relapse events, and higher frequency of abstinent days.

The COMBINE Study, a multisite study sponsored by NIAAA, is another example of research that directly tests the interaction between psychosocial and pharmacological treatments for alcoholism (COMBINE Study Research Group 2003a, 2003b). Patients were randomly assigned to receive placebo, naltrexone, acamprosate, or naltrexone plus acamprosate, and they were also randomly assigned to one of two psychosocial treatments: 1) a low-intensity medical management condition that addressed medication adherence, monitored side effects, and provided brief intervention or 2) a high-intensity condition that included elements of the low-intensity treatment plus counseling grounded in CBT and motivational and 12-step approaches (combined behavioral intervention; CBI). The primary article from this study reported that the groups that received naltrexone and medical management only (no CBI or acamprosate) or CBI and medical management only (no naltrexone or acamprosate) had the highest percentage of days abstinent scores during the 16-week treatment phase. Naltrexone also reduced the risk of experiencing a heavy drinking day during the trial. No combination of medications or treatments produced better outcomes than medical management plus naltrexone or CBI (Anton et al. 2006). These two interventions also reduced the likelihood of experiencing alcohol use trajectories characterized by very frequent drinking during the follow-up (Gueorguieva et al. 2010).

Longabaugh and colleagues (2009) conducted a study that crossed duration of naltrexone (12 vs. 24 weeks) with type of psychosocial treatment (MET vs. a version of CBT tailored to patients' needs). The combination of extended naltrexone and the tailored CBT intervention produced better scores on the two primary outcomes—time to first drink and time to first heavy drinking day—than on the other three conditions.

Some studies with cocaine and opioid abusers have also examined the interaction between pharmacotherapy and psychotherapy. Carroll et al. (1998) randomly assigned 122 patients who abused both cocaine and alcohol to receive one of five treatments: 1) CBT plus disulfiram, 2) 12-step facilitation plus disulfiram, 3) clinical management plus disulfiram, 4) CBT alone, or 5) 12-step facilitation alone. The patients who received disulfiram remained in treatment longer and achieved greater durations of cocaine and alcohol abstinence than did those who did not receive disulfiram. Furthermore, those who received CBT or 12-step facilitation had longer periods of abstinence from cocaine use and combined cocaine and alcohol use than did those who received clinical management. These data suggest a possible additive effect of certain forms of psychotherapy in conjunction with disulfiram in the treatment of concurrent cocaine and alcohol abuse, at least in the short run. However, differences between CBT, 12-step, and case management and between disulfiram and no medication were no longer statistically significant by the end of a 1-year follow-up period (Carroll et al. 2000).

Carroll et al. (2004) conducted another study examining psychotherapy and disulfiram treatment for cocaine dependence. In this randomized, double-blind, placebo-controlled study, patients (N=121) were assigned to one of four conditions: 1) disulfiram plus CBT; 2) disulfiram plus interpersonal therapy (IPT), which addressed psychiatric problems, interpersonal functioning, and supportive therapeutic exploration; 3) placebo plus CBT; or 4) placebo plus IPT. The patients who received disulfiram reduced their cocaine use relative to those who received placebo, and the patients who received CBT reduced their cocaine use relative to those who received IPT. Cocaine abstinence among the patients who received CBT plus placebo was not statistically different from that of the patients who received CBT or IPT in addition to disulfiram. These results are consistent with the findings of a prior study that confirmed the efficacy of CBT and disulfiram for treatment of cocaine dependence (Carroll et al. 1998).

In another double-blind, placebo-controlled study of treatment for cocaine dependence, Carroll and colleagues (1994a) focused on the interaction of CBT and desipramine (an antidepressant medication). Patients ($N=121$) were randomly assigned to one of four treatment conditions: 1) case management and placebo, 2) case management and desipramine, 3) CBT and placebo, or 4) CBT and desipramine. Case management involved providing nonspecific elements of psychotherapy (i.e., therapeutic relationship, empathy, education), medication management, and a convincing therapeutic rationale. Patients in each group improved over the 12-week study period, but no overall differences in retention or cocaine abstinence were found among the four treatment groups. However, the patients with more severe baseline cocaine use benefited more from CBT than from case management, although low-severity patients benefited more when taking desipramine than when taking placebo. Furthermore, depressed patients benefited more from CBT than from case management. These findings indicate that interaction effects may be complex and difficult to detect in studies that examine only medication or only psychotherapy.

At 1-year follow-up (Carroll et al. 1994b), 80% of the patients from the original study by Carroll et al. (1994a) were reassessed. Patients in all groups had maintained cocaine use reductions. However, CBT-treated patients had had a delayed improvement, relative to the case management patients, and they reported fewer cocaine-related symptoms. These results were similar to those of other CBT studies that have found delayed positive treatment effects (O'Malley et al. 1996). They were inconsistent, however, with the findings of Carroll et al. (2000) in a follow-up of disulfiram-treated cocaine-dependent patients, in which the long-term effects of CBT were similar to those of 12-step facilitation and clinical management.

Gruber et al. (2008) studied the interaction of methadone treatment (21-day detoxification vs. 6 months of maintenance) and counseling level in the methadone maintenance condition (minimal vs. standard). Six months of methadone maintenance, with either the minimal or the standard counseling level, produced better opiate use outcomes than did the 21-day detoxification program. The standard counseling level had no added advantage over minimal counseling.

Several CM studies have explored interactions between medication and psychosocial treatments for substance use disorders. In a 12-week randomized, double-blind study of buprenorphine-maintained opioid- and cocaine-dependent patients, Kosten et al. (2003a) found that desipramine and CM together led to greater abstinence from cocaine and heroin and more consecutive weeks of abstinence than either treatment individually or placebo. A later report on this same group of patients found that eliminating the escalating voucher reinforcement and replacing it with a fixed reinforcement value had a negative effect on abstinence, particularly in patients who were receiving both CM and desipramine (Kosten et al. 2003b). Therefore, reducing or changing this intervention in certain ways may have a detrimental effect on some patients, but such results need to be replicated.

In another CM study, Dallery et al. (2001) used a within-subject design to examine the effect of varying the contingency magnitude and methadone dose on treatment-resistant opiate and cocaine use in methadone-maintained patients. Baseline low-magnitude ($374) and high-magnitude ($3,369) voucher reinforcement schedules were compared in patients alternately receiving maintenance doses of 60 mg/day and 120 mg/day of methadone. Regardless of methadone dose, only 2% of urine samples were negative for both cocaine and heroin before contingencies were in place. During phase 1, when patients were maintained on 60 mg/day of methadone, 19% of the samples during low-magnitude reinforcement and 28% of the samples during high-magnitude reinforcement were negative for both opiates and cocaine. When the dosage of methadone was raised to 120 mg/day (phase 2), 32% of the low-magnitude samples and 46% of the high-magnitude samples tested negative for both drugs. These results suggest that methadone dose and increased reinforcement value had an additive effect on drug use.

In a double-blind methadone study, Preston et al. (2000) randomly assigned 120 methadone-maintained opioid-dependent patients to one of four conditions: 1) standard methadone treatment, 2) standard treatment plus CM vouchers, 3) standard treatment plus a 20 mg/day methadone dose increase, or 4) standard treatment plus CM and a 20 mg/day methadone dose increase. Standard treatment consisted of 50 mg/day of methadone, weekly individual counseling, and noncontingent vouchers. Contingent vouchers were associated with greater abstinence from heroin, regardless of whether the patient also received a methadone dose increase. The methadone dose increase was associated with reduced self-reported opioid use and fewer cravings. In contrast to the findings of Dallery et al. (2001), combining CM and the dose increase did not improve treatment outcome beyond either treatment presented alone.

Schottenfeld and colleagues (2005) conducted a 24-week, double-blind medication trial in which 162 opioid- and cocaine-dependent patients received manual-guided counseling and were randomly assigned to receive sublingual buprenorphine (12–16 mg/day) or methadone (65–85 mg/day). Patients were also randomly assigned to receive voucher-based CM or feedback on their treatment performance. The CM escalated during the first 12 weeks and was maintained at a lower nominal level for the second 12 weeks of the study. Patients receiving methadone stayed in treatment longer, had longer periods of abstinence from cocaine and opioids, and had a larger proportion of drug-free urine tests than did patients who received buprenorphine. Patients who received CM experienced more abstinence from cocaine and opioids during the first 12 weeks of the study (when voucher amounts escalated) than did patients in the performance-feedback condition, but this difference was not significant when results from the entire 24 weeks of the study were analyzed. No interaction effects were found between medication type and treatment condition. The authors concluded that adding CM to methadone or buprenorphine treatment may improve treatment outcomes for patients with co-occurring cocaine and opioid dependence.

Two studies have examined the interaction of medication and CM treatments for cocaine-dependent patients. Schmitz et al. (2008) examined the efficacy of levodopa compared with placebo across three behavioral treatment platforms (clinical management vs. clinical management+CBT vs. clinical management+CBT+CM). A significant main effect favored levodopa over placebo on all cocaine outcome measures, with the effect greatest in the condition that included CM. A second study (Schmitz et al. 2009) by the same group crossed medication (high-dose naltrexone vs. placebo) with psychosocial intervention (CBT+CM vs. CBT alone) in patients dependent on cocaine and alcohol. The four groups did not differ on cocaine urine toxicology or on drinks per day. However, naltrexone reduced frequency of heavy drinking days, as did CBT without CM. Adding CM to CBT did not improve outcomes over CBT alone.

Finally, the efficacy of bupropion and CM for cocaine dependence in methadone maintenance patients was evaluated by Poling et al. (2006). In this study, medication (bupropion vs. placebo) was crossed with CM (contingent vs. noncontingent on opioid and cocaine urine toxicology results). The contingent CM plus bupropion group had the best cocaine use outcomes of all four groups.

Some of the studies that combined psychosocial and pharmacological treatments indicated potential interactions or additive effects between the therapies tested. However, the interactions found were not consistent or reliable across studies, nor were many of them predicted. More research on the interactions between medication and psychosocial interventions will further inform our understanding of the most effective treatment combinations.

Conclusion

Many studies have examined the efficacy of a variety of psychosocial treatments for alcohol, cocaine, and opioid use disorders, alone and in conjunction with pharmacotherapy. However, only a handful of studies have explored how these two treatment approaches may interact. More research is needed to further explore the ways in which psychosocial interventions may be used in conjunction with pharmacotherapy to optimize outcomes for both treatments. Providing encouragement for abstinence, greater treatment retention, medication adherence, and coping with medication side effects are some potential applications of psychosocial therapies.

In some pharmacotherapy studies, psychotherapy exposure has been minimized because of concern that psychotherapy may produce a ceiling effect on improvement in drug or alcohol use, making medication effects difficult to detect. However, in this chapter, we have also noted instances when psychosocial and medication treatments have had beneficial additive effects. Minimization of psychotherapy in pharmacotherapy trials may be counterproductive, because psychosocial therapies that encourage the patient to remain engaged in treatment may positively affect patients' adherence to the medication regimen.

Although studies directed at measuring the interaction between psychotherapies and medications are complex, additional research in this area is needed. Such studies offer the methodological sophistication required to understand the complicated relations between interventions that can substantially affect treatment outcomes.

References

Adamson SJ, Sellman JD: Five-year outcomes of alcohol-dependent persons treated with motivational enhancement. J Stud Alcohol Drugs 69:589–593, 2008

Anton RF, Moak DH, Waid LR, et al: Naltrexone and cognitive behavioral therapy for the treatment of outpatient alcoholics: results of a placebo-controlled trial. Am J Psychiatry 156:1758–1764, 1999

Anton RF, Moak DH, Latham PK, et al: Posttreatment results of combining naltrexone with cognitive-behavior therapy for the treatment of alcoholism. J Clin Psychopharmacol 21:72–77, 2001

Anton RF, Pettinati H, Zweben A, et al: A multi-site dose ranging study of nalmefene in the treatment of alcohol dependence. J Clin Psychopharmacol 24:421–428, 2004

Anton RF, Moak DH, Latham P, et al: Naltrexone combined with either cognitive behavioral or motivational enhancement therapy for alcohol dependence. J Clin Psychopharmacol 25:349–357, 2005

Anton RF, O'Malley SS, Ciraulo DA, et al: Combined pharmacotherapies and behavioral interventions for alcohol dependence. JAMA 295:2003–2017, 2006

Azrin NH: Improvements in the community reinforcement approach to alcoholism. Behav Res Ther 14:339–348, 1976

Azrin NH, Sisson RW, Meyers R, et al: Alcoholism treatment by disulfiram and community reinforcement therapy. J Behav Ther Exp Psychiatry 13:105–112, 1982

Bernstein J, Bernstein E, Tassiopoulos K, et al: Brief motivational intervention at a clinic visit reduces cocaine and heroin use. Drug Alcohol Depend 77:49–59, 2005

Brown SE, Carmody TJ, Schmitz JM, et al: A randomized, double-blind, placebo-controlled pilot study of naltrexone in outpatients with bipolar disorder and alcohol dependence. Alcohol Clin Exp Res 33:1863–1869, 2009

Budney AJ, Moore BA, Rocha HL, et al: Clinical trial of abstinence-based vouchers and cognitive-behavioral therapy for cannabis dependence. J Consult Clin Psychol 74:307–316, 2006

Carroll KM: Relapse prevention as a psychosocial treatment: a review of controlled clinical trials. Exp Clin Psychopharmacol 4:46–54, 1996

Carroll KM, Rounsaville BJ, Gordon LT, et al: Psychotherapy and pharmacotherapy for ambulatory cocaine abusers. Arch Gen Psychiatry 51:177–187, 1994a

Carroll KM, Rounsaville BJ, Nich C, et al: One-year follow-up of psychotherapy and pharmacotherapy for cocaine dependence: delayed emergence of psychotherapy effects. Arch Gen Psychiatry 51:989–997, 1994b

Carroll KM, Nich C, Ball SA, et al: Treatment of cocaine and alcohol dependence with psychotherapy and disulfiram. Addiction 93:713–728, 1998

Carroll KM, Nich C, Ball SA, et al: One-year follow-up of disulfiram and psychotherapy for cocaine-alcohol users: sustained effects of treatment. Addiction 95:1335–1349, 2000

Carroll KM, Ball SA, Nich C, et al: Targeting behavioral therapies to enhance naltrexone treatment of opioid dependence: efficacy of contingency management and significant other involvement. Arch Gen Psychiatry 58:755–761, 2001

Carroll KM, Fenton LR, Ball SA, et al: Efficacy of disulfiram and cognitive behavior therapy in cocaine-dependent outpatients. Arch Gen Psychiatry 61:264–272, 2004

Chick J, Gough K, Faldowski W, et al: Disulfiram treatment of alcoholism. Br J Psychiatry 161:84–89, 1992

COMBINE Study Research Group: Testing combined pharmacotherapies and behavioral interventions in alcohol dependence: rationale and methods. Alcohol Clin Exp Res 27:1107–1122, 2003a

COMBINE Study Research Group: Testing combined pharmacotherapies and behavioral interventions in alcohol dependence (the COMBINE Study): a pilot feasibility study. Alcohol Clin Exp Res 27:1123–1131, 2003b

Dallery J, Silverman K, Chutuape MA, et al: Voucher-based reinforcement of opiate plus cocaine abstinence in treatment-resistant methadone patients: effects of reinforcer magnitude. Exp Clin Psychopharmacol 9:317–325, 2001

Davidson D, Gulliver SB, Longabaugh R, et al: Building a better cognitive-behavioral therapy: is broad spectrum treatment more effective than motivational-enhancement therapy for alcohol-dependent patients treated with naltrexone? J Stud Alcohol Drugs 68:238–247, 2007

Dutra L, Stathopoulou G, Basden SL, et al: A meta-analytic review of psychosocial interventions for substance use disorders. Am J Psychiatry 165:179–187, 2008

Epstein EE, McCrady BS: Behavioral couples treatment of alcohol and drug use disorders: current status and innovations. Clin Psychol Rev 18:689–711, 1998

Fals-Stewart W, O'Farrell TJ: Behavioral family counseling and naltrexone for male opioid-dependent patients. J Consult Clin Psychol 71:432–442, 2003

Fals-Stewart W, O'Farrell TJ, Birchler GR: Behavioral couples therapy for male methadone maintenance patients: effects of drug-using behavior and relationship adjustment. Behav Ther 32:391–411, 2001

Fals-Stewart W, O'Farrell TJ, Lam WK: Behavioral couple therapy for gay and lesbian couples with alcohol use disorders. J Subst Abuse Treat 37:379–387, 2009

Fleming M, Manwell LB: Brief intervention in primary care settings: a primary treatment method for at-risk, problem, and dependent drinkers. Alcohol Res Health 23:128–137, 1999

Goldstein MF, Deren S, Sung-Yeon K, et al: Evaluation of an alternative program for MMTP drop-outs: impact on treatment re-entry. Drug Alcohol Depend 66:181–187, 2002

Gossop M, Harris J, Best D, et al: Is attendance at Alcoholics Anonymous meetings after inpatient treatment related to improved outcomes? A 6-month follow-up study. Alcohol Alcohol 38:421–426, 2003

Gossop M, Stewart D, Marsden J: Attendance at Narcotics Anonymous and Alcoholics Anonymous meetings, frequency of attendance and substance use outcomes after residential treatment for drug dependence: a 5-year follow-up study. Addiction 103:119–125, 2008

Gruber VA, Delucchi KL, Kielstein A, et al: A randomized trial of six-month methadone maintenance with standard or minimal counseling versus 21-day methadone detoxification. Drug Alcohol Depend 94:199–206, 2008

Gueorguieva R, Wu R, Donovan D, et al: Naltrexone and combined behavioral intervention effects on trajectories of drinking in the COMBINE study. Drug Alcohol Depend 107:221–229, 2010

Heffner JL, Tran GQ, Johnson CS, et al: Combining motivational interviewing with compliance enhancement therapy (MI-CET): development and preliminary evaluation of a new, manual-guided psychosocial adjunct to alcohol-dependence pharmacotherapy. J Stud Alcohol Drugs 71:61–70, 2010

Higgins ST, Budney AJ, Bickel WK, et al: Incentives improve outcome in outpatient behavioral treatment of cocaine-dependence. Arch Gen Psychiatry 51:568–576, 1994

Higgins ST, Heil SH, Dantona R, et al: Effects of varying the monetary value of voucher-based incentives on abstinence achieved during and following treatment among cocaine-dependent outpatients. Addiction 102:271–281, 2007

Humeniuk R, Ali R, Babor T, et al: A randomized controlled trial of a brief intervention for illicit drugs linked to the Alcohol, Smoking and Substance Involvement Screening Test (ASSIST) in clients recruited from primary health-care settings in four countries. Addiction 107:957–966, 2012

Ingersoll KS, Farrell-Carnahan L, Cohen-Filipic J, et al: A pilot randomized clinical trial of two medication adherence and drug use interventions for HIV+ crack cocaine users. Drug Alcohol Depend 116:177–187, 2011

Johnson A, Jasinski DR, Galloway GP, et al: Ritanserin in the treatment of alcohol dependence: a multi-center clinical trial. Psychopharmacology 128:206–215, 1996

Johnson BA, Roache JD, Javors MA, et al: Ondansetron for reduction of drinking among biologically predisposed alcoholic patients: a randomized controlled trial. JAMA 284:963–971, 2000

Kadden RM: Behavioral and cognitive-behavioral treatments for alcoholism: research opportunities. Addict Behav 26:489–507, 2001

Kaner EF, Dickinson HO, Beyer FR, et al: Effectiveness of brief alcohol interventions in primary care populations. Cochrane Database of Systematic Reviews 2007, Issue 2. Art. No.: CD004148. DOI: 10.1002/14651858.CD004148.pub3.

Kelley ML, Fals-Stewart W: Treating paternal alcoholism with Learning Sobriety Together: effects on adolescents versus preadolescents. J Fam Psychol 21:435–444, 2007

Kosten T, Oliveto A, Feingold A, et al: Desipramine and contingency management for cocaine and opiate dependence in buprenorphine maintained patients. Drug Alcohol Depend 70:315–325, 2003a

Kosten T, Poling J, Oliveto A: Effects of reducing contingency management values on heroin and cocaine use for buprenorphine- and desipramine-treated patients. Addiction 98:665–671, 2003b

Kranzler HR, Burleson JA, Korner P, et al: Placebo-controlled trial of fluoxetine as an adjunct to relapse prevention in alcoholics. Am J Psychiatry 152:391–397, 1995

Kranzler HR, Armeli S, Tennen H, et al: Targeted naltrexone for early problem drinkers. J Clin Psychopharmacol 23:294–304, 2003

Kranzler HR, Wesson DR, Billot L, et al: Naltrexone depot for treatment of alcohol dependence: a multicenter, randomized, placebo-controlled clinical trial. Alcohol Clin Exp Res 28:1051–1059, 2004

Krystal JH, Cramer JA, Krol WF, et al: Naltrexone in the treatment of alcohol dependence. N Engl J Med 345:1734–1739, 2001

LaBrie JW, Huchting K, Tawalbeh S, et al: A randomized motivational enhancement prevention group reduces drinking and alcohol consequences in first-year college women. Psychol Addict Behav 22:149–155, 2008

Longabaugh R, Wirtz PW, Gulliver SB, et al: Extended naltrexone and broad spectrum treatment or motivational enhancement therapy. Psychopharmacology 206:367–376, 2009

Madras BK, Compton WM, Avula D, et al: Screening, brief interventions, referral to treatment (SBIRT) for illicit drug and alcohol use at multiple healthcare sites: comparison at intake and 6 months later. Drug Alcohol Depend 99:280–295, 2009

Magill M, Ray LA: Cognitive-behavioral treatment with adult alcohol and illicit drug users: a meta-analysis of randomized controlled trials. J Stud Alcohol Drugs 70:516–527, 2009

Martino S, Carroll KM, Nich C, et al: A randomized controlled pilot study of motivational interviewing for patients with psychotic and drug use disorders. Addiction 101:1479–1492, 2006

Mason BJ, Salvato, FR, Williams LD, et al: Double-blind, placebo-controlled study of oral nalmefene for alcohol dependence. Arch Gen Psychiatry 56:719–724, 1999

McCrady BS, Miller WR (eds): Alcoholics Anonymous: Opportunities and Alternatives. New Brunswick, NJ, Rutgers Center of Alcohol Studies, 1993

McCrady BS, Stout N, Noel N, et al: Effectiveness of three types of spouse-involved behavioral alcoholism treatments. Br J Addict 86:1415–1424, 1991

McKay JR, Alterman AI, McLellan AT, et al: Treatment goals, continuity of care, and outcome in a day hospital substance abuse rehabilitation program. Am J Psychiatry 151:254–259, 1994

McKee SA, Carroll KM, Sinha R, et al: Enhancing brief cognitive-behavioral therapy with motivational enhancement techniques in cocaine users. Drug Alcohol Depend 91:97–101, 2007

Miller WR, Rollnick S: Motivational Interviewing: Preparing People to Change Addictive Behavior, 2nd Edition. New York, Guilford, 2002

Miller WR, Brown JM, Simpson TL, et al: What works? A methodological analysis of the alcohol treatment outcome literature, in Handbook of Alcoholism Treatment Approaches: Effective Alternatives, 2nd Edition. Edited by Herster RK, Miller WR. Boston, MA, Allyn & Bacon, 1995, pp 12 44

Moyer A, Finney JW, Swearingen CE, et al: Brief interventions for alcohol problems: a meta-analytic review of controlled investigations in treatment-seeking and non-treatment-seeking populations. Addiction 97:279–292, 2002

Nunes EV, Rothenberg JL, Sullivan MA, et al: Behavioral therapy to augment oral naltrexone for opioid dependence: a ceiling on effectiveness? Am J Drug Alcohol Abuse 32:503–517, 2006

Nyamathi A, Shoptaw S, Cohen A, et al: Effect of motivational interviewing on reduction of alcohol use. Drug Alcohol Depend 107:23–30, 2010

O'Farrell TJ, Cutter HS, Choquette KA, et al: Behavioral marital therapy for male alcoholics: marital and drinking adjustment during the two years after treatment. Behav Ther 23:529–549, 1992

O'Farrell TJ, Choquette KA, Cutter HS: Couples relapse prevention sessions after behavioral marital therapy for alcoholics and their wives: outcomes during three years after starting treatment. J Stud Alcohol 59:357–370, 1998

Oliveto A, Poling J, Mancino MJ, et al: Randomized, double-blind, placebo-controlled trial of disulfiram for the treatment of cocaine dependence in methadone-stabilized patients. Drug Alcohol Depend 113:184–191, 2011

O'Malley SS, Jaffe AJ, Chang G, et al: Naltrexone and coping skills therapy for alcohol dependence: a controlled study. Arch Gen Psychiatry 49:881–887, 1992

O'Malley SS, Jaffe AJ, Chang G, et al: Six-month follow-up of naltrexone and psychotherapy for alcohol dependence. Arch Gen Psychiatry 53:217–224, 1996

O'Neill K, Baker A, Cooke M, et al: Evaluation of a cognitive-behavioural intervention for pregnant injecting drug users at risk for HIV infection. Addiction 91:1115–1125, 1996

Peirce JM, Petry NM, Stitzer ML, et al: Effects of lower-cost incentives on stimulant abstinence in methadone maintenance treatment: a National Drug Abuse Treatment Clinical Trials Network study. Arch Gen Psychiatry 63:201–208, 2006

Petry NM, Martin B, Cooney JL, et al: Give them prizes, and they will come: contingency management for treatment of alcohol dependence. J Consult Clin Psychol 68:250–257, 2000

Petry NM, Alessi S, Marx J, et al: Vouchers versus prizes: contingency management treatment of substance abusers in community settings. J Consult Clin Psychol 73:1005–1014, 2005a

Petry NM, Peirce JM, Stitzer ML, et al. Effect of prize-based incentives on outcomes in stimulant abusers in outpatient psychosocial treatment programs: a national drug abuse treatment clinical trials network study. Arch Gen Psychiatry 62:1148–1156, 2005b

Petry NM, Weinstock J, Alessi SM: A randomized trial of contingency management delivered in the context of group counseling. J Consult Clin Psychol 79:686–696, 2011

Petry NM, Rash CJ, Byrne S, Ashraf S, et al: Financial reinforcers for improving medication adherence: findings from a meta-analysis. Am J Med 125:888–896, 2012

Pettinati HM, Volpicelli JR, Luck G, et al: Double-blind clinical trial of sertraline treatment for alcohol dependence. J Clin Pharmacol 21:143–153, 2001

Poling J, Oliveto A, Petry N, et al: Six-month trial of bupropion with contingency management for cocaine dependence in a methadone-maintained population. Arch Gen Psychiatry 63:219–228, 2006

Powers MB, Vedel E, Emmelkamp PM: Behavioral couples therapy (BCT) for alcohol and drug use disorders: a meta-analysis. Clin Psychol Rev 28:952–962, 2008

Preston KL, Umbricht A, Epstein DH: Methadone dose increase and abstinence reinforcement for treatment of continued heroin use during methadone maintenance. Arch Gen Psychiatry 57:395–404, 2000

Prochaska JO, DiClemente CC: Toward a comprehensive model of change, in Treating Addictive Behaviors: Processes of Change. Edited by Miller WR, Heather N. New York, Plenum, 1986, pp 3–27

Project MATCH Research Group: Matching alcoholism treatments to client heterogeneity: Project MATCH posttreatment drinking outcomes. J Stud Alcohol 58:7–29, 1997

Rawson RA, McCann MJ, Flammino F, et al: A comparison of contingency management and cognitive-behavioral approaches for stimulant-dependent individuals. Addiction 101:267–274, 2006

Rohsenow DJ, Monti PM, Martin RA, et al: Motivational enhancement and coping skills training for cocaine abusers: effect on substance use outcomes. Addiction 99:862–874, 2004

Rosenblum A, Magura S, Palij M, et al: Enhanced treatment outcomes for cocaine-using methadone patients. Drug Alcohol Depend 54:207–218, 1999

Rotunda RJ, O'Farrell TJ, Murphy M, et al: Behavioral couples therapy for comorbid substance use disorders and combat-related posttraumatic stress disorder among male veterans: an initial evaluation. Addict Behav 33:180–187, 2008

Ruff S, McComb JL, Coker CJ, et al: Behavioral couples therapy for the treatment of substance abuse: a substantive and methodological review of O'Farrell, Fals-Stewart, and colleagues' program of research. Fam Process 49:439–456, 2010

Rychtarik RG, Connors GJ, Dermen KH, et al: Alcoholics Anonymous and the use of medications to prevent relapse: an anonymous survey of member attitudes. J Stud Alcohol 61:134–138, 2000

Schmitz JM, Mooney ME, Moeller FG, et al: Levodopa pharmacotherapy for cocaine dependence: choosing the optimal behavioral therapy platform. Drug Alcohol Depend 94:142–150, 2008

Schmitz JM, Lindsay JA, Green CE, et al: High-dose naltrexone therapy for cocaine-alcohol dependence. Am J Addict 18:356–362, 2009

Schottenfeld RS, Chawarski MC, Pakes JR, et al: Methadone versus buprenorphine with contingency management or performance feedback for cocaine and opioid dependence. Am J Psychiatry 162:340–349, 2005

Smith JE, Meyers RJ, Delaney HD: Community reinforcement approach with homeless alcohol-dependent individuals. J Consult Clin Psychol 66:541–548, 1998

Stein MD, Herman DS, Anderson BJ: A motivational intervention trial to reduce cocaine use. J Subst Abuse Treat 36:118–125, 2009

Stotts AL, Schmitz JM, Rhoades HM, et al: Motivational interviewing with cocaine-dependent patients: a pilot study. J Consult Clin Psychol 69:858–862, 2001

Sullivan LE, Tetrault JM, Braithwaite RS, et al: A meta-analysis of the efficacy of non-physician brief interventions for unhealthy alcohol use: implications for the patient-centered medical home. Am J Addict 20:343–356, 2011

Timko C, DeBenedetti A: A randomized controlled trial of intensive referral to 12-step self-help groups: one-year outcomes. Drug Alcohol Depend 90:270–279, 2007

Walitzer KS, Dermen KH, Barrick C: Facilitating involvement in Alcoholics Anonymous during out-patient treatment: a randomized clinical trial. Addiction 104:391–401, 2009

Winters J, Fals-Stewart W, O'Farrell TJ, et al: Behavioral couples therapy for female substance-abusing patients: effects on substance use and relationship adjustment. J Consult Clin Psychol 70:344–355, 2002

Yahne CE, Miller WR, Irvin-Vitela L, et al: Magdalena Pilot Project: motivational outreach to substance abusing women street sex workers. J Subst Abuse Treat 23:49–53, 2002

Ye Y, Kaskutas LA: Using propensity scores to adjust for selection bias when assessing the effectiveness of Alcoholics Anonymous in observational studies. Drug Alcohol Depend 104:56–64, 2009

Index

Page numbers printed in *boldface* type refer to figures or tables.